PRAISE FOR *COME AS YOU ARE*

Goodreads Choice Awards, Top 5 Science and Technology Books
Buzzfeed's 17 Things that Changed Our Sex Lives in 2015
Book Riot's Best of 2015
Autostraddle's Top 10 Queer and Feminist Books
SSTAR's 2017 Consumer Book Award

"This is the best book I have ever read exploring the science of female sexuality. I am a total evangelist for Nagoski's work. . . . You think you know how women's sexuality works? I can guarantee that you do not. Not until you read this, anyway. The book is definitely great for college students and for bright high schoolers as well."

—Peggy Orenstein, author of *Girls and Sex*

"This is the best book I have ever read about sexual desire and why some couples just stop having sex, and what they can do about it. *Come As You Are* is an absolutely necessary guide for all couples who want to understand the ups and downs in their own sex life. It is a must-read!"

—John Gottman, Ph.D., author of *The Seven Principles for Making Marriage Work*

"Emily Nagoski has written one of the most important books about sex any woman (or anybody else) could ever pick up, full of insights that are both fascinating and deeply useful. Synthesizing new research and theory about sexuality with old-school sex-positive information of the sort you didn't learn in sex ed (unless, perhaps, you are a Unitarian, or Scandinavian, or lucky enough to be in Dr. Nagoski's class), I guarantee *Come As You Are* will open minds and change lives."

—Carol Queen, Ph.D., founding director of the Center for Sex & Culture

"Emily Nagoski is worth her weight in TED Talks, and *Come as You Are* is a master class in the science of sex."

—Ian Kerner, sex therapist and bestselling author of *She Comes First*

"It's the science of sex, decoded and demystified. Want to be educated on the latest findings about female genitalia? Of course you do. Empowering and sex-positive at best, this informative read makes for an enticing bedfellow."

—Refinery29

"Lots of books—and articles and experts—claim to have the keys to transform your sex life. This one actually has it. It isn't as fast as taking a pill, but it will last a whole lot longer. You will find no hot new bedroom moves—it's that deeper-level soul stuff. You know, the stuff that actually works."

—Salon.com

"Wonderful new language to help us articulate to women (and their lovers) what is going on."

—*Huffington Post*

"Like a punch to the gut. When I read the passage that made me realize—after all these years—that I was not actually broken, I began to cry. . . . I wished [Nagoski] was someone who was actively in my life, someone I could reach out to for grounding every time I momentarily forgot the lessons in her book."

—Book Riot

"Nagoski's book deserves plaudits for the rare achievement of merging pop science and the sexual self-help genre in prose that's not insufferably twee. . . . [*Come As You Are*] offers up hard facts on the science of arousal and desire in a friendly and accessible way."

—*The Guardian* (UK)

come
as you are

The Surprising New Science that
Will Transform Your Sex Life

Emily Nagoski, Ph.D.

Simon & Schuster Paperbacks

New York   London   Toronto   Sydney   New Delhi

Simon & Schuster Paperbacks
An Imprint of Simon & Schuster
1230 Avenue of the Americas
New York, NY 10020

This Simon & Schuster trade paperback edition March 2021

SIMON & SCHUSTER PAPERBACKS and colophon
are registered trademarks of Simon & Schuster, Inc.

For information about special discounts for bulk purchases, please contact
Simon & Schuster Special Sales at 1-866-506-1949 or business@simonandschuster.com.

The Simon & Schuster Speakers Bureau can bring authors to your live event.
For more information or to book an event, contact the Simon & Schuster Speakers
Bureau at 1-866-248-3049 or visit our website at www.simonspeakers.com.

Illustrated by Erika Moen
Interior design by Ruth Lee-Mui

Manufactured in the United States of America

9   10

Library of Congress Cataloging-in-Publication Data

Names: Nagoski, Emily, author.
Title: Come as you are : the surprising new science that will transform
your sex life / Emily Nagoski, Ph.D.
Description: Simon & Schuster trade paperback edition, revised and updated. |
New York : Simon & Schuster Paperbacks, 2021. | Includes
bibliographical references and index.
Identifiers: LCCN 2020043421 (print) | LCCN 2020043422 (ebook) |
ISBN 9781982165314 (paperback) | ISBN 9781982165321 (ebook)
Subjects: LCSH: Sex instruction for women. | Sexual health. | Women—Sexual
behavior. | Women—Health and hygiene.
Classification: LCC HQ46 .N32 2021 (print) | LCC HQ46 (ebook) |
DDC 306.7082—dc23
LC record available at https://lccn.loc.gov/2020043421
LC ebook record available at https://lccn.loc.gov/2020043422

ISBN 978-1-9821-6531-4
ISBN 978-1-9821-6532-1 (ebook)

For my students

contents

part 2 sex in context

part 3 sex in action

part 4 ecstasy for everybody

introduction

To be a sex educator is to be asked questions. I've stood in college din-
ing halls with a plate of food in my hands, answering questions about
orgasm. I've been stopped in hotel lobbies at professional conferences
to answer questions about vibrators. I've sat on a park bench, checking social media on my phone, only to find questions from a stranger
about her asymmetrical genitals. I've gotten emails from students, from
friends, from their friends, from total strangers, about sexual desire,
sexual arousal, sexual pleasure, sexual pain, orgasm, fetishes, fantasies,
bodily fluids, and more.

Questions like . . .

- *Once my partner initiates, I'm into it, but it seems like it never even*
  occurs to me to be the one to start things. Why is that?
- *My boyfriend was like, "You're not ready, you're still dry." But I*
  was so *ready. So why wasn't I wet?*
- *I saw this thing about women who can't enjoy sex because they worry*
  about their bodies the whole time. That's me. How do I stop doing
  that?

- *I read something about women who stop wanting sex after a while in a relationship, even if they still love their partner. That's me. How do I start wanting sex with my partner again?*
- *I think maybe I peed when I had an orgasm . . . ?*
- *I think maybe I've never had an orgasm . . . ?*

Under all these questions, there's really just one question:

Am I normal?

(The answer is nearly always: Yes.)

This book is a collection of answers. They're answers that I've seen change women's lives, answers informed by the most relevant science and by the personal stories of women whose growing understanding of sex has transformed their relationships with their own bodies. These women are my heroines, and I hope that by telling their stories, I'll empower you to follow your own path, to reach for and achieve your own profound and unique sexual potential.

the true story of sex

After all the books that have been written about sex, all the podcasts and TV shows and magazine articles and radio Q&As, how can it be that we all still have so many questions?

Well. The frustrating reality is we've been lied to—not deliberately, it's no one's fault, but still. We were told the wrong story.

For a long, long time in Western science and medicine, women's sexuality was viewed as Men's Sexuality Lite—basically the same but not quite as good.

For instance, it was just sort of assumed that since men have orgasms during penis-in-vagina sex (intercourse), women should have orgasms with intercourse, too, and if they don't, it's because they're broken.

In reality, about a quarter of women orgasm reliably with intercourse. The other 75 percent sometimes, rarely, or *never* orgasm with intercourse, and they're all healthy and normal. A woman might orgasm lots of other ways—manual sex, oral sex, vibrators, breast stimulation, toe sucking, pretty much any way you can imagine—and still not orgasm during intercourse. That's normal.

It was just assumed, too, that because men's genitals typically behave the way their minds are behaving—if a penis is erect, the person attached to it is feeling turned on—a woman's genitals should also match her emotional experience.

And again, some women's do, many don't. A woman can be perfectly normal and healthy and experience "arousal nonconcordance," where the behavior of her genitals (being wet or dry) may not match her mental experience (feeling turned on or not).

And it was also assumed that because men experience spontaneous, out-of-the-blue desire for sex, women should also want sex spontaneously.

Again it turns out that's true sometimes, but not necessarily. A woman can be perfectly normal and healthy and never experience spontaneous sexual desire. Instead, she may experience "responsive" desire, in which her desire emerges only in a highly erotic context.

In reality, women and men are different.

But wait. Women and men both experience orgasm, desire, and arousal, and men, too, can experience responsive desire, arousal nonconcordance, and lack of orgasm with penetration. Women and men both can fall in love, fantasize, masturbate, feel puzzled about sex, and experience ecstatic pleasure. They both can ooze fluids, travel forbidden paths of sexual imagination, encounter the unexpected and startling ways that sex shows up in every domain of life—and confront the unexpected and startling ways that sex sometimes declines, politely or otherwise, to show up.

So . . . are women and men really that different?

The problem here is that we've been taught to think about sex in terms of behavior, rather than in terms of the biological, psychological, and social processes underlying the behavior. We think about our physiological behavior—blood flow and genital secretions and heart rate. We think about our social behavior—what we do in bed, whom we do it with, and how often. A lot of books about sex focus on those things; they tell you how many times per week the average couple has sex or they offer instructions on how to have an orgasm, and they can be helpful.

But if you really want to *understand* human sexuality, behavior alone won't get you there. Trying to understand sex by looking at behavior is like trying to understand love by looking at a couple's wedding portrait . . . and their divorce papers. Being able to describe *what* happened—two people got married and then got divorced—doesn't get us very far. What we want to know is *why* and *how* it came to be. Did our couple fall out of love after they got married, and that's why they divorced? Or were they never in love but were forced to marry, and finally became free when they divorced? Without better evidence, we're mostly guessing.

Until very recently, that's how it's been for sex—mostly guessing. But we're at a pivotal moment in sex science because, after decades of research describing *what happens* in human sexual response, we're finally figuring out the *why* and *how*—the process underlying the behavior.

In the last decade of the twentieth century, researchers Erick Janssen and John Bancroft at the Kinsey Institute for Research in Sex, Gender, and Reproduction developed a model of human sexual response that provides an organizing principle for understanding the true story of sex. According to their "dual control model," the sexual response mechanism in our brains consists of a pair of universal components—a sexual accelerator and sexual brakes—and those components respond to broad categories of sexual stimuli—including genital sensations, visual stimulation, and emotional context. And the sensitivity of each component varies from person to person.

The result is that sexual arousal, desire, and orgasm are nearly universal experiences, but when and how we experience them depends largely on the sensitivities of our "brakes" and "accelerator" and on the kinds of stimulation they're given.

This is the mechanism underlying the behavior—the why and the how. And it's the rule that governs the story I'll be telling in this book:

We're all made of the same parts, but in each of us, those parts are orga-nized in a unique way that may change over our life span.

No organization is better or worse than any other, and no phase in our life span is better or worse than any other; they're just different. An apple tree can be healthy no matter what variety of apple it is—though one variety may need constant direct sunlight and another might enjoy some shade. And an apple tree can be healthy when it's a seed, when it's a seedling, as it's growing, and as it fades at the end of the season, as well as when, in late summer, it is laden with fruit. But it has different needs at each of those phases in its life.

You, too, are healthy and normal at the start of your sexual develop-ment, as you grow, and as you bear the fruits of living with confidence and joy inside your body. You are healthy when you need lots of sun, and you're healthy when you enjoy some shade. That's the true story. We are all the same. We are all different. We are all normal.

the organization of this book

The book is divided into four parts: (1) The (Not-So-Basic) Basics; (2) Sex in Context; (3) Sex in Action; and (4) Ecstasy for Everybody. The three chapters in the first part describe the basic hardware you were born with—a body, a brain, and a context. In chapter 1, I talk about genitals—their parts, the meaning we impose on those parts, and the science that proves definitively that yes, your genitals are perfectly healthy and beau-tiful just as they are. Chapter 2 details the sexual response mechanism in the brain—the dual control model of inhibition and excitation, or brakes and accelerator. Then in chapter 3, I introduce the ways that your sexual brakes and accelerator interact with the many other systems in your brain and environment, to shape whether a particular sensation or person turns you on, right now, in this moment.

In the second part of the book, "Sex in Context," we think about how all the basic hardware functions within the reality of your actual life—your emotions, your relationship, your feelings about your body, and your attitudes toward sex. Chapter 4 focuses on two primary emotional systems, love and stress, and the surprising and contradictory ways they can influence your sexual responsiveness. Then chapter 5 describes the cultural forces that shape and constrain sexual functioning, and how you can maximize the good things about this process and overcome the destructive things. What we'll learn is that *context*—your external circumstances and your present mental state—is as crucial to your sexual wellbeing as your body and brain. Master the content in these chapters and your sexual life will transform—along with, quite possibly, the rest of your life.

The third part of the book, "Sex in Action," is about sexual response itself, and I bust two long-standing and dangerous myths. Chapter 6 lays out the evidence that sexual pleasure and desire may or may not have anything to do with what's happening in your genitals. This is where we learn why arousal nonconcordance, which I mentioned earlier, is normal and healthy. And after you read chapter 7, you will never again hear someone say "sex drive" without thinking to yourself, *Ah, but sex is* not *a drive*. In this chapter I explain how "responsive desire" works. If you (or your partner) have ever experienced a change in your interest in sex—increase or decrease—this is an important chapter for you.

And the fourth part of the book, "Ecstasy for Everybody," explains how to make sex entirely *yours*, which is how you create peak sexual ecstasy in your life. Chapter 8 is about orgasms—what they are, what they're not, how to have them, and how to make them like the ones you read about, the ones that turn the stars into rainbows. And finally, in chapter 9, I describe the single most important thing you can do to improve your sex life. But I'll give it away right now: It turns out what matters most is not the parts you are made of or how they are organized, but *how you feel* about those parts. When you embrace your sexuality precisely as it is right now, that's the context that creates the greatest potential for ecstatic pleasure.

Several chapters include worksheets or other interactive activities and exercises. A lot of these are fun—like in chapter 3, I ask you to think about times when you've had great sex and identify what aspects of the context helped to make that sex great. All of the exercises turn the science into something practical that can genuinely transform your sex life.

Throughout the book, you'll follow the stories of four women—Olivia, Merritt, Camilla, and Laurie. These women don't exist as individuals; they're composites, integrating the real stories of the many women I've taught, talked with, emailed, and supported in my two decades as a sex educator. You can imagine each woman as a collage of snapshots—the face from one photograph, the arms from another, the feet from a third . . . each part represents someone real, and the collection hangs together meaningfully, but I've invented the relationships that the parts have to each other.

I've chosen to construct these composites rather than tell the stories of specific women for two reasons. First, people tell me their stories in confidence, and I want to protect their identities, so I've changed details in order to keep their story *their* story. And second, I believe I can describe the widest possible variety of women's sexual experiences by focusing not on specific stories of one individual woman but on the larger narratives that contain the common themes I've seen in all these hundreds of women's lives.

And finally, at the end of each chapter you'll find a "tl;dr" list—"too long; didn't read," the blunt internet abbreviation that means, "Just get to the point." Each tl;dr list briefly summarizes the four most important messages in the chapter. If you find yourself thinking, "My friend Alice should totally read this chapter!" or "I really wish my partner knew this," you might start by showing them the tl;dr list. Or, if you're like me and get too excited about these ideas to keep them to yourself, you can follow your partner around the house, reading the tl;dr list out loud and saying, "See, honey, arousal nonconcordance is a thing!" or "It turns out I have responsive desire!" or "You give me great context, sweetie!"

a couple of caveats

First, there are times when I discuss what trans sex educator S. Bear Bergman calls "factory-installed parts"—the anatomical details that make doctors declare a baby a "girl" or a "boy." For clarity and simplicity, when I'm talking about those parts, I'll use the words "female" or "male," referring to the biological categories that can describe many sexually reproducing species, not just humans. When I'm talking about a whole person, I'll use the words "woman" or "man," referring to the person's identity and social role.

A further gender caveat: Because this book is grounded in the existing science, most of the time when I say "women" in this book, I mean cisgender women—that is, people who were born in bodies that made the adults around them declare, "It's a girl!" and then they were raised as girls and now feel comfortable in the social role and psychological identity of "woman." There are plenty of women who don't have one or more of these characteristics, and there are plenty of people who don't identify as "woman" who do fit one or more of these characteristics. Trans and nonbinary people deserve excellent, science-based, pleasure-oriented sex education, too . . . and there's still (still!) too little research on trans sexual functioning for me to say with certainty whether what's true about cisgender women's sexual wellbeing is also true for trans folks'. I think it probably is, and as more research emerges over the coming decades, we'll find out. I am totally sure that people of any gender—including cisgender men—can learn a lot from the existing science, incomplete though it is. But while we wait for more and better research, I want to acknowledge that this book relies on science that is almost entirely based on cisgender people.

Third, I am passionate about the role of science in promoting women's sexual wellbeing, and I have worked hard in this book to encapsulate the research in the service of teaching women to live with confidence and joy inside their bodies. But I've been very intentional about the empirical details I've included or excluded. I asked myself, "Does this fact help women have better sex lives, or is it just a totally fascinating and important empirical puzzle?"

And I cut the puzzles.

I kept only the science that has the most immediate relevance in women's everyday lives. So what you'll find in these pages isn't the whole story of women's sexuality—I'm not sure the whole story would actually fit in one book. Instead, I've included the parts of the story that I've found most powerful in my work as a sex educator, promoting women's sexual wellbeing, autonomy, and pleasure.

The purpose of this book is to offer a new, science-based way of thinking about women's sexual wellbeing. Like all new ways of thinking, it opens up a lot of questions and challenges much preexisting knowledge. If you want to dive deeper, you'll find references in the notes, along with details about my process for boiling down a complex and multifaceted body of research into something practical.

if you feel broken, or know someone who does

One more thing before we get into chapter 1. Remember how I said we've all been lied to? I want to take a moment to recognize the damage done by that lie.

So many women come to my workshops or to my class or to my public talks convinced that they are sexually broken. They feel dysfunctional. Abnormal. And on top of that, they feel anxious, frustrated, and hopeless about the lack of information and support they've received from medical professionals, therapists, partners, family, and friends.

"Just relax," they've been told. "Have a glass of wine."

Or, "Women just don't want sex that much. Get over it."

Or, "Sometimes sex hurts—can't you just ignore it?"

I understand the frustration these women experience, and the despair—and in the second half of the book I talk about the neurological process that traps people in frustration and despair, shutting them off from hope and joy, and I describe science-based ways to get out of the trap.

Here's what I need you to know right now: The information in this book will show you that whatever you're experiencing in your sexuality—whether it's challenges with arousal, desire, orgasm, pain, no sexual sensations, whatever—is the result of your sexual response mechanism functioning appropriately . . . in an inappropriate world. *You* are normal; it is the world around you that's broken.

That's actually the bad news.

The good news is that when you understand how your sexual response mechanism works, you can begin to take control of your environment and your brain in order to maximize your sexual potential, even in a broken world. And when you change your environment and your brain, you can change—and heal—your sexual functioning.

This book contains information that I have seen transform women's sexual wellbeing. I've seen it transform men's understanding of their women partners. I've seen same-sex couples look at each other and say, "Oh. So *that's* what was going on." Students, friends, blog readers, and even fellow sex educators have read this book or heard me give a talk and said, "Why did no one tell me this before? It explains *everything*!"

I know for sure that what I've written in this book can help you. It may not be enough to heal all the wounds inflicted on your sexuality by a culture in which it sometimes feels nearly impossible for a woman to "do" sexuality right, but it will provide powerful tools in support of your healing.

How do I know?

Evidence, of course!

At the end of one semester, I asked my 187 students to write down one really important thing they learned in my class. Here's a small sample of what they wrote:

I am normal!

I AM NORMAL

I learned that everything is NORMAL, making it possible to go through the rest of my life with confidence and joy.

I learned that I am normal! And I learned that some people have spontaneous desire and others have responsive desire and this fact helped me really understand my personal life.

Women vary! And just because I do not experience my sexuality in the same way as many other women, that does not make me abnormal.

Women's sexual desire, arousal, response, etc., is incredibly varied.

The one thing I can count on regarding sexuality is that people vary, a lot.

That everyone is different and everything is normal; no two alike.

No two alike!

And many more. More than half of them wrote some version of "I am normal."

I sat in my office and read those responses with tears in my eyes. There was something urgently important to my students about feeling "normal," and somehow my class had cleared a path to that feeling.

The science of women's sexual wellbeing is young, and there is much still to be learned. But this young science has already discovered truths about women's sexuality that have transformed my students' relationships with their bodies—and it has certainly transformed mine. I wrote this book to share the science, stories, and sex-positive insights that prove to us that, despite our culture's vested interest in making us feel broken, dysfunctional, unlovely, and unlovable, we are in fact fully capable of confident, joyful sex.

The promise of *Come as You Are* is this: No matter where you are in your sexual journey right now, whether you have an awesome sex life and want to expand the awesomeness, or you're struggling and want to find solutions, you will learn something that will improve your sex life and transform the way you understand what it means to be a sexual being. And you'll discover that, even if you don't yet feel that way, you are already sexually whole and healthy.

The science says so.

I can prove it.

part 1

the (not-so-basic) basics

one

anatomy

NO TWO ALIKE

Olivia likes to watch herself in the mirror when she masturbates.

Like many women, Olivia masturbates lying on her back and rubbing her clitoris with her hand. Unlike many women, she props herself up on one elbow in front of a full-length mirror and watches her fingers moving in the folds of her vulva.

"I started when I was a teenager," she told me. "I had seen porn on the internet, and I was curious about what I looked like, so I got a mirror and started pulling apart my labia so I could see my clit, and what can I say? It felt good, so I started masturbating."

It's not the only way she masturbates. She also enjoys the "pulse" spray on her showerhead, she has a small army of vibrators at her command, and she spent several months teaching herself to have "breath" orgasms, coming without touching her body at all.

This is the kind of thing women tell you when you're a sex educator.

She also told me that looking at her vulva convinced her that her sexuality was more like a man's, because her clitoris is comparatively large—"like a baby carrot, almost"—which, she concluded, made her more masculine; it must be bigger because she had more testosterone, which in turn made her a horny lady.

I told her, "Actually there's no evidence of a relationship between an adult woman's hormone levels, genital shape or size, and sexual desire."

"Are you sure about that?" she asked.

"Well, some women have 'testosterone-dependent' desire," I said, pondering, "which means they need a certain very low minimum of T, but that's not the same as 'high testosterone.' And the distance between the clitoris and the urethra predicts how reliably orgasmic a woman is during intercourse, but that's a whole other thing.[1] I'd be fascinated to see a study that directly asked the question, but the available evidence suggests that variation in women's genital shapes, sizes, and colors doesn't predict anything in particular about her level of sexual interest."

"Oh," she said. And that single syllable said to me: "Emily, you have missed the point."

Olivia is a psychology grad student—a former student of mine, an activist around women's reproductive health issues, and now doing her own research, which is how we got started on this conversation—so I got excited about the opportunity to talk about the science. But with that quiet, "Oh," I realized that this wasn't about the science for Olivia. It was about her struggle to embrace her body and her sexuality just as it is, when so much of her culture was trying to convince her there is something wrong with her.

So I said, "You know, your clitoris is totally normal. Everyone's genitals are made of all the same parts, just organized in different ways. The differences don't necessarily mean anything, they're just varieties of beautiful and healthy. Actually," I continued, "that could be the most important thing you'll ever learn about human sexuality."

"Really?" she asked. "Why?"

This chapter is the answer to that question.

Medieval anatomists called women's external genitals the "pudendum," a word derived from the Latin *pudere*, meaning "to make ashamed." Our genitalia were thus named "from the shamefacedness that is in women to have them seen."[2]

Wait: *What?*

The reasoning went like this: Women's genitals are tucked away between their legs, as if they wanted to be hidden, whereas male genitals face forward, for all to see. And why would male and female genitals be different in this way? If you're a medieval anatomist, steeped in a sexual ethic of purity, it's because: shame.

Now, if we assume "shame" isn't really why women's genitals are under the body—and I hope it's eye-rollingly obvious that it's not—why, biologically, are male genitals in front and female genitals underneath?

The answer is, they're not! The female equivalent to the penis—the clitoris—is positioned right up front, in the equivalent location to the penis. It's less obvious than the penis because it's smaller—and it's smaller not because it's shy or ashamed, but because females don't have to transport our DNA from inside our own bodies to inside someone else's body. And the female equivalent of the scrotum—the outer labia—is also located in very much the same place as the scrotum, but because the female gonads (the ovaries) are internal, rather than external like the testicles, the labia don't extend much past the body, so they're less obvious. Again, the ovaries are not internal because of shame, but because we're the ones who get pregnant.

In short, female genitals appear "hidden" only if you look at them through the lens of cultural assumptions rather than through the eyes of biology.

We'll see this over and over again throughout the book: Culture adopts a random act of biology and tries to make it Meaningful, with a capital "Mmmh." We metaphorize genitals, seeing what they are like rather than what they are, we superimpose cultural Meaning on them, as Olivia superimposed the meaning of "masculine" on her largish clitoris, to conclude that her anatomy had some grand meaning about her as sexually masculine.

When you can see your body as it is, rather than what culture proclaims it to Mean, then you experience how much easier it is to live with and love your genitals, along with the rest of your sexuality, precisely as they are.

So in this chapter, we'll look at our genitals through biological eyes, cultural lenses off. First, I'll walk you through the ways that male and female genitals are made of the same parts, just organized in different ways. I'll point out where the biology says one thing and culture says something else, and you can decide which makes more sense to you. I'll illustrate how the idea of all the same parts, organized in different ways extends far beyond our anatomy to every aspect of human sexual response, and I'll argue that this might be the most important thing you'll ever learn about your sexuality.

In the end, I'll offer a new central metaphor to replace all the wacky, biased, or nonsensical ones that culture has tried to impose on women's bodies. My goal in this chapter is to introduce an alternative way of thinking about your body and your sexuality, so that you can relate to your body on its own terms, rather than on terms somebody else chose for you.

the beginning

Imagine two fertilized eggs that have just implanted in a uterus. One is XX—genetically female—and the other is XY—genetically male. Fraternal twins, a sister and a brother. Faces, fingers, and feet, the siblings will develop all the same body parts, but the parts will be organized differently, to give them the individual bodies that will be instantly distinguishable from each other as they grow up. And just as their faces will each have two eyes, one nose, and a mouth, all arranged in more or less the same places, so their genitals will have all the same basic elements, organized in roughly the same way. But unlike their faces and fingers and feet, their genitals will develop before birth into configurations that their parents will automatically declare to be "boy" or "girl."

Here's how it happens. About six weeks after the fertilized egg implants in the uterus, there is a wash of masculinizing hormones. The male

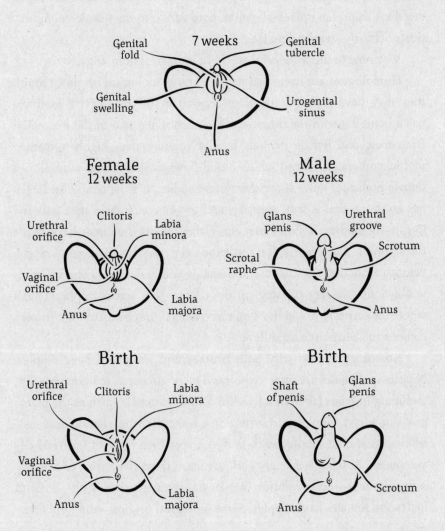

All the same parts, organized in different ways. Every body's genitals are the same until six weeks into gestation, when the universal genital hardware begins to organize itself into either the female configuration or the male configuration.

embryo responds to this by developing its "prefab" universal genital hardware into the male configuration of penis, testicles, and scrotum. The female embryo does not respond to the hormone wash at all, and instead develops its prefab universal genital hardware into the female configuration of clitoris, ovaries, and labia.

Welcome to the wonderful world of biological homology.

Homologues are traits that have the same biological origins, though they may have different functions. Each part of the external genitalia has a homologue in the other sex. I've mentioned two of them already: Both male and female genitals have a round-ended, highly sensitive, multichambered organ to which blood flows during sexual arousal. On female bodies, it's the clitoris; on male bodies, it's the penis. And each has an organ that is soft, stretchy, and grows coarse hair after puberty. On female bodies, it's the outer lips (labia majora); on male bodies, it's the scrotum. These parts don't just look superficially alike; they are developed from the equivalent fetal tissue. If you look closely at a scrotum, you'll notice a seam running up the center—the scrotal raphe. That's where the scrotum would have split into labia if the chemistry or chromosomes had been a little bit different.

Homology is also why both brother and sister will have nipples. Nipples on females are vital to the survival of almost all mammal species, including humans (though a handful of old mammals, such as the platypus, don't have nipples, and instead just leak milk from their abdomens), so evolution built nipples in right at the very beginning of our fetal development. It takes less energy to just leave them there than to actively suppress them—and evolution is as lazy as it can get away with—so both males and females have nipples. Same biological origins—different functions.

the clit, the whole clit, and nothing but the clit

The clitoris and penis are the external genital organs most densely packed with nerve endings. The visible part of the clitoris, the glans clitoris, is located right up at the top of the genitals—some distance from the vagina, you'll notice. (This fact will be crucial when I talk about orgasm, in chapter 8.) The clitoris is . . .

The hokey pokey—it's what it's all about.

Two turntables and a microphone—it's where it's at.

A Visa card—it's everywhere you want to be.

It is your Grand Central Station of erotic sensation. Averaging just one-eighth the size of a penis yet loaded with nearly double the nerve endings, it can range in size from a barely visible pea to a fair-sized gherkin, or anywhere in between, and it's all normal, all beautiful.

Unlike the penis, the clitoris's only job is sensation. The penis has four jobs: sensation, penetration, ejaculation, and urination.

Two different ways of functioning, one shared biological origin.

The external part of the clitoris—the glans—is actually just the head of the clit, just as the glans penis—the vaguely acorn-shaped cap at the end of the penile shaft—is just the head. There's a lot more to it, though. The shaft of the penis is familiar to many. It is constructed of three chambers: a pair of cavernous bodies (corpora cavernosa) and a spongy body (corpus spongiosum), through which the urethra passes. All three of these chambers extend deep into the body. The corpus spongiosum ends in the bulb of the penis deep inside the pelvis. The corpora cavernosa taper away from each other and attach the pelvic bone.

The cultural understanding of clitoris is "the little nub at the top of the vulva." But the biological understanding of clitoris is more like "far-ranging mostly internal anatomical structure with a head emerging at the top of the vulva." Like the penis, the clitoris is composed of three chambers: a pair of legs (crura), which are homologous to the corpora cavernosa, and the bulbs of the vestibule, homologous to the corpus spongiosum, including its bulb of the penis. The vestibule is the mouth of the vagina; the bulbs extend from the head of the clitoris, deep inside the tissue of the vulva, then split to straddle the urethra and the vagina. That's right: The clitoris extends all the way to the vaginal opening.

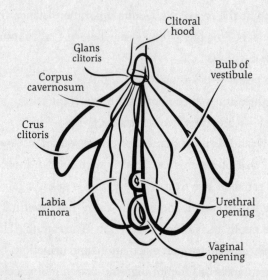

The anatomy of the clitoris. The cultural meaning of "clitoris" is often limited to the external part, the glans. The biological meaning includes a vast range of internal erectile tissue that extends all the way to the vaginal opening.

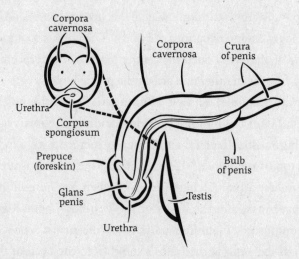

The anatomy of the penis. As with the clitoris, the cultural meaning of "penis" is limited to the external part—the glans and shaft. And, like the clitoris, the penis has internal erectile tissue. All the same parts, organized in different ways.

The clitoral hood covers the head of the clitoris, as its homologue, the foreskin, covers the head of the penis. And the male frenulum—the "Y-spot" near the glans, where the foreskin attaches to the shaft—is the homologue of the female fourchette (the French word for "fork"), the curve of tissue on the lower edge of the vagina. This is a highly sensitive and undervalued piece of real estate on all bodies.

meet your clitoris

If you've never met your clitoris "face-to-face," now is the time. (Even if you've had some good chats with your clitoris in the past, feel free to take this opportunity to get reacquainted.) You can find it visually or manually. After you've read the next two paragraphs, put down the book and try either method.

To find it visually, get a mirror, spread your labia (the soft, hairy outer lips of your vulva), and actually *look at it*. You'll see a nub at the top of your vulva.

Or you can find it with your fingers. Start with the tip of your middle finger at the cleft where your labia divide. Press down gently, wiggle your finger back and forth, and scoot your fingertip slowly down between your labia until you feel a rubbery little cord under the skin. It might help to pull your skin taut by tugging upward on your mons with your other hand. It might also help to lubricate your finger with spit, commercial lube, some allergen-free hand cream, or even a little coconut oil.

I have a specific reason for asking you to actually *look* at your clitoris:

A student came up to me after class one night and told me that she had been Skyping with her mom, talking about her classes that semester, including my class, "Women's Sexuality." The student mentioned to her mom that my lecture slides included actual photos of vulvas, along with diagrams and illustrations. And her mom told her the most astonishing thing. She said, "I don't know where the clitoris is."

The mom was fifty-four.

So my student emailed her mom my lecture slides.

That story is why the first chapter in this book is about anatomy. That story makes me want to print T-shirts with a drawing of a vulva and an arrow pointing to the clitoris, saying IT'S RIGHT HERE. It makes me want to hand out pamphlets on street corners with instructions for locating your own clitoris, both manually and visually. I want an animated GIF of a woman pointing to her clitoris to go viral on the internet. I want a billboard in Times Square. I want everyone to know.

But even more, it makes me want every single person who reads this to stop right now and look directly at their clitoris. Knowing where the clitoris is is important, but knowing where *your* clitoris is . . . that's power. Get a mirror and look at your clitoris, in honor of that student and her brave, amazing mom.

When I first looked at my clitoris, during my earliest training as a sex educator, I cried. I was eighteen and in a bad relationship and looking for answers. And my instructor had said, "When you go home tonight, get a mirror and find your clitoris." So I did. And I was stunned to tears to find that there was nothing gross or weird about it, it was just . . . part of my body. It belonged to me.

That moment set the stage for a decade of discovering and rediscovering that my best source of knowledge about my sexuality was my own body.

So go look at your clitoris.

And as long as you're in the neighborhood, check out the rest of your vulva, too.

I love having nontraditional students in my class—those who aren't in that eighteen-to-twenty-two age range—and Merritt was as nontraditional as they come: a perimenopausal lesbian author of gay erotica, with a teenage daughter whom she was raising with her partner of nearly twenty years. I was uninformed enough when I first met her to be surprised when she told me that her Korean parents were Fundamentalist Christians and that she grew up with quintessential socially conservative values. Which made her outness as a lesbian, her writing, and her presence in my classroom all the more remarkable.

At forty-two, Merritt had never considered looking at her clitoris. It didn't even cross her mind as a possibility until I suggested it during the first lecture, as I always do. She came up to me after class and said, "Is it really a good idea to suggest that kids this young look at their bodies? What if they just . . . shut down?"

"That's a really important question," I said. "No one has ever told me of an experience like that, but it's not a requirement, so maybe the folks most likely to have that experience don't try it. Still, it's something I recommend, especially for students who plan to continue on in public health or medicine, but it's entirely up to each person whether or not they want to look."

Merritt didn't do it.

Instead, she had her partner, Carol, look—which in some ways is even braver than looking herself—and she looked at her partner's. And they talked about what they saw and about how they had never before taken the time to deliberately look at and talk about their sexual bodies. And Merritt learned something remarkable, which she told me about the following week:

"Carol told me she'd looked at her vulva! She was part of a feminist consciousness-raising group in the '80s, and they all got together in a circle with their hand mirrors."

"Wow!" I said, and meant it.

She held her hands out, palms up, weighing her feelings. "I don't know why this kind of thing is so much harder for me than it is for her. When it comes to sex, I always feel like I'm teetering at the edge of a cliff with my arms windmilling around me."

The ambivalence Merritt experienced is absolutely normal for anyone whose family of origin taught them that sex should fit into a certain prescribed place in life and nowhere else. But it made sense for Merritt for other reasons, too, having to do with the way her brain is wired. I'll talk about that in chapter 2.

lips, both great and small

Female inner labia (labia minora or "small lips") may not be very "inner" at all, but extend out beyond the big lips—or they may tuck themselves away, hidden inside the vulva until you go looking for them. And the inner labia may be all one homogeneous color, or they may show a gradient of color, darkening toward the tips. All of that is normal and healthy and beautiful. Long, short, pink, beige, brown—all normal.

The outer labia, too, vary from person to person. Some are densely hairy, with the hair extending out onto the thigh and around the anus, while others have very little hair. Some lips are quite puffy while others are relatively flush with the body. Some are the same color as the surrounding skin, and some are darker or lighter than the surrounding skin. All normal, all beautiful.

As with the clitoris, the cultural view of labia doesn't match the biological reality. Vulvas in soft-core porn may be digitally edited to conform to a specific standard of "tucked-in" labia and homogeneous coloring, to be "less detailed."[3] This means that cultural representations of vulvas are limited to a pretty narrow range. In reality, there is a great deal of variety among genitals—and there is no medical condition associated with almost any of the variability. But such limited representations of women's bodies may actually be changing women's perceptions of what a "normal" vulva looks like.[4]

So if you decide to have a look at someone else's vulva—which I highly recommend, by the way, but only with their enthusiastic consent—you'll notice how very, very different they all are from each other. Only rarely do you find the tidily tucked-in vulvas you see in *Playboy*.

Unless you're experiencing pain (and if you are, check with your medical provider!), your genitals are perfect exactly as they are.

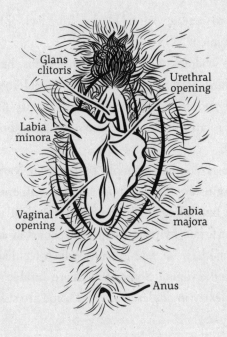

One example of a vulva.

hymen truths

You may or may not have a hymen—a thin membrane along the lower edge of your vaginal opening. Whether you have one or not, I guarantee that virtually everything you were taught about the hymen is wrong.[5]

The closest thing to true is that during intercourse the hymen can be painful if it's not used to being stretched—that's one of a number of potential causes of pain with penetration, but it is by no means the most common. (The most common is lack of lubrication.)

But the hymen doesn't break and stay broken forever, like some kind of freshness seal. If a hymen tears or bruises, it *heals*. And the size of a hymen doesn't vary depending on whether the vagina has been penetrated. Also, it usually doesn't bleed. Any blood with first penetration is more likely due to general vaginal tearing from lack of lubrication than to damage to the hymen.

What does change when a woman begins having the hymen stretched regularly is that it grows more flexible. And as hormones change with the end of adolescence (around twenty-five years old), the hymen is likely to atrophy and become much less noticeable—if it was noticeable at all.

The hymen is another example of the wide variability in female genitals. Some of us are born without hymens. Others have imperforate hymens (a thin but solid membrane covering all of the vaginal opening) or microperforate hymens (many tiny holes in an otherwise solid membrane). Some have septate hymens, which feel like a strand of skin stretching across the vagina. Some hymens are durable, others are fragile. Some disappear early in adolescence, and some are still in evidence past menopause.

Hymens vary because, as far as science has been able to discover, the hymen was not selected for by evolution. It has no reproductive or any other function. It's a byproduct, a little bonus left behind by the juggernaut of evolutionary selection pressure, like male nipples. It's the homologue of the seminal colliculus, a crest in the wall of the urethra where the male urethra passes through the prostate and joins with the seminal ducts.

The hymen is a profound example of the way humans metaphorize anatomy. Here is an organ that has no biological function, and yet Western culture made up a powerful story about the hymen a long time ago. This story has nothing to do with biology and everything to do with controlling women. Culture saw a "barrier" at the mouth of the vagina and decided it was a marker of "virginity" (itself a biologically meaningless idea). Such a weird idea could have been invented only in a society where women were literally property, their vaginas their most valuable real estate—a gated community.

Even though the hymen performs no physical or biological

function, many cultures have created myths around the hymen so profound that there are actually surgeries available to "reconstruct" the hymen, as if it were a medical necessity. (Where is the surgery to perfect men's nipples?)

In a sense, the hymen can be relevant to women's health: Some women are beaten or even killed for not having a hymen. Some women are told they "couldn't have been raped" because their hymen is intact. For them, the hymen has real impact on their physical wellbeing, not because of their anatomy but because of what their culture believes about that anatomy.

a word on words

One more thing about genitals: The name for the whole package of female external genitalia is "vulva." "Vagina" refers to the internal reproductive canal that leads up to the uterus. People often use "vagina" to refer to the vulva, but now you know better. And if you are standing up naked in front of a mirror and you see the classic triangle? That's your mons ("mound"), or mons pubis.

Got that?

Vagina = reproductive canal
Vulva = external genitalia
Mons = area over the pubic bone where hair grows

I'm not suggesting that you go around correcting people who use the wrong words, or picket *The Vagina Monologues* with signs saying, "Actually, they're *The Vulva Monologues*," but now you know what words *you* should use. You wouldn't call your face or your forehead your throat, right? So let's not call the vulva or mons the vagina. Let's make the world a better place for vulvas.

the sticky bits

Vulvas have a set of glands at either side of the mouth of the vagina, called Bartholin's glands, which release fluid during sexual arousal— maybe to reduce the friction of vaginal penetration, maybe to create a scent that communicates health and fertility status. When female genitals "get wet," this is what's happening. And it turns out, both male and female bodies "get wet." The male homologue, the Cowper's gland, just below the prostate, produces preejaculate.

Why do we talk about penises "getting hard" and vaginas "getting wet," when from a biological perspective both male and female genitals get both hard and wet? It's a cultural thing again. Male "hardness" (erection) is a necessary prerequisite for intercourse, and "wetness" is taken to be an indication that a body is "ready" for intercourse (though in chapter 6, we'll see how wrong this can be). Since intercourse is assumed to be the center of the sexual universe, we've metaphorized male hardness and female wetness as the Ultimate Indicators of Arousal. But like our anatomies, our physiologies are all made of the same components—changes in blood flow, production of genital secretions, etc.—organized in different ways. We put a spotlight on male hardness and a spotlight on female wetness, but male wetness is happening, too, and so is female hardness.

Vulvas also have a set of glands at the mouth of the urethra, the orifice we pee out of, called Skene's glands. These are the homologue of the male prostate. The prostate does two things: It swells around the urethra so that it's difficult or impossible to urinate during sexual arousal, and it produces about half of the seminal fluid in which sperm travels. In other words, it makes ejaculate. The Skene's glands also swell around the urethra, making it difficult to urinate when you're very aroused. If you've ever tried to pee right after having an orgasm, you've confronted this directly—you have to take deep, cleansing breaths to give your genitals time to relax.

Sometimes, the Skene's glands produce fluid, which is probably a source of "female ejaculate." Female ejaculation—"squirting"—has gotten some attention lately, in part because more science has been done and in part because it's been featured in porn. As a result, I get asked about it pretty regularly. In fact, one day I was visiting a student residence hall to answer anonymous questions out of a box, only to find that one student had put in the question, "How do I learn to squirt?" while another student had put in, "How do I stop squirting?"[7]

Needless to say, our culture sends mixed messages to women about their genital fluids . . . or their lack thereof. On the one hand, ejaculation is viewed as a quintessentially masculine event and women's genitals are, ya know, shameful, so for a female body to do something so emphatic and wet is unacceptable. On the other hand, it's a comparatively rare event, and the perpetual pursuit of novelty, coupled with basic supply-and-demand dynamics, means that the rare commodity of a female body that ejaculates is prized and put on display. So if they're paying attention to cultural messages about ejaculation, women are understandably confused.

The biological message is simple: Female ejaculation is a byproduct, like male nipples and the hymen. No matter how big a deal culture makes of it, people just vary. One woman I know never ejaculated in her life until shortly after menopause, when she got a new partner. All of a sudden she was ejaculating a quarter of a cup of fluid with every orgasm. Was it the change in partner? Was it the hormonal shift of menopause? None of the above? I have no idea. Some research has found that the number of Skene's glands orifices (that is, the number of holes exiting the Skene's glands) predicts whether someone ejaculates.[8] Does the presence of more openings increase the likelihood of ejaculation? Does ejaculation lead to the development of more openings? Again, no idea.

But this brings me to an important point about genitals: They get wet sometimes, and they have a fragrance. A scent. A rich and earthy bouquet, redolent of grass and amber, with a hint of woody musk. Genitals are aromatic, sometimes, and sticky sometimes, too. Ellen Støkken Dahl and Nina Brochmann, authors of the women's sexuality book *The Wonder Down Under*, introduced the phrase "disco mouse" to describe the vulva after a long, sweaty day. Your genital secretions are probably different at different phases in your menstrual cycle, and they change as you age, and they change with your diet—women vary.

If you don't find the smell or sensation of genital wetness to be completely beautiful and entrancing, that's unsurprising given how we teach people to feel about their genitals. But *how you feel* about your genitals and their secretions is learned, and loving your body just as it is will give you more intense pleasure and desire and bigger, better orgasms. More on that in chapter 5.

intersex parts

Intersex folks,[9] whose genitals are not obviously male or female at birth, also have all the same parts; theirs happen to be organized somewhere between the standard female and standard male configurations. The size of the phallus, the location of the urethral opening, or the split of the labioscrotal tissue may be anywhere in between.

Homology goes a long way in explaining how intersex genitals come to be. People whose genitals are "somewhere in between" experienced some slight variation in the hugely complex cascade of biochemical events involved in the growth of a fetus, from egg fertilization through embryonic development and gestation. This small change results in slightly different genitals in about one in sixty newborns.[10] There's nothing wrong with their genitals any more than there's anything wrong with a person whose labia are uniquely large or small.[11] It's still all the same parts, just organized in a different way. For example, the male urethral opening may be anywhere on the head of the penis; rarely, it is somewhere along the shaft of the penis, but that too is just fine, as long as it doesn't impede urination or cause chronic infection (which it usually does not). As long as the genitals don't cause pain and aren't prone to infection or other medical issues, they're healthy and don't require any kind of medical intervention. We're all made of the same parts, just organized in different ways.

This is why I don't need to see your genitals to tell you that they're normal and healthy. You've got all the same parts, just organized in your own unique way.

Like many sex educators, I include photographs of a variety of vulvas in my anatomy lecture slides.

Where do I find these photographs? On the internet, of course.

My only difficulty is getting a diverse range—mostly I find images of the vulvas of young, thin, white, completely shaved vulvas. I have to search carefully to find great sex-positive images of older vulvas, vulvas of people of color and people of size, surgically constructed vulvas, and vulvas with all their pubic hair.

One day I was sitting around a busy comics convention talking about this challenge with Camilla, who, like me, is a nerd and a former college peer sex educator. Unlike me, she has a degree in gender studies and studio art, is African American, and makes her living as an illustrator—all of which gave her insight into my little challenge.

She said, "Seriously, Emily? You're googling, what, like, 'black vulva'? At work?"

I shrugged apologetically. "Sausages, laws, and sex education lectures. You don't want to know how any of them are made."

And Camilla said, "Let me guess: All you find is porny images, nothing artistic or empowered or body positive?"

"Porn and graphic medical pictures," I agreed. "I tried searching 'feminist vulvas of color,' but all I got was embroidery projects from Pinterest and Etsy."

Camilla laughed at that, but said, "Now think if you were a young woman trying to see what a normal, healthy vulva looks like. If you're white, you're all set, Tumblr is full of those. But if you're Black or Asian or Latina, what is there? Porn and medical pictures. What does that tell you?"

I said, "But I can't say, 'Hey, women of color, post more pictures of your vulvas on the web, so that other women will know they're normal.'"

"No, but still," Camilla said, "the images we see—or don't see—matter. You know those Escher girls?"

"No, what's an Escher girl?"

"They're the female characters in comics with abdomens so flat there's no room for their internal organs, and their spines are impossibly twisted so that you can see both boobs and both butt cheeks at the same time. Their poses are so anatomically absurd that they're named after an artist famous for impossible illusions."

"Sounds like some bad porn I've seen," I said.

"Right," said Camilla. "I saw those as a teenager and I felt like that said everything about what a 'female' was supposed to be, and because that wasn't what being female felt like to me, I decided my first identity is 'geek.' Not woman, not Black: geek. Gamer. It took a long time to integrate the other parts of my identity, because I couldn't see how they all fit together. Images matter. They tell us what's possible, what things go together, what belongs and what doesn't belong. And we're all just trying to belong somewhere."

This statement was such a gift to me. I go back to this idea over and over now, as I write my lectures. I spend hours searching the internet for sex-positive images of a wide variety of vulvas, because my students vary—no two alike—and I want them to know that their bodies are normal and that they belong there in my classroom.

why it matters

Why might the seemingly simple fact that all human genitals are made of the same parts, organized in different ways be the most important thing you'll ever learn about human sexuality?

Two reasons:

First, because it means your genitals are normal—and not just normal, but amazing and beautiful and captivating and delicious and enticing, on down the alphabet, all the way to zesty—regardless of what they look like. They are unique to you. The entire range is normal. Beautiful. Perfect.

And second, because it is true for each and every facet of human sexual expression. As we'll see in the chapters that follow, from genital response to spanking fetishes, our sexual physiology, psychology, and desires are all made of the same parts, just organized in different ways.

If we embrace this simple, profound idea—all the same parts, organized in different ways—it answers that ever-popular question: Are men's and women's sexualities the same, or are they different?

Answer: Yes.

They're made of the same parts, organized differently.

While we can see obvious group differences when we look at populations—male and female bodies—there's at least as much variability within those groups as there is between those groups.

I can illustrate with a non-sex example. The average height of adult women is five feet four and the average height of adult men is five feet ten, a six-inch difference between the two groups' averages. But height varies more within each group than between the groups. If you measured the heights of a thousand random people—five hundred men and five hundred women—you'd find that nearly all the women would be between five feet and five feet eight—an eight-inch difference within the group—and nearly all the men would be between five feet four and six feet four—a twelve-inch difference. Notice three things: There's more difference *within* each group (eight or twelve inches) than *between* the two groups (six inches); there are four inches of overlap between the groups; and one or two hundred people among the thousand would be outside even these wide ranges![12]

The same goes for sex. Within each group we find a vast range of diversity—and I don't mean just anatomically. I mean in sexual orientation, sexual preferences, gender identity and expression, and—the subject of the rest of this book—sexual functioning: arousal, desire, pleasure, and orgasm. We also find overlap between the two groups, and we find folks who vary wildly from the "average" while still being perfectly normal and healthy.

Some authors argue that the differences between men and women are more important than the similarities. Others say that the similarities are more important than the differences. My view is that the basic fact of homology—all the same parts, organized in different ways—is more important than either.

And *variety* may be the one and only truly universal characteristic of human sexuality. From our bodies to our desires to our behaviors, there are as many "sexualities" as there are humans alive on Earth. No two alike.

Here's the kind of conversation you have when you're a sex educator out drinking with your friends:

LAURIE: "This woman I know told me if she ever has kids, she'll have plastic surgery on her ladybusiness right after she gives birth, because she thinks it won't look good anymore."

CAMILLA: "Did you tell her that the cosmetic medical-industrial complex paid a lot of money to make sure she felt that way about her body, so that they could profit from her needless self-criticism, despite the fact that there's no unbiased evidence that it improves sexual functioning?"[13]

LAURIE: "No, I told her that once you have kids, your partner is just glad if they ever get to see your business, whatever it looks like."

EMILY: "Let's invent a ritual where women celebrate the transition into their postpartum bodies. I mean, it's not just its appearance that changes, it's what your body means, *to yourself and to the world."*

Laurie was the only mom in the group, and she was the only one who didn't look at me like I was on drugs. She said, "I totally want a ritual. Anything to make it easier to live in a body that feels like a deflated balloon."

"But you're so beautiful!" everyone said instantly.

The compliments to Laurie's indisputable beauty flowed even faster than the wine, but a few days later, Laurie told me that was the opposite of what she needed.

"What I need is to hear that it's okay to feel sad that my body will never be what it used to be. I put a lot of effort into learning to love that body, and now I've got to start all over again learning to love this one."

So I said, "It's okay to feel sad that your body has permanently changed."

Laurie burst into tears—which is something she does a lot lately, sudden quiet little storms that pass through her anytime she finds herself on the receiving end of the affection and attention she lavishes on others.

"It shouldn't even be about whether I like my body or not," she sniffed. "That's really what changed after I had Trev. Now it should really be about whether or not it does what I need it to do."

By "what she needs it to do," Laurie means giving birth—at home, squatting in the tub, like a boss—breast-feeding for more than a year, and never sleeping more than four hours in a row for almost three years—the sentence "Trevor is a bad sleeper" doesn't even begin to cover the dark circles under Laurie's eyes. Laurie's body is amazing.

But she doesn't feel that way.

The notion of "all the same parts, organized in different ways" is as true for the ways a woman's body changes over the course of her life as it is for the ways people's genitals vary. And just as everyone's genitals are normal and beautiful, so all women's bodies are normal and beautiful.

But mostly that's not what women are taught. Mostly we're taught that our bodies are supposed to be one specific shape, otherwise there's something wrong *with us. I'll talk about that—and how to overcome it—in chapter 5.*

change how you see[14]

I realize that just saying "Your genitals are perfect and beautiful" won't change anything if you feel uncomfortable with your genitals, but if seeing the beauty of your unique and healthy genitals is something you struggle with, there are two things I'd like you to do:

1. Get a hand mirror and look at your vulva, as I described earlier in the chapter. (Sometimes people use their cell phone with the camera in self-portrait mode. That works, too!) As you look, make note of all the things you *like* about what you see. Write them down. You'll notice that your brain tries to list all the things you don't like, but don't include those. Do it again every week. Or twice a week. Or more. Each time, the things you like will become a little more salient and the noise will get a little quieter. Maybe even consider telling someone else about what you see and what you like. Better still, tell someone who also did the exercise!

    This activity gets labeled "cognitive dissonance" because it forces us to be aware of good things, when mostly we tend to be aware of the "negative" things. Try it.

2. Ask your partner, if you have one, to have a close look. Turn on the light, take off your clothes, get on your back, and let them look. Ask them to tell you what they see, how they feel about what they see, what memories they have of your vulva. Let your partner know what you've felt worried about, and ask them to help you see what they see. Listen to what they say—listen with your heart, not with your fear.

a better metaphor

We started this chapter thinking about the ways we metaphorize anatomy, creating meaning from random acts of biology in ways that end up making us feel uncomfortable with our bodies. To help undo all that, I like to use a different metaphor: a garden. It's a metaphor I use a lot—remember the apple tree from the introduction?—because it offers a judgment-free way of thinking about how the sexual hardware we're born with (our bodies and brains) and the families and culture we're born into interact to give rise to the individual sexual self that emerges in adulthood.

It goes like this: On the day you're born, you're given a little plot of rich and fertile soil, slightly different from everyone else's. And right away, your family and your culture start to plant things and tend the garden for you, until you're old enough to take over its care yourself. They plant language and attitudes and knowledge about love and safety and bodies and pleasure. And they teach you how to tend your garden, because as you transition through adolescence into adulthood, you'll take on full responsibility for its care.

And you didn't choose any of that. You didn't choose your plot of land, the seeds that were planted, or the way your garden was tended in the early years of your life.

As you reach adolescence, you begin to take care of the garden on your own. And you may find that your family and culture have planted some beautiful, healthy things that are thriving in a well-tended garden. And you may notice some things you want to change. Maybe the strategies you were taught for cultivating the garden are inefficient, so you need to find different ways of taking care of it so that it will thrive (that's in chapter 3). Maybe the seeds that were planted were not the kind of thing that will thrive in your particular garden, so you need to find something that's a better fit for you (that's in chapters 4 and 5).

Some of us get lucky with our land and what gets planted. We have healthy and thriving gardens from the earliest moments of our awareness. And some of us get stuck with some pretty toxic crap in our gardens, and we're left with the task of uprooting all the junk and replacing it with something healthier, something we choose for ourselves.

Your physical body—including your genitals—is one part of the basic hardware of your sexuality, the plot of land. Your brain and your environment are the rest of the hardware, and they're the subject of chapters 2 and 3.

what it *is*, not what it *means*

Olivia used her idea about her hormones, her "masculine" genitals, and her high sexual interest as a shield against the cultural criticisms that said she was . . . well, all kinds of things for which she "ought to be ashamed." A slut. A nymphomaniac. Trying to "get attention," "get a man," or "control people" with her body—none of which were true, but all of which had been flung at her at various times in her life. The world had tried to convince her that her sexuality was toxic, dangerous to both herself and the people around her.

She had fought hard against these messages, in defense of her own sexual wellbeing. The shield of "It's my hormones, so it's natural" was an important part of that defense.

But as she absorbed the idea of "all the same parts, organized in different ways," she didn't need the shield anymore. She realized that the shield was actually blocking her off from other people, while "all the same parts" actively connected her with other people—it meant she wasn't different or separate. She was the same—unique, but still connected in the continuum of human sexuality.

This is what science can do for us, if we let it. It offers us an opportunity to lower our defenses and experience the ways that we are all connected.

I know for a fact that Olivia was not born feeling uncomfortable with her genitals or her sexuality, and neither were you. When you were born, you were deeply, gloriously satisfied with (and curious about) each and every part of your body. But decades of sex-negative culture have let in weeds of dissatisfaction. Chapters 3 and 4 explain precisely how this can influence your sexual wellbeing, and chapter 5 describes how to undo that process and get back to living wholly inside your body, to return to that state you were born into, of deep, warm affection for and curiosity about your own body.

But before we get there, let's spend a chapter talking about the most important of all your sex organs and how it, too, is made of all the same parts as everyone else's but organized in a unique way.

I refer, of course, to your brain.

tl;dr

- Everyone's genitals are made of the same parts, organized in different ways. No two alike.
- Are you experiencing pain? If so, talk to a medical provider. If not, then your genitals are normal and healthy and beautiful and perfect just as they are.
- The genitals you see in soft-core porn images may have been digitally altered to appear more "tucked in"; don't let that fool you into believing that all vulvas look that way.
- Find a mirror (or use the self-portrait camera on your phone) and actually look at your clitoris. Knowing where the clitoris is is important, but knowing where *your* clitoris is is *power*.

two

the dual control model

YOUR SEXUAL PERSONALITY

Laurie hadn't actually wanted *sex with her husband, Johnny—I mean, really* craved *it—since before their son Trev was born. At first she figured it was the pregnancy. Then she figured it was a postpartum thing.*

Then she figured she was just tired.

Or depressed.

Or maybe she didn't actually love her husband.

Or maybe she was broken.

Or maybe humans just aren't meant to stay erotically connected after the months of cleaning baby puke off each other's shirts.

They'd had a great run. Right up until she got pregnant, their sex life was the kind of thing you find in romance novels—hot, hungry, passionate, sweet, loving, and just kinky enough to give them something wicked to think about as they locked eyes over his parents' Thanksgiving dinner table.

So maybe that was all they got. Maybe the rest of their lives would be sexless.

Still, they'd been trying. They'd bought some toys and massage oil.

They'd tried tying her up, tying him up, using flavored lube, videoing themselves, playing games . . . and sometimes it worked, all this exploration.

But mostly it didn't. Mostly Laurie wound up feeling sad and lonely because she loved Johnny, loved him so much it hurt, yet she couldn't make herself want him, not even with all the novelty and adventure available to them in a twenty-first-century world of technology, fantasy, and permissiveness.

One side benefit of this whole situation was that Laurie found she could have an orgasm in about five minutes with the vibrator, and that made falling asleep easier. So she'd go to bed early and buzz herself to sleep. But she hid it from Johnny, because she was pretty sure he'd be unhappy to learn that she was having orgasms on her own but not with him. It puzzled her, this interest in solo orgasm, when hardly anything could prompt her to want sex with her husband.

So she felt stuck and confused and crazy when she sat down to talk with me about it.

Her perception of the situation—and her sense of hopelessness—changed completely when she learned what's in this chapter: Your sexual brain has an "accelerator" that responds to sexual stimulation, but it also has "brakes," which respond to all the very good reasons not to be turned on right now.

Imagine it's 1964 and you're working in the laboratory of groundbreaking sex researchers William Masters and Virginia Johnson, at Washington University in St. Louis. You're on the cutting edge of science, working to understand what has never been studied before, and you spend a lot of time posting want ads in the local paper. You're looking for people, ordinary people, who are not only willing but also able to have orgasm in a laboratory ("research quarters") while connected to machines that measure their heart rate, blood pressure, blood flow, and genital response, with you and the team of scientists in the room, observing.

When a woman responds to the ad, you invite her to the lab, where you take a detailed medical and sexual history, you conduct a physical exam to check for any health issues, and you introduce her to the research quarters and its equipment. Next time she comes in, she practices having an orgasm in the research quarters, first on her own and then with the research team there in the room with her.

Now she'll be observed, measured, and assessed as she stimulates herself with the equipment in the research quarters, all the way to orgasm. For science.

This is what you'll observe:[1]

Excitement. As stimulation begins, her heart rate, blood pressure, and respiration rate increase, and her labia minora and the clitoris darken and swell, separating the outer labia. The walls of the vagina begin to lubricate and then lengthen. Her breasts swell and the nipples become erect. Late in excitement, she may begin to sweat.

Plateau. Lubrication begins at the mouth of the vagina, from the Bartholin's glands. Her breasts continue to swell, so much that the nipples seem to retract into the breasts. She may experience "sex flush," a concentration of color over the chest. By now her inner labia have doubled in size from their resting state. The internal structures of the clitoris lift, drawing the external portion up and inward, so that it retracts from the surface of the body. The vagina itself "tents" around the cervix, open and wide deep inside the body. She experiences the involuntary muscle contraction known as myotonia, including carpopedal spasms (contraction of muscles in the hands and feet). She may begin to pant or hold her breath, as the thoracic and pelvic diaphragms contract in unison.

Orgasm. All the sphincters of her pelvic diaphragm (the "Kegel" muscle) contract in unison—urethra, vagina, and anus. She experiences rapid breathing, rapid heartbeat, and increased blood pressure. Her pelvis may rock, various muscle groups may tighten involuntarily. She experiences the sudden release of the tension that has accumulated in the muscles throughout her body.

Resolution. Breasts return to baseline, clitoris and labia return to baseline, heart rate, respiration rate, blood pressure all return to baseline.

This four-phase model of sexual response quickly became the foundation of sex therapists', educators', and researchers' understanding of the human sexual response. As the first scientific description of the physiology of sexual response, it would become the basis for defining sexual health and also sexual problems.

Now imagine you're a sex therapist in the 1970s, using the four-phase model to understand and treat clients with sexual dysfunction. Some of them you can help. Clients with anorgasmia (lack of orgasm) can learn to have orgasms, those with premature ejaculation can learn to control orgasm, those with vaginismus (vaginal spasms) can learn to relax those muscles. But there's a group of clients who just don't seem to respond to therapy informed by the four-phase model.

This is what happened to psychotherapist Helen Singer Kaplan. Reviewing treatment failures among her own and her colleagues' patients, she found that the clients with the least successful outcomes were those who lacked interest in sex. Kaplan realized something important was entirely missing from the four-phase model: *desire*. The entire concept of sexual desire was utterly missing from the dominant theory of human sexual response.

It seems like a glaring oversight in retrospect, but of course it was missing—people who come to a laboratory to masturbate for science don't have to *want* sex before they begin; they just have to get aroused for the purpose of the experiment.

So Kaplan took the four-phase model out of the laboratory and adapted it to the lived experience of her clients. Her "triphasic" model of the sexual response cycle begins with desire, which she conceptualized as "interest in" or "appetite for" sex, much like hunger or thirst.[2] The second phase is arousal, which combines excitement and plateau into one phase, and the third phase is orgasm.

For decades, Kaplan's new triphasic model of sexual response served as the foundation for diagnostic criteria in the American Psychiatric

Association's *Diagnostic and Statistical Manual*. You could have normal or problematic desire, normal or problematic arousal, and normal or problematic orgasm. A number of these diagnoses now have effective treatments, including cognitive-behavioral therapy, mindfulness, sensorimotor therapies, and medications.

Fast-forward two more decades. Now, low desire and desire discrepancy are the most common reasons people seek sex therapy, while other clients experience "hypersexuality," where they feel out of control of their desire and behaviors. What's going on? How can so many people struggle with lack of desire, while others struggle with too much? Why does desire level change? What controls whether and when we're interested in sex? Exactly how much desire is the "right amount" of desire?

At the turn of the twenty-first century, a pair of sex researchers at the Kinsey Institute proposed a model of sexual response that answered these questions. It wasn't just a description of what happens in the body, like Masters and Johnson's work, or even a description of what happens in a sexual relationship, like Kaplan's. It was a description of the brain mechanism that governs sexual response. And it's the topic of this chapter.

In the first section of the chapter, I'll describe the basic theory of the "dual control model" of sexual response, which proposes a sexual "accelerator" and sexual "brakes." And like desire, once someone points it out, it's obvious . . . and it changes your entire understanding of how sex works.

In the second section of this chapter, I'll talk about individual differences in the sensitivity of the brakes and accelerator. This variation impacts how a person responds to the sexual world. We'll find that while yes, as you'd expect, men often have more sensitive accelerators and women have more sensitive brakes, there's far more variation within those groups than between them. What's more interesting than just how sensitive the mechanisms are is how these mechanisms relate to your mood and to your environment.

And that's what the third section is about: what the brakes and accelerator respond to. What on earth is a "sex-related stimulus"? What kind of "potential threat" causes our brains to hit the brakes? How does our brain know what to respond to and what not to respond to? And can we change that?

I bet that before you picked up this book, you already knew that female genitals include a vagina and a clitoris, and you already knew that arousal, desire, and orgasm are things people generally experience as part of sexual response. Once you've read this chapter, I want you to feel that your accelerator and your brakes are as basic, as integral to your sexual functioning, as your clitoris and your desire. If I do my job in the next few pages, you'll be telling everyone you know: "OMG, everybody, *there's a brake!*"

turn on the ons, turn off the offs

Allow me to introduce you to the dual control model.

Developed in the late 1990s by Erick Janssen and John Bancroft at the Kinsey Institute, the dual control model of sexual response goes far beyond earlier models of human sexuality, by describing not just "what happens" during arousal—erection, lubrication, etc.—but also the central mechanism that governs sexual arousal, which controls how and when you respond to sex-related sights, sounds, sensations, and ideas.[3]

The more I learned about the dual control model during my graduate education, the more I felt the lights come on in my understanding of human sexuality. I've been teaching about it for decades now, and the more I teach it, the more I see how valuable it is in helping people to understand their own sexual functioning.

Here's how it works:

Your central nervous system (your brain and spinal cord) is made up of a series of partnerships of accelerator and brakes—like the pairing of your sympathetic nervous system ("accelerator") and your parasympathetic nervous system ("brakes"). A core insight of the dual control model is that what's true for other aspects of the nervous system must also be true for the brain system that coordinates sex: a sexual accelerator

and sexual brakes. (Daniel Kahneman wrote of his own Nobel Prize–
winning research in economics, "You know you have made a theoretical
advance when you can no longer reconstruct why you failed for so long
to see the obvious." So it was with Kahneman's prospect theory, and so it
is with the dual control model. I stand ready to send Erick and John large
fruit baskets on the day the Nobel committee gets its act together and
recognizes the importance of their insight.) So the dual control model of
sexual response, as the name implies, consists of two parts:

Sexual Excitation System (SE). The accelerator of your sexual
response. It receives information about sex-related stimuli in the
environment—things you see, hear, smell, touch, taste, or imagine—and
sends signals from the brain to the genitals to tell them, "Turn on!" SE
is constantly scanning your context (including your own thoughts and
feelings) for things that are sex-related. It is always at work, far below
the level of consciousness. You aren't aware that it's there until you find
yourself turned on and pursuing sexual pleasure.

Sexual Inhibition System (SI). Your sexual brakes. "Inhibition" here
doesn't mean "shyness" but rather neurological "off" signals. Research
has found that there are actually two brakes, reflecting the different functions of an inhibitory system. One brake works in much the same way as
the accelerator. It notices all the potential threats in the environment—
everything you see, hear, smell, touch, taste, or imagine—and sends
signals saying, "Turn off!" It's like the foot brake in a car, responding to
stimuli in the moment. Just as the accelerator scans the environment for
turn-ons, this brake scans for anything your brain interprets as a good
reason not to be aroused right now—risk of STI transmission, unwanted
pregnancy, social consequences, etc. And all day long it sends a steady
stream of "Turn off!" messages. This brake is responsible for preventing
us from getting inappropriately aroused in the middle of a business meeting or at dinner with our family. It's also the system that throws the off
switch if, say, in the middle of some nookie, your grandmother walks in
the room.

The second brake is a little different. It's more like the hand brake in a car, a chronic, low-level "No thank you" signal. If you try to drive with the hand brake on, you might be able to get where you want to go, but it'll take longer and use a lot more gas. Where the foot brake is associated with "fear of performance consequences," the hand brake is associated with "fear of performance failure," like worry about not having an orgasm.

For the rest of the book, I'll be referring to the brakes generally, without differentiating between the two kinds, since, so far, effective strategies for turning off the brakes aren't different depending on which brake is being hit. As more science emerges, we might develop behavioral strategies or even medications that target a specific system, but in the meantime, you don't need to know for sure which brake is being hit in order to figure out how to stop hitting it.

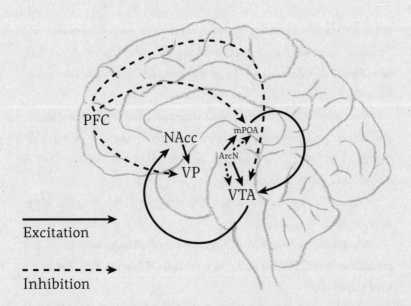

A highly simplified illustration of some excitatory (accelerator) and inhibitory (brakes) signals in the brain. ArcN = arcuate nucleus; mPOA = media preoptical area; NAcc = nucleus accumbens; PFC = prefrontal cortex; VP = ventral pallidum; VTA = ventral tegmental area. Notice signals from the ArcN are both excitatory and inhibitory.

In essence, that's all the dual control model is: the brakes and the accelerator. And it's not a metaphor, it's a literal description of the excitatory and inhibitory activity of the central nervous system.[4] The details are more complex, obviously, but the implications of even this basic idea are powerful, because you can immediately conceptualize all sexual functioning—and all sexual dysfunction—as a balance between brakes and accelerator. If you're having trouble with any phase of sexual response, is it because there's not enough stimulation to the accelerator? Or is there too much stimulation to the brakes? Indeed, a common mistake made by people who are struggling with orgasm or desire is assuming that the problem is a lack of accelerator; it's more likely that the problem is too much brakes (more on that in chapters 7 and 8). And once you know whether it's a problem with the accelerator or the brakes, you can figure out how to create change.

> When Olivia (the exuberant masturbator from chapter 1) answered my "excitors" questions [in the worksheets on pages 54–55] with, "I can feel turned on doing the dishes," I had a pretty good idea what her sexual brain was like.
>
> She told me, "I love sex. I love my partner. I love trying new things, new places, new positions, new toys, new porn, new everything. I'm One Big Yes." And I could see it in her face: the joy, the confidence of a woman living fully inside her body.
>
> I asked, "Have you sometimes done things and then thought, 'Why did I do that?'"
>
> She winced and nodded. "That's happened. Rarely, but . . . when I get super stressed, I'll just go out and be like, 'Whatever. Go.' I've done some stupid shit."
>
> "And are there times when you feel like you need to masturbate several times a day?" I asked, and she blinked at me like she wondered if I had a camera in her bedroom.
>
> "Usually I can ignore it," she said. "But every once in a while it

just makes me crazy. It's like having an itch that no amount of scratching will help. I have this out-of-control feeling."

"Yeah," I said. "A sensitive accelerator can make people more prone to risk-taking and compulsivity—that 'out-of-control' feeling."

"That's why? A sensitive accelerator?" she said. "I'm not high testosterone, I'm high SE?"

"It would explain both your 'One Big Yes' and the occasional out-of-control feeling."

It's easy to assume that having a sensitive accelerator is fun—and it can be, in the right context. Olivia has a partner she delights in and a wide-open attitude that allows her to explore without worry or fear. She dives right in. And then sometimes, especially when she's stressed or anxious, Olivia said, "It can feel like my sex drive is constantly demanding my attention and won't leave me alone."

There's another level, too, to the risks that can accompany a sensitive accelerator. Because she sometimes feels like her own sexuality is bossing her around, Olivia finds herself worried that she, in turn, is bossing her partner around, being too pushy, too demanding, too sexual, just plain too much.

"I have to wield my powerful sexuality carefully, for the betterment of humanity," she announced—mostly kidding.

Mostly.

your sexual temperament

According to the dual control model, sexual arousal is really two processes: activating the accelerator and deactivating the brakes. So your level of sexual arousal at any given moment is the product of how much stimulation the accelerator is getting and how little stimulation the brakes are getting.

But it's also a product of *how sensitive* your brakes and accelerator are to that stimulation.

The brakes and accelerator are *traits*. We all have them and they're more or less stable over time, but, like introversion/extroversion, they vary from individual to individual.[5] Just as we all have phalluses and urethras, as we saw in chapter 1, we all have a sexual accelerator and sexual brakes in our central nervous systems (we're all the same!). But we all have *different sensitivities* of brakes and accelerator (we're all different!), which leads to different sexual temperaments or personalities.

Some people are high on both brakes and accelerator, others are low on both, some have high brakes but low accelerator, and some have high accelerator but low brakes. And most of us are average. The variation is distributed on a nice bell curve; the majority of people are heaped up in the middle and a few people are at the extreme ends.

Let's take a look at what happens if brakes or accelerator is especially sensitive (or not).

Suppose you're high on SE and low on SI—sensitive accelerator and hardly any brakes. What kind of sexual response do you have?

You respond readily to sex-related stimuli but not to potential threats, so you're easily turned on and have a difficult time turning off. Which isn't always as fun as it might sound, and it can, under some circumstances, be related to inconsistent condom use, more partners, more one-night stands, and feeling "out of control" of your sexuality, which are higher risk for unwanted consequences.[6]

The sensitive accelerator plus not-so-sensitive brakes combination describes between roughly 2 and 6 percent of women, and it's associated with sexual risk-taking and compulsivity.[7] Because the brain mechanism responsible for noticing sex-related stimuli is very sensitive, you're highly motivated to pursue sex, and because the brain mechanism responsible for stopping you from doing higher-risk things is less responsive, you may sometimes feel "out of control" of your sexuality, especially when you're stressed. You're likely to have more partners, use less protection, and feel less "in control." You might also be more likely to want sex when you are stressed ("redliners"), whereas other folks are likely to find that their interest in sex plummets when they're stressed ("flatliners").

What if you have the opposite combination—sensitive brakes plus not-so-sensitive accelerator? This describes about 1 to 4 percent of women and is associated with problems with getting aroused, lack of interest or desire, and difficulty with orgasm. If you have sensitive brakes, you're very responsive to all the reasons *not* to be aroused, and if you have a relatively insensitive accelerator, it takes a lot of concentration and deliberate attention to tune in to sex.

Sensitive brakes, regardless of the accelerator, is the strongest predictor of sexual problems of all kinds. In a 2008 survey of 226 women age eighteen to eighty-one, low interest in sex, arousal difficulties, and orgasm difficulty were significantly correlated with inhibition factors, especially "arousal contingency" ("Unless things are 'just right' it is difficult for me to become sexually aroused") and concerns about sexual function ("If I am worried about taking too long to become aroused or to orgasm, this can interfere with my arousal").[8]

You can complete the Sexual Temperament Questionnaire that follows to get an idea of how sensitive your own brakes and accelerator are. Don't mistake this for actual science! It's a *Cosmo* quiz adaptation of the science, intended to guide you in your understanding of how your internal sexual response mechanism may influence your response to sexual stimulation, but it is just an approximation.[9] Remember, especially, that there are actually two different brakes. Some people's arousal is shut down more because of internal fears (e.g., taking too long to become aroused), and others are more affected by fears about external factors (e.g., getting an STI or getting caught having sex). Both can decrease your arousal, or prevent you from becoming aroused in the first place.

Inhibitors

Sometimes I have so many worries that I am unable to get aroused.

0	1	2	3	4
Not at all like me	Not much like me	Somewhat like me	A lot like me	Exactly like me

Unless things are "just right," it is difficult for me to become sexually aroused.

0	1	2	3	4
Not at all like me	Not much like me	Somewhat like me	A lot like me	Exactly like me

If I am uncertain how my partner feels about me, it is harder for me to get aroused.

0	1	2	3	4
Not at all like me	Not much like me	Somewhat like me	A lot like me	Exactly like me

If I am worried about taking too long to become aroused or to orgasm, this can interfere with my arousal.

0	1	2	3	4
Not at all like me	Not much like me	Somewhat like me	A lot like me	Exactly like me

Sometimes I feel so "shy" or self-conscious during sex that I cannot become fully aroused.

0	1	2	3	4
Not at all like me	Not much like me	Somewhat like me	A lot like me	Exactly like me

Total (out of 20) _____

Excitors

Seeing a partner doing something that shows their talent or intelligence, or watching them interacting well with others can make me very sexually aroused.

0	1	2	3	4
Not at all like me	Not much like me	Somewhat like me	A lot like me	Exactly like me

When I think about someone I find sexually attractive or fantasize about sex, I easily become sexually aroused.

0	1	2	3	4
Not at all like me	Not much like me	Somewhat like me	A lot like me	Exactly like me

If it is possible someone might see or hear us having sex, it is more difficult for me to get aroused.

4	3	2	1	0
Not at all like me	Not much like me	Somewhat like me	A lot like me	Exactly like me

Particular scents are very arousing to me.

0	1	2	3	4
Not at all like me	Not much like me	Somewhat like me	A lot like me	Exactly like me

I think about sex a lot when I am bored.

0	1	2	3	4
Not at all like me	Not much like me	Somewhat like me	A lot like me	Exactly like me

Total (out of 20) _____

Score Your Sexual Temperament Questionnaire

Low SI (0–6)

You're not so sensitive to all the reasons not to be sexually aroused. You don't tend to worry about your own sexual functioning, and body image issues don't interfere too much with your sexuality. When you're sexually engaged, your attention is not very distractible, and you wouldn't be inclined to describe yourself as "sexually shy." Most circumstances can be sexual for you. You may find that your main challenge around sexual functioning is holding yourself back, reining yourself in. Staying aware of potential consequences can help with this. Around 15 percent of the women I've asked fit in this range.

Medium SI (7–13)

You're right in the middle, along with more than half the women I've asked. This means that whether or not your brakes engage will be largely dependent on context. Risky or novel situations, such as a new partner, might increase your concerns about your own sexual functioning, shyness, or your distractibility during sex. Contexts that easily arouse you are likely to be low risk and more familiar, and anytime your stress—which includes anxiety, depression, overwhelm, and exhaustion—escalates your brakes will reduce your interest in and response to sexual signals.

High SI (14–20)

You're pretty sensitive to all the reasons not to be sexually aroused. You need a setting of trust and relaxation in order to be aroused, and it's best if you don't feel rushed or pressured in any way. You might be easily distracted from sex. High SI, regardless of SE, is the most strongly correlated factor with sexual problems, so if this is you, pay close attention to the "sexy contexts" worksheets in the chapters that follow. About a quarter of the women I've asked fall into this range.

Low SE (0–6)

You're not so sensitive to sex-related stimuli and need to make a more deliberate effort to tune your attention in that direction. Novel situations are less likely to be sexy to you than familiar ones. You're a person whose sexual functioning will benefit from adding a greater intensity of stimulation (like a vibrator) and daily practice of paying attention to sensations. Lower SE is also associated with asexuality, so if you're very low SE, you might resonate with some components of the asexual identity. The women I ask are probably higher SE than the overall population— they're women who are interested enough in sex to take a class, attend a workshop, or read a sex blog—but still about 8 percent of those women fall into this range.

Medium SE (7–13)

You're right in the middle, so whether or not you're sensitive to sexual stimuli probably depends on the context. In situations of high romance or eroticism, you tune in readily to sexual stimuli; and in situations of low romance or eroticism, it may be pretty challenging to move your attention to sexual things. Recognize the role that context plays in your arousal and pleasure, and take steps to increase the sexiness of your life's contexts. Seventy percent of the women I've asked fall into this range.

High SE (14–20)

You're pretty sensitive to sex-related stimuli, maybe even to things humans aren't generally very sensitive to, like smell and taste. A fairly wide range of contexts can be sexual for you, and novelty may be really exciting. You may be a person who likes having sex as a way to de-stress. Your sexual functioning may benefit from making sure you create lots of time and space for your partner; because you're sensitive, you can derive intense satisfaction from your partner's pleasure, so you'll both benefit! About 16 percent of the women I ask fall into this group.

what "medium" means

Did you score right in the middle on both? More than half of people do. Scoring very high or very low on these traits is comparatively rare, so for the majority of people the value of the dual control model lies not in the discovery that, "Wow, my brain is extra sensitive/not sensitive to this kind of input, so I need to pay attention to that!" The value instead lies in the insight that the brakes and the accelerator are *two separate systems*. Some things in the world activate your accelerator. Other things hit your brakes. Some things even hit both at once! One blog reader emailed me that "brakes and accelerator at the same time" exactly described her experience while reading the best-selling sexually explicit novel *Fifty Shades of Grey*.

Medium means you can say to yourself, "Hey, I'm normal!" and start thinking about what hits your brakes or activates your accelerator, and how to recalibrate your life to suit your brain. I'll discuss how to do that in chapters 3, 4, and 5.

If you scored high or low on either scale—especially if your score is at an extreme end—you can say to yourself, "Hey, I'm normal and also comparatively rare!" And as you consider what engages your brakes and accelerator, you'll begin to realize that you relate to the sexual world around you in ways most other people don't experience.

Camilla, the artist, is smart—smart and curious. One of the things she's curious about is sex. She doesn't just read books about it; she reads the original research.

And she has struggled to reconcile her intellectual hunger for knowledge about sex with her contrastingly small desire to actually have any sex. That day when we were talking about images of women, she mentioned this puzzle, especially noting that she never seemed to experience "out of the blue" desire.

I wondered if she might have sensitive brakes, so I asked her "inhibitors" questions: Do things have to be "just right" in order for you to get aroused? Do you need total trust in your partner? Do you worry about sex while you're having it?

Not really, not really, and not really.

Then I asked the "excitors" questions. Do you sometimes get aroused just by watching your partner do something (nonsexual) that they're good at, or by their smell, or when you feel sexually "wanted"? Are you aroused by new situations? Do you feel turned on by fantasies?

Not really, heck no, and . . . what fantasies?

Camilla's low SE. This doesn't mean she's not interested in the idea of sex; it means her brain requires a bunch of stimulation in order to cross the threshold into active desire for sex.

I asked about orgasm.

"Few in number and slow to come," she said, "and they don't often seem worth the effort." She finds she's most reliably orgasmic with a vibrator, and that makes perfect sense—mechanical vibration can provide an intensity of stimulation that no organic stimulation can match. But for her, orgasm is sometimes more of a distraction than a goal with sex. She loves being with her partner, she loves playing and exploring. But sometimes she's just as happy cooking with him as having sex.

"Henry isn't the most sexually driven guy in the world," she said. (Henry is her husband. He's a super-nice guy.) "But he'd love it if I initiated sex a little more often. Is this something a person can change?"

Yes it is.

Part of Camilla's solution is in chapter 3, but we'll have to wait until chapter 7 to get to the heart of it.

different for girls . . . sometimes

If you had to guess which group, men or women, has higher SE on average—a more sensitive accelerator—which would you pick?

Men, right? Yep. At the population level, on average, men have more sensitive accelerators.[10]

And which group has higher SI—more sensitive brakes?

Uh-huh. Women, on average, as a population, tend to have more sensitive brakes.

But remember from chapter 1 how height varies between men and women, but it varies more within each group than between the groups? Women in particular vary from one another in terms of their brakes and accelerator. A lot. Ask a thousand women how often they would ideally like to have sex and their answers will range from *never* to *multiple times a day*, and all of those answers are normal.

A more important difference than simply the sensitivity of the accelerators and brakes of men and women is the relationships of these two mechanisms with other aspects of men's and women's psychologies—especially mood and anxiety.

For example, about 10 to 20 percent of both men and women report an increase in their sexual interest when they're anxious or depressed.[11] But a guy who wants sex more when he's anxious or depressed may have *less sensitive brakes*. A woman who wants sex more when she's anxious or depressed may have a *more sensitive accelerator*.

What this shows us is that there's more than just a population-level difference in the average sensitivities of brakes and accelerator between men and women; there also seem to be a difference in how these two systems relate to the other motivational systems in the brain, particularly the stress response system. (We'll really get into this in chapter 4.)

But hey, look: It's all too easy to metaphorize the population-level differences in brakes and accelerator, the way previous generations metaphorized our genitals. Like, "Women are easily turned off and difficult to turn on." Or, "Women want sex less than men." As we'll see in the chapters that follow, the reality is nothing like that—for most people, sexual response depends as much on *context* as on brain mechanism.

Your own brakes and accelerator, and their relationship to your mood or anxiety, are unique and individual. The goal of understanding your brakes and accelerator is not to understand "what men are like" versus "what women are like," but to understand what *you* are like. Unique, with great potential for awesomeness.

what turns you on?

Huge, beautiful bathtubs at a B and B
Watching a partner put the kids to bed
"Slash fiction" of Harry Potter and Draco Malfoy
A fantasy about having sex in public
Actually having sex in public

No one was born responding sexually to any of these, but they're all things that women have told me turn them on. The dual control model tidily explains how the brain responds to stimuli, to increase or decrease your arousal. The brain notices sex-related stimuli (like fantasies or an attractive partner) and potential threats (like an unappreciative audience), and sends signals accordingly; sexual arousal is the dual process of turning on the ons and turning off the offs. But that doesn't tell us anything about how your brain figures out what counts as a sex-related stimulus or a potential threat.

The process of learning what is sex-related and what is a threat works sort of like learning a language. We're all born with the innate capacity to learn any human language, but we don't learn a random language, right? If you grow up surrounded by people who speak only English, there is no way you'll get to kindergarten speaking French. You learn the language you are surrounded by.

Similarly, you learn the *sexual* language you're surrounded by. Just as there are no innate words, there appear to be almost no innate sexual stimuli. What turns us on (or off) is learned from culture, in much the same way children learn vocabulary and accents from culture.

I'll illustrate this with three rat studies from the lab of researcher Jim Pfaus.

Imagine you're a male lab rat. Your mother raises you with everything a young rat needs, normal and healthy. In addition to that normal, healthy development, the researchers train you to associate the smell of lemons with sexual activity.[12] Ordinarily, lemons mean as much to rat sexuality as they do to human sexuality: nothing. But you've been trained to link lemons and sex in your brain. So when you're presented with two receptive female rats, one of whom smells like a healthy, receptive female rat and the other smells like a healthy, receptive female rat plus lemons, you'll prefer the one who smells like lemons—and by "prefer," I mean you'll copulate with both females, but 80 percent of your ejaculations will be with the lemony partner, and only about 20 percent of your ejaculations will be with the nonlemony partner. Your ratty sexual accelerator learned that lemons are sex-related, so the lemony partner hits your accelerator more.

Let's look at another experiment. This time, imagine that your brother was raised in the normal, healthy rat way, without the lemon thing. But during his first opportunity to copulate with a receptive female, the researchers put him into a rodent harness, a comfortable little jacket.[13]

If your brother is wearing his little rat jacket the first time he copulates with the receptive female, then the next time he's with a receptive female but not wearing the jacket, he'll actually self-inhibit. His brakes will stay on because during that single first experience, his brain learned that "jacket + female in estrus = sexytimes." It did not learn simply "female in estrus = sexytimes."

What these two experiments show us is that both the accelerator and the brakes learn what to respond to based on experience. Neither lemons nor jackets are innate; both were learned.

But it gets even more basic:

Now imagine once more that you're a male lab rat, raised healthy and happy by your mother. Then when you get to late adolescence and are still "sexually naïve" (aka a virgin), the experimenters introduce you to a female rat in estrus. This is about as erotic as it gets for a male rat on his first venture! But the researchers don't give you an opportunity to copulate with her.[14] You never actually get to have sex with this ready and willing female.

Result: You don't develop a preference for the smell of a fertile female over the smell of an infertile female or even of another male. It requires a sexy (i.e., copulatory) experience to teach the male rat's brain that a female in estrus is "sex-related." The instinct to attempt copulation is there, and he'll attempt copulation with everybody—but if he doesn't have the experience, he can't learn how to turn that instinct into successful action.

What is innate is the mechanism by which this learning takes place: ratty accelerator and brakes and the ability to learn through experience and association. But rats need experience to teach their brakes and accelerator what's a threat and what's sex-related.

In a rat's natural environment, outside the lab, he would never need a jacket in order to feel sexy, and the smell of lemons wouldn't make him ejaculate. The rats learned these things because humans created an environment where those were salient features of their sexual environment. But even things you would assume are innate—fertile female rats—must be learned by experience.

"Years of struggle."

That's how Merritt described her sex life. After she graduated, we became friends, which is when she told me that the most important thing she had taken away from my class was that there is a brake, *as well as an accelerator. It helped her understand why she felt desire for sex . . . but it seemed to be trapped. She realized she had sensitive brakes: Things had to be "just right" for her to get aroused, and she needed total trust in her partner. And she worried about sex while she was having it. She called this "noisy brain."*

"Yep, totally high SI. The noise is your sexual brakes, metaphori-

cally squealing," I said. "It would explain the 'windmilling on a cliff'
sensation you described to me a million years ago—your accelerator and
your brakes are activated at the same time."

With sensitive brakes, Merritt's sexual motivation system is the
highest risk for problems with desire, arousal, and orgasm—and she had
struggled with all three at some point in her life, she told me. Lately, it
was orgasm.

"I can get so close, and then it's like there's all this noise in my head."

She has a great relationship, she and her partner have loving and
playful sex on a pretty regular basis, but her arousal bottlenecks inside
her and then orgasm just isn't there for her, and then she gets frustrated,
and basically sex is turning into more of a hassle than a pleasure. We'll
hear more about the cause of Merritt's challenge in chapter 4, and a
great deal about the solution in chapter 8.

can you change your brain?

If a woman is experiencing sexual difficulties, the dual control model demands that we ask four questions:

- How sensitive is her accelerator?
- What's activating it?
- How sensitive are her brakes?
- What's hitting them?

So far in this chapter, you've been a sex researcher in the '60s, and
you've been a male lab rat with a lemon fetish. Now imagine you're a sex
educator, armed with the dual control model to help people understand
how their sexuality works. People ask you frustrated questions, dissatisfied with their sexual response mechanism—it doesn't behave the way
they want or expect it to, and they want to change it.

So can we change it?

The answer has two parts, both equally important.

First, accelerator and brakes are traits you're born with that remain more or less stable over time, and so far the only variable that seems to impact either is *partner characteristics* (see chapter 3).[15] In general, though, it seems there's very little we can do to deliberately change the mechanism in your brain.

And anyway, the sensitivities of most people's accelerator and brakes are "medium"—neither overly sensitive nor problematically insensitive. Changing the accelerator and brakes if you're medium isn't even desirable.

But then there's the second part of the answer: You may not be able to change the mechanism itself, but you probably can change what the mechanism responds to. You can often change what your brakes consider a potential threat, and you can reduce those threats, like unwanted pregnancy, STIs, stress, etc.

You also can change what your accelerator considers sex-related, and you can increase the sex-related things in your life. In other words, you can change the context—your external circumstances and your internal state. The why and how of these changes is the main topic of the next three chapters, but here's the short version:

You know that almost nothing your accelerator and brakes respond to is innate; your brain learned to associate particular stimuli with excitation or inhibition. Through a process of "tuning" your context—both your brain and your environment—you can maximize your sexual potential.

I thought Laurie, with her low desire, might be high SI. We wrote a list of things that activate her brakes: kid, full-time job with a rotten boss, her parents—not to mention the ways her body had changed since her pregnancy, which made her unhappy, and she also felt unhappy about feeling unhappy, since the feminist in her made her judge herself for not being able to let go of the arbitrary cultural ideal and just Love Her Body. Oh, and also? She was going back to school for a master's degree. So no big deal.

She didn't have particularly sensitive brakes—she had an ava-lanche of stuff constantly putting pressure on very average brakes.

"Just seeing all this written down makes me need a massage," she groaned.

"So ask Johnny to give you a massage," I suggested.

"Sure, and then I feel guilty if we don't have sex after that."

"Oooh, good insight! Add that to the list of things that hit your brakes: feeling like you're expected to have sex."

She did. And that's when I saw the lights go on for her. She said, "So all the toys and games were hitting the accelerator, but at the same time all these things in my life were hitting the brakes in my brain . . . and it doesn't matter how hard you hit the accelerator if the brake is on the floor. Huh."

"Right."

"So how do I stop hitting the brakes?"

The million-dollar question.

The short answer is: Reduce your stress, be affectionate toward your body, and let go of the false ideas about how sex is "supposed" to work, to create space in your life for how sex actually works.

The full answer is . . . the rest of this book.

My suggestion to Laurie was to stop trying to make herself want sex for a while. Take away the performance pressure.

She did not follow my advice—not right away, anyway. What she tried instead was a clever shift in context, which is what the next chapter is about.

To put it in terms of the garden metaphor I used in chapter 1, your accelerator and brakes are characteristics of the soil in your garden. So are your genitals and the rest of your body and brain. The innate sensitivity of your accelerator and brakes influences how your garden grows—which species of plants will thrive, how densely you can plant them—but other factors can have at least as much influence. Water, sun, choice of plants, even the addition of fertilizer—in other words, everything from stress to love to trust to a vibrator—can all influence the abundance of your garden. You can't change the soil itself, but you can augment it and you can make smart decisions about how to manage it.

And that's what chapter 3 is about.

tl;dr

- Your brain has a sexual "accelerator" that responds to "sex-related" stimulation—anything you see, hear, smell, touch, taste, or imagine that your brain has learned to associate with sexual arousal.
- Your brain also has sexual "brakes" that respond to "potential threats"—anything you see, hear, smell, touch, taste, or imagine that your brain interprets as a good reason not to be turned on right now. These can be anything from STIs and unwanted pregnancy to relationship·issues or social reputation.
- There's virtually no "innate" sex-related stimulus or threat; our accelerators and brakes learn when to respond through experience.
- People vary in how sensitive their brakes and accelerator are. Take the little quiz on page 54 to find out how sensitive yours are—and remember that most people score in the medium range, and all scores are normal.

three

context

AND THE "ONE RING" (TO RULE THEM ALL) IN YOUR EMOTIONAL BRAIN

You'd like Henry if you met him—he's polite, with a sweet smile and a soft voice, handsome, a little old-fashioned. He stands up when a lady enters the room. Henry is almost as geeky as Camilla, his wife. Their ideal Friday night involves Settlers of Catan, anything by Joss Whedon, or Cards Against Humanity—or possibly all three.

And they have a nice sex life, he and Camilla. Henry is pretty much always the initiator, and though he'd certainly enjoy being the object of his wife's sexual pursuit, he's an easygoing guy who feels lucky to have a life partner who shares both his sense of humor and his need to have the bathroom kept organized at all times. They're careful, thoughtful, introverted sweethearts.

When they first met—I mean, when they first met in person, which doesn't include the weeks of online flirting—their eyes met and both of them experienced an instantaneous, "Yes. This is it. You're it."

But they're careful, thoughtful people, and they took it slow.

They told each other, "I'm not really ready for a relationship. We should just be friends."

And they nodded solemnly at each other.

And they became friends.

For a year.

Gradually, Henry began to court her. He brought flowers . . . made of Legos. He commissioned her favorite webcomic artist to draw a portrait of her. He wrote RPG scenarios for her. He wore ties. He held her hand.

By the time they kissed, they were both in love—though neither had said so. And by the time they first made love, they had committed their lives to each other, and they told each other so over and over, urgent whispers in the dark.

Camilla, you'll remember, is a low SE woman—she represents about 4–8 percent of women whose sensitivity to sex-related stimuli is fairly low.[1] *And yet on the day she got married, oh, she was sensitive.*

Five years later . . . not so much.

She told me, "It used to be, I'd be in the kitchen and he'd come up behind me and start kissing my neck and I'd just melt instantly. But now he'll do the same thing and I'll just be like, 'I'm trying make dinner.' I don't understand what's wrong with me now."

"Nothing's wrong, the context is just different," I said.

"How is it different? I still love him exactly as much as I did the day we got married; I just seem to have emptied my 'lust tank.' Do people have a 'lust tank' that can be empty?"

"No . . . well . . . sort of? Not really. It's not so much a tank as . . . a . . . a shower," I said. "A shower where sometimes there's tons of hot water, and the water pressure and the showerhead are great, and other times there's hardly any water pressure or the showerhead is all gummed up with schmutz. You can always take a shower, but all these contextual factors influence whether that shower is fantastic or frustrating."

"Contextual factors. So what is that in real life? Candles and flowers?" She was grimacing. "Bodice ripping?"

"Those are circumstances. Situations. That's part of it, but when I say 'context,' I also mean, like, brain states."

"Oh!" she said, brightening. "That sounds much more interesting than candles."

It is. And it's what this chapter is about: how to get the water nice and hot and build up the water pressure.

In their survey research on "cues for sexual desire factors," Katie McCall and Cindy Meston asked women what turned them on, and found that the results divided into four general categories.[2]

Love/Emotional Bonding Cues, such as feeling a sense of love, security, commitment, emotional closeness, protection, and support in your relationship, and feeling a kind of "special attention" from your partner. Example: A woman told me the extraordinarily romantic story of a boyfriend who flew halfway around the globe to surprise her for their second anniversary of dating. Talk about closeness, commitment, and special attention. Yeah, that man got *laid*.

Explicit/Erotic Cues, such as watching a sexy movie, reading an erotic story, watching or hearing other people having sex, anticipating having sex, knowing your partner desires you, or noticing your own or your partner's sexual response. Example: A woman in her twenties told me of a time when she woke up in the middle of the night in her boyfriend's apartment, to the sound of the upstairs neighbors having sex. The rhythmic squeaking and grunting instantly turned her on. She kissed her boyfriend awake and they listened together, then had fast, intense sex.

Visual/Proximity Cues, such as seeing an attractive, well-dressed potential partner, with a well-toned body and lots of confidence, intelligence, and class. Example: A friend once said to me rhetorically, "What is it about the white cuffs of a shirt peeking out under a suit jacket?" I suggested, "Maybe a marker of a social status?" And she added, "That, and grooming. A man with pristine white cuffs is a man whose skin will taste good."

Romantic/Implicit Cues include intimate behaviors such as dancing closely, sharing a hot tub or massages or other intimate touch (like touching the face or hair), watching a sunset, laughing or whispering together, or smelling pleasant. Example: A woman in her thirties told me that she and her husband were saving up to remodel their bathroom, after they realized that a reason she was so keen for sex when they went on vacation was that they took long, hot (in every sense) baths together in the giant tubs at the B and Bs where they stayed. More baths, more sex.

None of this is too surprising, but it's always great to have data to back up our intuitions: A blend of erotic and romantic cues increases desire in women. McCall and Meston's work tells us what activates the accelerator.

In a series of nine focus groups with eighty women, Cynthia Graham, Stephanie Sanders, Robin Milhausen, and Kimberly McBride cataloged women's thoughts on things that cause them to turn on or to "keep the brakes on."[3] These researchers found themes that have interesting parallels with McCall and Meston's work. Here are the themes, with a quote from the research participants to illustrate each:

- *Feelings About One's Body.* "It's much easier for me to feel aroused when I'm feeling really comfortable with myself . . . it's not as easy to feel aroused when I'm not feeling good about myself and my body."

- *Concerns About Reputation.* "Being single and you know, wanting to be sexual with another person and thinking 'okay, am I going to be too much?' or 'am I going to be not enough?' or 'what are they going to think of me because I'm doing these things?' . . . "

- *Putting on the Brakes.* "I think it's like you might have some inclinations and then you're like, 'wait a minute, you can't do that,' you're in a relationship or that guy's a loser . . . and all of a sudden you just [think] 'okay, fine, forget it, I can't. That's a bad idea,' and just walk away from it."

- *Unwanted Pregnancy/Contraception.* "Unwanted pregnancy is a big turn off and if you're with a partner who seems unconcerned about that, then it really feels like a danger."

- *Feeling Desired Versus Feeling Used by Partner.* "I like it when [men] caress not only, like, your body parts that get sexually

aroused but just, like, your arms . . . it feels like he's encompass-
ing you and appreciating your whole body."

- *Feeling "Accepted" by Partner.* "Even with my second husband,
and we were together 16 years, he was not accepting of my sexual
responses . . . I make a lot of noise or [with] my favorite way to
orgasm, he felt left out . . . That was just the beginning of just
really shutting down."

- *Style of Approach/Initiation and Timing.* "His 'game' . . . you know,
how the man approached you, how did he get me to talk to him longer than like, five minutes? . . . [It's] the ways he went about it."

- *Negative Mood.* "If you're very upset with your intended sexual
partner, if you're very upset with him about something, there's no
way that you are going to be aroused."

These two studies help us begin to understand that women's sexual
interest depends on a wide range of factors. When we ask them, "What
gets you in the mood?" women tell us:

- Having an attractive partner who respects them and accepts them
as they are
- Feeling trusting and affectionate in their relationship
- Being confident and healthy—both emotionally and physically
- Feeling desired by their partner, being approached in a way that
makes them feel special
- Explicit erotic cues, like erotica or porn, or hearing or seeing other
people having sex

But what these answers tell us, too, is *it depends*. A woman who feels
confident in herself, and who is in a great relationship with a partner she
loves, trusts, and feels attracted to, still may not want sex if she has the flu,
worked seventy hours that week, or prefers that both she and her partner
be freshly showered before sex and they've just come in from doing yard
work together.

Another thing these answers tell us is that what women say on surveys and in focus groups can't tell us everything that happens in real life. In *The Science of Trust*, relationship researcher John Gottman recounts the stories of women in abusive relationships, in which they habitually were targets of physical violence.[4] These women astonished him and his research partner by telling them that some of the best sex they had followed immediately after the acts of violence. And in *What Do Women Want?* Daniel Bergner describes Isabel, who couldn't get herself into a hot and bothered state about her respectful, cherishing boyfriend, yet she had felt magnetically drawn to the objectifying jerk who wanted her to dress trashy and, she knew, would never commit to a relationship with her.[5] I've heard similar stories from many women, and nothing in this research explains it. Nothing tells us why make-up and breakup sex have earned a reputation for intensity.

So what gives?

What gives is the dual control mechanism's relationship with your many other motivational systems. What gives is *context*.

Context is made of two things: the circumstances of the present moment—whom you're with, where you are, whether the situation is novel or familiar, risky or safe, etc.—and your brain state in the present moment—whether you're relaxed or stressed, trusting or not, loving or not, right now, in this moment. The evidence is mounting that women's sexual response is more sensitive than men's to context, including mood and relationship factors, and women vary more from each other in how much such factors influence their sexual response.[6]

So this chapter is about context: how your external circumstances and your internal brain state can influence your sexual responsiveness.

We'll start with the idea that your experience or perception of all kinds of sensations varies, depending on a number of factors, including external circumstances, mood, trust, and life history. Then we'll get deep into the nitty-gritty of why this is true and unchangeable: When your brain is in a stressed state, almost everything is perceived as a potential threat. And then I'll show you the specific brain mechanism that governs this whole process. Understanding this mechanism—I call it your emotional "One Ring"—is central to figuring out how context affects your sexual responsiveness.

I want to warn you ahead of time: This is the nerdiest, scienciest chapter in the book. Dust off your thinking cap. It's worth it. The payoff is that anytime you hear someone complain, "Women are so complicated—yesterday she liked one thing, today she wants something completely different," or wonder, "Why don't I respond the way I used to?" you'll be able to say, "Context! What you want and like changes based on your external circumstances and your internal state." This chapter tells you how to crack the code and make sense of it all.

Laurie's dissatisfaction with her sex life wasn't a result of a challenging accelerator and brakes; it was a result of a challenging context. But she didn't like my suggestion that she just let herself not want sex for a while. To her, that felt like giving up. She wanted *to want sex, and, darn it all, she was going to try.*

So she thought about times in the past when she had pleasurable sex and remembered a particularly excellent pre-baby anniversary vacation at a fancy hotel in the mountains.

"Aha! Context!" she thought, and she and Johnny made a reservation and planned a trip to recapture the passion.

The plan failed utterly. The drive was long and exhausting, they argued on the way there, and by the time they finished dinner, the pressure of expectation was totally overwhelming. Laurie felt herself shut down, and she just said no, no to everything. She took a hot bath, had a glass of wine, and went to sleep. Johnny watched a movie.

And then in the morning, she felt too guilty about the previous night to try again.

So one afternoon soon after that, Laurie and Johnny sat down and tried to figure out what had worked on that first trip that was missing the second time.

Well, their whole lives were different now: They were parents, she had a frustrating job, she was a student . . . They had replicated the external circumstances but not the context.

"Great, so all you have to do is quit your job, quit school, and sell Trevor to the circus. Problem solved," Johnny teased. More constructively, he said, "Maybe we're thinking about it the wrong way. Maybe it's about what it feels *like*, rather than where we are or what we're doing. When you think about the great sex we had on that anniversary, what did it feel like?"

She thought about it for a minute.

And then she burst into tears.

She began talking about how much she loved him, how she relied on him for her sanity in a life that seemed specifically designed to make her crazy, how she wanted to show him, not just tell him, how important he is to her, but every time she considered initiating sex, she just felt swamped and overwhelmed and her body shut down on her. Undifferentiated grief flowed from her as she talked—grief for her lost sexuality, but also for her lost peace of mind, her lost sense of self, independent of her roles as mother, daughter, wife, boss, employee, student . . .

And then, when the tide of her grief ebbed, they had great sex.

After that, Laurie came to me and said, "What the hell?! We go on a romantic getaway, nothing—worse than nothing! But I ugly cry about how much I love him and how exhausting my life is, and we have hot and dirty sex. This context thing makes no sense!"

So I explained.

sensation in context

Suppose you're flirting with a certain special someone, and they start tickling you. You can imagine some situations where that's fun, right? Flirtatious. Potentially leading to some nookie.

Now imagine that you are feeling annoyed with that same special someone and they try to tickle you.

It feels irritating, right? Like maybe you'd want to punch that person in the face.

It's the same *sensation*, but because the context is different, your *perception* of that sensation is different.

It's true for all our sensory domains. A smell that seems pleasant when it's labeled "cheese" smells gross when it is labeled "body odor." [7] Same smell + different context = different perception. Mood changes your perception of taste, too: feeling sad, as you do at the end of a weepy movie, reduces your ability to taste fat in food. [8]

It's true in all your other senses, too, not just the basic five you learned in elementary school. We've all experienced it with thermoreception: Imagine your car has run out of gas one mile from the gas station, on a scorching-hot, sauna-humid day. You walk the mile through the sludgy air. You get to the air-conditioned gas station, chilled to seventy-two degrees, and it feels like a frigid blast, a powerful relief from the heat. Now imagine your car runs out of gas in the same place six months later, and it's a bitterly cold, bitingly windy day, and you trudge the same mile to the gas station. That same seventy-two degrees now feels like a warmed oven, a powerful relief from the painful cold. Context.

It's also true for equilibrioception (sense of balance): Anyone who's gotten off a ship after a week-long cruise knows that our brains adapt to movement—you spend two days wondering why the ground is moving under your feet. Nociception (sense of pain): People who've experienced serious pain develop a higher tolerance for future pain. [9] And chronoception (sense of time): Time does indeed seem to fly when you're having fun—or rather, when you're in a state of "flow." [10]

These changes in perception are not "just in your head." People who are given a drug that will relax them and are told, "This is a drug that will relax you," not only feel more relaxed compared to those who got the drug but not the information, they also *have more of the drug in their blood plasma*. [11] Context changes more than how you feel; it can change your blood chemistry.

It's also true for sexual stimuli. In chapter 2, I described how the dual control mechanism responds to stimuli that are either sex-related or a threat, and I talked about how we learn what stimuli goes into which category—remember the rat with a lemon fetish? But just as the smell of cheese or the taste of fat is influenced by our mental state and the external circumstances, whether a particular stimulus is interpreted as sex-related or a threat depends on the context in which we perceive it.

Tickling is one example of this. Watching your partner do chores is another. If you feel overall supported and connected in your relationship, then seeing your partner doing the laundry may act as a cue for erotic thoughts. But if you've been feeling resentful because you've been doing a disproportionate amount of the chores lately, then seeing your partner do laundry may feel satisfying—"It's about time!"—without feeling sexy.

The same goes for whether something hits the brakes. For example, the extent to which a person's sexual brakes are engaged because of fear of an STI changes depending on the perceived likelihood of infection and the perceived impact of that STI. Using a condom? Know your partner's health history and sexual history? Trust that you're both being monogamous? Less threat. No condom? No history? Potential for betrayal? More threat. It's the same with social consequences, too: Potential damage to your social status, your reputation, or your relationship all act as threats, depending on how likely they seem and how negative they would be if they happened.

Learning to recognize the contexts that increase your brain's perception of the world as a sexy place, and having skills to maximize the sexy contexts, is key to increasing your sexual satisfaction. At the end of this chapter, you'll find worksheets to help you think through what aspects of context influence your perception of sensations. On those worksheets, you'll recall three amazing sexual experiences you've had and three not-so-great sexual experiences, and think concretely and specifically about what made those experiences what they were, in terms of both external circumstances and your internal state. Do take the time to do this. Thinking through even just one amazing experience and one not-so-great experience can give you a sense of which contexts increase your brain's tendency to interpret the world as sexy and which reduce that tendency.

Painful or Erotic?

If your partner spanks your butt while you're in the middle of tying your toddler's shoes, it's annoying. But if your partner spanks your butt in the middle of sex, it can feel very, very sexy indeed. Context can cause sensations that are typically perceived as painful, like spanking or whipping, to be erotic. Sexual "submission" requires relaxing into trust—turning off the offs—and allowing your partner to take control. In this explicitly erotic, highly trusting, and consensual context, your brain is open and receptive, ready to interpret any and all sensations as erotic. And in a culture where women have to spend so much time with the brakes on, saying *no*, it's no wonder we have fantasies about abandoning all control, relaxing into absolute trust (turning off the brakes), and allowing ourselves to experience sensation.

sex, rats, and rock 'n' roll

What is the ultimate nerd evidence of the power of context to influence your brain's perception of a sensation? Look at what happens to rat brains when you play them Iggy Pop:

Imagine you're a lab rat, and you're in a three-chambered box.[12] The researchers have painlessly implanted a tiny probe in your brain so that they can zap your nucleus accumbens (NAc), which is a tiny region deep within your brain; its job is to tell you which direction to go—toward or away from something in the environment. In the first chamber, you're surrounded by the ordinary setup that you always encounter in the lab— the lights are on, but it's fairly quiet. Here, if the researcher zaps the top region of the NAc, you engage in approach behaviors, like sniffing and exploration. Psychologist John Gottman calls these *"What's this?"* behaviors.[13] Curious. Exploring. Moving toward. And when the researchers stimulate the bottom region of your NAc, you exhibit avoidance—*"What the hell is that?"* behaviors, like stamping your paws and turning away your head. Fearful. Avoidant. Moving away. And all of that is normal and exactly what you would expect, as a sort of bionic, semiremote-controlled rat.

So now you go into the next chamber, where the lights are off, it's quiet and calm, and it smells like home. You love it here, it's like a spa for rats. In this context, when the researcher zaps your top NAc, the same thing happens—approach behaviors. But this is where it gets interesting: When the researcher zaps your bottom NAc . . . approach behaviors! In a safe, relaxing environment, almost the entire NAc activates approach motivation!

As soon as you move into the third chamber, ultrabright lights turn on and suddenly Iggy Pop is blaring—imagine *Live at the King Biscuit Flower Hour* playing at randomly varying volumes, so you can't even get used to it. Everything about this environment stresses you out. You're like an introverted bookworm at a bad nightclub. Now when the researchers zap your top NAc, it doesn't activate curiosity or approach behaviors, as it has in the previous environments; no, in the new, stressful environment, zapping almost anywhere on the NAc generates avoidant, *"What the hell is that?"* behavior.

When I say that perception of sensation is context dependent, this is the deepest sense in which I mean it. I mean that evolutionarily old parts of your brain (your "monkey brain") can respond in opposite ways, approach or avoidance, depending on the circumstances in which they are functioning.[14] In a safe, comfortable environment, it hardly matters where you stimulate; you'll activate approach, curiosity, *desire*. And in a stressful, dangerous environment, it hardly matters where you stimulate; you'll activate avoidance, anxiety, *dread*.

"Context changes how your brain responds to sex" doesn't just mean "Set the mood," like with candles, corsets, and a locked bedroom door. It also means that when you're in a great sex-positive context, almost everything can activate your curious "What's this?" desirous approach to sex. And when you're in a not-so-great context—either external circumstances or internal brain state—it doesn't matter how sexy your partner is, how much you love them, or how fancy your underwear is, almost nothing will activate that curious, appreciative, desirous experience.

It's completely normal that context changes how you perceive sensations. It's just how brains work.

Here's a puzzle:

Merritt, with her sensitive brakes, struggled mightily with sex in real life. Yet she had an active sexual imagination and had been both a reader and author of erotic fiction for a decade. Her favorite stories to read and to write were gay male BDSM—she jokingly calls it "Fifty Shades of Gay." There just seemed to be something about the idea of two men tangled in an intense power dynamic that really captured her erotic imagination.

"Getting turned on by stories about two men having kinky sex, but being so easily shut down during sex with the woman I love? How does that make sense? A noise. A fingernail when I'm not expecting it. A stray thought, even. And yet I spend hours every day writing about men having sex in public or on a rack or tied to trees."

Learning about her sexual brakes helped some, but it was when she and Carol talked about context—What contexts arouse you? What contexts hit the brakes?—that they discovered that fantasies were great for Merritt, while real life was . . . a challenge.

Which makes lots of sense for a woman with sensitive brakes. The context—external circumstances and internal brain state—of a fantasy is very different from the context of real life. When you're alone in bed fantasizing about being dominated by five big, unknown men, you are actually safe, there is no threat to activate your stress response, and the novelty of the fantasy adds fuel to the fire. Great context!

But if in real life you were surrounded by five big, unknown men, your brain would probably react with a stress response—Run! Fight!

or Freeze!—*and that stress response would most likely hit your sexual brakes. Not a great context.*

"So what do we do about that?" Merritt asked me.

"Trust," I said. "Letting go of the brakes is about trust."

Merritt shook her head and looked at Carol. "I trust you one hundred fifty percent. I'd jump off a cliff blindfolded if you said there was a crash pad at the bottom, no hesitation."

And then Carol said, "That only leaves one other person for you not to trust, huh?"

Merritt blinked at us both and said, "Me. I don't trust me. Is that what you're saying?"

I said, "Do you?"

"I trust myself to pay bills on time. I trust myself as a parent. As a writer. Yeah, I . . . huh." She stopped and frowned thoughtfully at me.

"You trust your intellect," Carol said, "and your heart. But do you trust your body?"

Merritt rubbed a hand hard against her forehead and said, "Honestly, no—and for good reason."

And then we talked about the good reason.

I'd like to spend some time with the mesolimbic cortex. It gets pretty nerdy right here—in terms of the garden metaphor, these next two sections are like describing how the soil transforms a seed into a seedling. It's not something the gardener has much control over, and it happens well below the surface, beyond our ability to observe directly. But especially if you have found cultivating your (or your partner's) sexuality kind of challenging, the next few pages could really enrich your entire understanding of what's happening in the deep, subconscious parts of your sexual response.

Ready? Okay.

liking, wanting, and learning

You've probably read about exciting research findings related to "the pleasure centers of the brain." Put food in your mouth, and these systems get to work. Drink water, they respond. Listen to music, look at art, shoot heroin, or read a novel, and your mesolimbic cortex is busily evaluating, learning, and motivating. Watch porn, hear your neighbors having sex, or feel your partner's hand gripping lightly in your hair, and these brain systems answer—assessing, planning, and encouraging you to move closer . . . or farther away.

For those of you who keep a map of the midbrain on your wall and would like to follow along at home, the organs involved in these systems are the ventral pallidum, the nucleus accumbens body and shell (this is the part from the Iggy Pop study), the amygdala, and the brain stem parabrachial nucleus, among others. (There's a great tidbit for cocktail parties—nothing like the phrase "brain stem parabrachial nucleus" to impress sexy singles over a dirty martini.)

The thing is, these are not really the "pleasure centers"—or not *just* pleasure centers.

What we often describe as the "pleasure centers" or "reward centers" of the brain are in fact crucially more subtle and interesting than that. Calling it "reward" or "pleasure" is like saying "vagina" when you mean "vulva": Pleasure is part of it, certainly, but only part, and to deny the other parts their names is to deny their significance and misunderstand the nature of the multifaceted beast.

There are actually three intertwined but separable functions in these deep, evolutionarily old parts of the brain: *liking*, *wanting*, and *learning*. These three mechanisms form the universal mammalian hardware that make, as Kent Berridge and Morten Kringelbach geekily put it, "One hedonic brain system to mediate them all." [15]

This is a reference to the One Ring from *The Lord of the Rings* mythology; in the original context, the One Ring has the power to control all the other Rings of Power. In the context of your emotional brain, the

One Ring processes *all* of your emotional/motivational systems, including stress responses (fear, aggression, and shutdown), disgust, all forms of pleasure from physical to artistic, love and social connection, and of course sex.[16] All these emotions function, all at once, all in the same place: in your emotional One Ring.

So don't be too impressed when you read a pop science article that says, "The same parts of your brain light up when you have sex as when you take cocaine." Of course they do. That's the One Ring. It mediates them all.

When I say "One Ring" for the rest of the book, I mean this cluster of *liking*, *wanting*, and *learning*, where all your emotional responses—sex, stress, love, disgust, etc.—compete and interact and influence each other.

Here's how the three systems work.

Liking is perhaps the closest to what we generally think of as "reward." The *liking* mechanism is the "Yes!" or "No!" in your brain—it assesses the "hedonic impact" of a stimulus: Does it feel good? How good? Does it feel bad? How bad? When you put a drop of sugar water on the tongue of a newborn, their *liking* system sets off fireworks; sugar is innately rewarding—we're born ready to enjoy sweet tastes. Salt is not. This one system manages all forms of pleasure, including sweet tastes, sexual sensations, the perception of beauty, the joy of love, and the thrill of winning.

Learning is the process of linking what's happening now with what should come next. Pavlov's dogs salivated when a bell rang because their *learning* system connected the bell with food. The rats in chapter 2 linked lemons or jackets with sex because of the *learning* system. This is implicit learning—a different experience from explicit learning. Explicit learning is how you memorize a poem with spaced repetition and conscious effort. Implicit learning is (in part) the *learning* system linking stimuli across time and space. We don't have to study or memorize anything to learn which foods taste delicious and which people are mean. We learn these kinds of emotional things implicitly.

Wanting—more technically known as "incentive salience"—is the generic accelerator of the emotional brain. It fuels the desire to move toward something or away from it. When *wanting* is activated with the stress response mechanism, we search for safety. When *wanting* is activated with the attachment mechanism (see the next chapter), we seek affection. And of course when *wanting* is activated with our sexual accelerator, we pursue sexual stimulation.

When *wanting* is activated, we experience what Kent Berridge calls "a moment of special temptation."[17] The experience of urgent craving or yearning is powered by the *wanting* system.

And it's context dependent. Remember the rat in the spa environment versus the nightclub environment? The *"What's this?"* and *"What the hell is that?"* behaviors triggered by stimulation of the NAc were *wanting* behaviors—*wanting* to get closer . . . or farther away. Which set of behaviors was elicited depended on how calm or stressed the rat was.

How do these systems work in human sexuality? If something activates your sexual accelerator—say, your partner kissing you—*learning* has done its job. Like the rats in jackets, your accelerator has learned that kissing is sex-related.

But *learning* is neutral, neither nice nor nasty, just . . . relevant. But when the cue that activates *learning* is not only sex-related but also nice (which depends on context), it activates *liking*, too. And when it's nice enough, it gives rise to *wanting*.

The sequence works this way: Something sex-related happens, and your brain goes, "Hey, that's sex-related." That's *learning*. And if the context is right, your brain also goes, "Hey, that's nice!" That's *liking*. And if the stimulus is nice enough, your brain goes, "Ooh, go get more of that!" That's *wanting*.

Did you make it? Phew! That was the hard part. Nice job. I'll be referring to the One Ring of *liking*, *wanting*, and *learning* throughout the rest of the book—like in chapter 6 we'll learn that genital response is *learning* while the conscious experience of being "turned on" is *learning* + *liking*. And in chapter 8 we'll learn how focusing the One Ring on sexual pleasure, and releasing it from all other motivations, is the path to ecstatic orgasms.

The research measuring how the three systems function in human sexuality has barely begun. I include them here not because I've already seen definitive proof of how they affect sexual wellbeing but because when I teach about them, I see how helpful people find it to know that desire, pleasure, and genital response are not the same thing. Your brain can *like* something without *wanting* more. It can *learn* that a kind of stimulation may lead to sex, and *learning* may activate desire—movement toward—but it may also activate dread—movement away—depending on the context. Your brain can even *want* something without particularly *liking* it, as we'll see with Olivia.

And all three are context dependent: If your *wanting*, *liking*, and *learning* substrates are busy coping with stress or attachment issues (which are the topic of the next chapter), then sex-related stimuli may not be perceived as sexy at all.

Understanding that these systems are separable is as powerful as learning there are brakes! Let's walk through the three systems in different contexts to see how they can change sexual responsiveness:

Context 1: Before you get pregnant. Your partner lies down in bed next to you and you enjoy your usual end-of-the-day cuddle while you talk through plans for tomorrow. Your partner's hands begin to wander over your body, which activates *learning* and *liking*, since you're in a relaxed, affectionate state of mind, and pretty soon *wanting* joins the party. So you start kissing and letting your hands wander, too, and one thing leads to another.

Context 2: Two months after you give birth. Your partner lies down in bed next to you, waking you up from a rare and precious sound sleep, wanting to cuddle and talk through plans for tomorrow. You turn into their arms and talk for a while, and their hands begin to wander over your body—your sleep-deprived, lactating, different-shaped body with its still-healing vagina and feet half a size bigger than they were a year ago, a body that has been constantly pawed by little baby hands. Your partner's touch on this strange new body of yours activates *learning* . . . which fills you with dread—*wanting* to avoid sex. So you turn back over and say, "Honey, not tonight."

And your partner thinks—and maybe you do, too—"I don't understand. This used to be great."

Same stimulation, different context. Different response by your emotional One Ring, leading to different outcomes.

We could replace "give birth" in that example with "put your parent into hospice care," "learn your partner was cheating on you," or "get laid off from your job," and get a somewhat similar outcome. On the other hand, we could replace it with "decide to try to get pregnant," "renew your vows," or "win the lottery," and get a pretty different outcome.

As we saw with the rats who had Iggy Pop blasted at them, when your stress levels are high, practically anything will cause your *wanting* to activate in an avoidant, "What the hell is that?" mode. But if you're in a sex-positive context, almost anything can activate *wanting* in curious, "What's this?" mode.

Exactly what context a woman experiences as sex positive varies both from woman to woman and also across a woman's life span, but generally it's a context that's

- low stress
- high affection
- explicitly erotic

Remember the studies of what women say turns them on, from the start of the chapter. That stuff, and more. Because of the One Ring, which mediates all of your different emotions at once, binding them together.

Olivia and Patrick are fabulous together—hilarious, charming, the kind of couple whose love is contagious; when you see them together, you fall a little in love yourself. They hug and laugh affectionately even while they're fighting. Though only in their twenties, you can tell these two will still be making out like teenagers when they're 103.

Their main conflict was about sex: Patrick, like about 80–90 percent of people, finds that stress hits his brakes, shutting down all interest in sex—he's a "flatliner" (more on that in chapter 4). But for Olivia, with her sensitive accelerator, stress is like fuel—she's a "redliner." And since they're both graduate students, they get stressed at the same time during the semester (final exams), which means that right when Olivia's most interested in sex, Patrick is least interested.

Same context—opposite experiences.

And when you put it in the context of a relationship, it gets worse, because the two styles escalate each other—when Patrick feels stressed about the fact that Olivia wants sex and he doesn't, that increases his stress, which hits his brakes even harder. And when Olivia feels stressed about the fact that she wants sex and Patrick doesn't, that increases her stress, which activates her accelerator even more. I call this "the chasing dynamic" (more about it in chapter 7), but Olivia had her own term for it:

"Shit show."

Patrick added, "And it comes at a time in the semester when we're both already stretched too thin and can barely feed ourselves, much less talk about our feelings. How can we fix it?"

I shrugged. "Easy. Work out a plan when you're both calm, and then use the plan when you're stressed."

Olivia said, "Oh."

There it was again—the disappointment that waved a giant red flag over a big emotional . . . something. Last time I missed it. This time I caught it.

"You were hoping for a different answer?" I asked.

"I was sort of hoping we could fix me."

"Fix you? Are you broken?"

"I guess not," she said, "but I just . . . it doesn't feel good, the out-of-controlness. I was hoping I could rein that part in, both for my own sake and so that I don't drive Patrick up the wall."

Which is normal. The context of stress plus sex doesn't bring with it an increase in pleasure. On the contrary, when she's stressed, anxious, or overwhelmed, Olivia said, "I feel this drive to orgasm, but it's a drive that disconnects me from my body and from Patrick. I hate it. It's like I'm a visitor in my body. Out of control."

It's a perfect example of wanting *without* liking.

"Ah, so it's a challenge in your relationship and also it's uncomfortable for you individually," I said. "It's pretty simple to change— simple, though not always easy."

They both said, "How?"

you can't make them

I use italics when I describe *wanting*, *liking*, and *learning* in order to be clear that I don't mean wanting, liking, or learning in the usual sense of, "Hey, what do you want for dinner?" or "Did you like the movie?" There is no deliberate intention—and often not even any awareness— accompanying the activation of these brain systems.[18]

On the contrary. In a study of cocaine addicts, research participants' mesolimbic systems responded to images related to cocaine that flashed on a screen for thirty-three milliseconds. If you asked them what they saw, they wouldn't be able to tell you, because the images flashed too fast to be "seen" consciously, but it was long enough to light up the addicts' *wanting* systems.[19] The research subjects were not aware of having seen the images, yet their emotional brains responded.

In terms of the garden, this is the difference between what the gardener does to the garden . . . and what the garden does all on its own. The gardener can weed and water and fertilize, but she doesn't actually make the plants grow. Your *wanting*, *liking*, and *learning* systems are what make the plants grow. All kinds of things influence them, including how well you tend them, the weather (that is, the external circumstances of your life), and how well suited your plants are to your particular soil (your body and your brakes and accelerator). But the gardener can't grit her teeth and make the garden grow; she can only create the best possible environment for the garden to thrive, and then let the garden do its thing. Chapters 4, 5, and 9 are about how to create that sex-positive context.

"is something wrong with me?" (answer: nope)

Sexual arousal, desire, and orgasm change all the time. Sometimes they change in ways that delight us, and sometimes they change in ways that puzzle or worry us. Sometimes these changes happen in response to a change in our sexual hardware—our genitals and the dual control mechanism. But more often they change in response to a change in our context—our environment and our mental states. Our mood. Our relationships. Our lives.

This may be the most important consequence of understanding the way context influences how your brain processes sex-related stimuli: When sex doesn't feel great, it doesn't mean there's something wrong with you. Maybe there's been a change in your external circumstances or your other motivational systems (like stress) that's influencing your sexual response. Which means that you can create positive change without changing *you*.

Another important consequence of understanding context is that it helps us understand why women are so different from each other. For many women, the most sex-positive contexts may not be the culturally sanctioned or readily available ones—such as hookups when you're in college or the same old sex for the 1,287th time when you've been married for ten years. For some women, those are great contexts, but for other women a great, sex-positive context might be an anonymous one-night hookup against a wall of other people's coats in a stranger's closet at a party. For others it's the warmly affectionate sex of a long-term, committed relationship. For some women, it's a wide range of contexts, and for others, it's a narrow window. As long as a woman is attending to her wellbeing and her partner's, it doesn't matter what the context is, as long as it brings her pleasure.

But if we ignore context, then anyone who finds sex unfun or whose desire diminishes may be tempted to conclude they're broken or they don't like sex . . . when really all they need is a better context.

In the right context, sexual behavior is arguably the most pleasurable experience a human can have. It can bond us with our partners, flood us with happy chemicals, satisfy deep biological urges, and transport us to spiritual heights. In the wrong context, though, it can literally feel like death. Depending on the context, sex can vary almost infinitely, from delicious to disgusting, from playful to painful—and because of the dual control mechanism, sometimes it's two conflicting things at the same time.

As she learned about the relationship between context and her insensitive accelerator, Camilla decided to think of her low-sensitivity accelerator in terms of the shower metaphor—the garden metaphor never really worked for her, but something about the shower metaphor felt like a good fit. She noticed that romantic, affectionate contexts, exciting and novel contexts, and low-stress contexts increased her brain's sensitivity to sexual cues.

Or, as she put it, "They heat up the water and build up the pressure."

And the very best context of all, she thought, was when she felt pursued. The extended courtship that characterized the earliest part of her relationship with Henry might have been specifically organized around the contextual factors that maximized her wanting for sex.

She and Henry talked about it, and they decided to try an experiment: He would create entire evenings where he courted Camilla, wooed her, and—eventually—won her. And they learned something from this that surprised them both: It wasn't the pursuing. It was the waiting that turned her on.

The first time they tried it, it was a little awkward because she knew what was coming, so she kept trying to move things along, to show that she was on board with the plan. When he held her hand as they walked home from the movie, she tried to kiss him. But Henry stopped her, slowed her down. When he kissed her, she tried to deepen the kiss, but again he slowed her down. "I'm chasing you, remember?" he said. "I can't chase you if you're moving toward me."

This was the lightbulb moment.

Camilla recognized that what she really needed was time for her liking to grow and expand until finally it activated her wanting. They had been working with the hypothesis that it was feeling pursued that made her feel desire, but it turned out the real trick was not the experience of being chased but the amount of accelerator activation that comes with going slowly, delaying gratification. For her, the process of getting from liking to wanting is a bit like the ticking pilot light on a gas stove—not quite enough gas, not quite enough, not quite, until phoof! *she crosses from liking into wanting.*

Or—going back to the shower analogy—her accelerator was like a hot-water heater that took a lot of time to heat the whole tank. It worked great, it just needed more patience, but it was so worth the wait.

Camilla and Henry are both careful, thoughtful people, methodical and slow paced, and this approach appeals to them deeply. It wouldn't work for everyone. But great sex isn't about doing what works for everyone, it's about what works for you and your partner.

In this first part of the book, we've looked at how your sexual hardware—your body, your brain, and the context—influence your overall sexual wellbeing. We've learned that all three elements are made of the same basic parts in everyone, but each person's brain, body, and context are unique. In other words, we each have a unique "garden" in which we grow our sexual wellbeing.

The next part of the book is about what specific factors influence your context, in terms of your environment and your brain state. These are like the sun and the rain and—sometimes—compost of your garden. Some you have control over, some you don't, and all of them influence how your garden thrives. In chapter 4, I'll talk about two primary motivational systems—stress and love—and how they can influence sexual response in surprising ways. And in chapter 5, I'll show how cultural factors in the environment—like social pressure to look or act a certain way, or moral and media messages about what's "right" or "wrong" sexually—can influence sexual functioning, and how to untangle the knots that a sex-negative culture ties in our sexual psychologies.

tl;dr

- Your brain's perception of a sensation is context dependent. Like tickling: If your partner tickles you when you're already feeling turned on, it can be fun. But if they tickle you when you're angry, it's just irritating. Same sensation, different context—therefore different perception.
- When you're stressed out, your brain interprets just about everything as a potential threat. When you're turned on, your brain could interpret just about anything as sex-related. Because: context!
- *Wanting*, *liking*, and *learning* are separate functions in your brain. You can want without liking (craving), anticipate without wanting (dread), or any other combination.
- For most people, the best context for sex is low stress + highly affectionate + explicitly erotic. Think through your contexts with the worksheets that follow.

sexy contexts

Think of a positive sexual experience from your past. Describe it here, with as many relevant details as you can recall:

Now consider what aspects of that experience made it positive:

Category	Description
Mental and physical wellbeing	
• Physical health	
• Body image	
• Mood	
• Anxiety	
• Distractibility	
• Worry about sexual functioning	
• Other	
Partner characteristics	
• Physical appearance	
• Physical health	
• Smell	
• Mental state	
• Other	

Relationship characteristics

- Trust
- Power dynamic
- Emotional connection
- Feeling desired
- Frequency of sex

Setting

- Private/public (at home, work, vacation, etc.)
- Distance sex (phone, chat, etc.)
- See partner do something positive, like interact with family or do work

Other life circumstances

- Work-related stress
- Family-related stress
- Holiday, anniversary, "occasion"

Ludic factors/play

- Self-guided fantasy
- Partner-guided fantasy ("talking dirty")
- Body parts that were touched or not
- Oral sex on you/on partner
- Intercourse, etc.

Other

sexy contexts

Think of a positive sexual experience from your past. Describe it here, with as many relevant details as you can recall:

Now consider what aspects of that experience made it positive:

Category	Description
Mental and physical wellbeing	
• Physical health	
• Body image	
• Mood	
• Anxiety	
• Distractibility	
• Worry about sexual functioning	
• Other	
Partner characteristics	
• Physical appearance	
• Physical health	
• Smell	
• Mental state	
• Other	

Relationship characteristics

- Trust
- Power dynamic
- Emotional connection
- Feeling desired
- Frequency of sex

Setting

- Private/public (at home, work, vacation, etc.)
- Distance sex (phone, chat, etc.)
- See partner do something positive, like interact with family or do work

Other life circumstances

- Work-related stress
- Family-related stress
- Holiday, anniversary, "occasion"

Ludic factors/play

- Self-guided fantasy
- Partner-guided fantasy ("talking dirty")
- Body parts that were touched or not
- Oral sex on you/on partner
- Intercourse, etc.

Other

sexy contexts

Think of a positive sexual experience from your past. Describe it here, with as many relevant details as you can recall:

Now consider what aspects of that experience made it positive:

Category	Description
Mental and physical wellbeing	
• Physical health	
• Body image	
• Mood	
• Anxiety	
• Distractibility	
• Worry about sexual functioning	
• Other	
Partner characteristics	
• Physical appearance	
• Physical health	
• Smell	
• Mental state	
• Other	

Relationship characteristics
- Trust
- Power dynamic
- Emotional connection
- Feeling desired
- Frequency of sex

Setting
- Private/public (at home, work, vacation, etc.)
- Distance sex (phone, chat, etc.)
- See partner do something positive, like interact with family or do work

Other life circumstances
- Work-related stress
- Family-related stress
- Holiday, anniversary, "occasion"

Ludic factors/play
- Self-guided fantasy
- Partner-guided fantasy ("talking dirty")
- Body parts that were touched or not
- Oral sex on you/on partner
- Intercourse, etc.

Other

not-so-sexy contexts

Think of a not-so-great sexual experience from your past—not a terrible one, just a not-so-great one. Describe it here, with as many relevant details as you can recall:

```



```

Now consider what aspects of that experience made it not-so-great:

Category	Description
Mental and physical wellbeing	
• Physical health	
• Body image	
• Mood	
• Anxiety	
• Distractibility	
• Worry about sexual functioning	
• Other	
Partner characteristics	
• Physical appearance	
• Physical health	
• Smell	
• Mental state	
• Other	

Relationship characteristics
- Trust
- Power dynamic
- Emotional connection
- Feeling desired
- Frequency of sex

Setting
- Private/public (at home, work, vacation, etc.)
- Distance sex (phone, chat, etc.)
- See partner do something positive, like interact with family or do work

Other life circumstances
- Work-related stress
- Family-related stress
- Holiday, anniversary, "occasion"

Ludic factors/play
- Self-guided fantasy
- Partner-guided fantasy ("talking dirty")
- Body parts that were touched or not
- Oral sex on you/on partner
- Intercourse, etc.

Other

not-so-sexy contexts

Think of a not-so-great sexual experience from your past—not a terrible one, just a not-so-great one. Describe it here, with as many relevant details as you can recall:

Now consider what aspects of that experience made it not-so-great:

Category	Description
Mental and physical wellbeing	
• Physical health	
• Body image	
• Mood	
• Anxiety	
• Distractibility	
• Worry about sexual functioning	
• Other	
Partner characteristics	
• Physical appearance	
• Physical health	
• Smell	
• Mental state	
• Other	

Relationship characteristics

- Trust
- Power dynamic
- Emotional connection
- Feeling desired
- Frequency of sex

Setting

- Private/public (at home, work, vacation, etc.)
- Distance sex (phone, chat, etc.)
- See partner do something positive, like interact with family or do work

Other life circumstances

- Work-related stress
- Family-related stress
- Holiday, anniversary, "occasion"

Ludic factors/play

- Self-guided fantasy
- Partner-guided fantasy ("talking dirty")
- Body parts that were touched or not
- Oral sex on you/on partner
- Intercourse, etc.

Other

not-so-sexy contexts

Think of a not-so-great sexual experience from your past—not a terrible one, just a not-so-great one. Describe it here, with as many relevant details as you can recall:

Now consider what aspects of that experience made it not-so-great:

Category	Description
Mental and physical wellbeing	
• Physical health	
• Body image	
• Mood	
• Anxiety	
• Distractibility	
• Worry about sexual functioning	
• Other	
Partner characteristics	
• Physical appearance	
• Physical health	
• Smell	
• Mental state	
• Other	

Relationship characteristics

- Trust
- Power dynamic
- Emotional connection
- Feeling desired
- Frequency of sex

Setting

- Private/public (at home, work, vacation, etc.)
- Distance sex (phone, chat, etc.)
- See partner do something positive, like interact with family or do work

Other life circumstances

- Work-related stress
- Family-related stress
- Holiday, anniversary, "occasion"

Ludic factors/play

- Self-guided fantasy
- Partner-guided fantasy ("talking dirty")
- Body parts that were touched or not
- Oral sex on you/on partner
- Intercourse, etc.

Other

sexual cues assessment

Read through all your sexy and not-so-sexy contexts. What do you notice as reliable contexts for great sex and reliable contexts for not-so-great sex?

Contexts That Make Sex Great

Contexts That Make Sex Not-So-Great

Identify five things you and/or your partner could do if you decided to work toward creating more frequent and easier access to the contexts that improve your sexual functioning.

Things to do	How much impact?	How easy?	How soon can you do it?
1. _____	_____	_____	_____
_____	_____	_____	_____
2. _____	_____	_____	_____
_____	_____	_____	_____
3. _____	_____	_____	_____
_____	_____	_____	_____
4. _____	_____	_____	_____
_____	_____	_____	_____
5. _____	_____	_____	_____
_____	_____	_____	_____

Now select the two or three that feel like the right combination of impact, ease, and immediacy, and list all the things that would have to happen in order for this change to occur. Be as CONCRETE AND SPECIFIC as you can. These should be ACTIONS rather than abstractions or ideas or attitudes. Ask yourself, "If we decide to create this change, what goes on our to-do list?"

Change 1

```



```

Change 2

```



```

Change 3

```



```

Finally, select just one change that you will actually implement. Choose a start date together that feels like good timing. Ideally this will be within the next month. Make your plan. AND DO IT!

part 2

sex in context

four

emotional context

SEX IN A MONKEY BRAIN

Women ask me questions, and then they tell me their stories. I have a whole mental library full of them—hilarious stories of sex adventures gone awry, sad stories of relationships that couldn't be healed, awe-inspiring stories of survival and transcendence. Every single one is a story of discovery.

Merritt's story is about survival.

"Why should I trust my body?" she said. "My whole adult life, my body has been unreliable and falling apart. When I get stressed, everything just shuts down—I get sick, I get injured, none of my systems work. And that includes sex."

This made some sense, given her sensitive brakes, but it seemed to me there was more going on.

"It sounds like your body is opting for the 'freeze' stress response, where it just shuts down instead of trying to escape or fight," I said. "It's what happens when a person has either long-term, high-intensity stress, or is in the process of healing after trauma. Does either of those sound like you?"

"Both," Carol and Merritt said together.

"You think stress explains why I have a hard time trusting my body?" Merritt asked me.

I definitely do.

This chapter is about stress and love and how they affect sexual pleasure.

Trust your body. Listen to it—not to the specific circumstances of the moment but to the deep, primal messages of your evolutionary heritage:

I am at risk/I am safe.

I am broken/I am whole.

I am lost/I am home.

If you're already skilled at listening to these messages in your body, feel free to skip this chapter. But if, like most of us, you could use help translating the signals your body is sending, you'll find this chapter informative. Because it's not just the sexual aspects of a context that influence whether you get turned on. It's all the other emotional aspects, including your preexisting emotional state.

And of all the emotional systems managed by your emotional One Ring, the two that may have the most immediate impact on sexual pleasure are *stress* and *love*. Stress is the physiological and neurological process that helps you deal with threats. Love is the physiological and neurological process that draws you to your tribe.

Stress underlies worry, anxiety, fear, terror, all the variants of "Run away!" But it also underlies anger—irritation, annoyance, frustration, rage. And to a great extent it underlies the shutdown that characterizes depression. In the first section of this chapter, I'll present a view of stress different from those you may have heard before: The key to managing stress (so that it doesn't mess with your sex life) is not simply "relaxing" or "calming down." *It's allowing the stress response cycle to complete.* Allow it to discharge fully. Let your body move all the way from "I am at risk" to "I am safe."

In the second part of this chapter, I'll discuss love. Love, for our purposes, is attachment, the innate biological mechanism that bonds humans together. It underlies passion, romance, and the joy of finding a partner you can connect with. But it also underlies grief, jealousy, and heartbreak. Sometimes it's joyful, like when you're falling in love. Sometimes it's agonizing, like when you're breaking up. But always attachment pushes us from "I am broken" to "I am whole."

And finally, in the third part of this chapter, I'll talk about the place where stress and attachment and sex overlap—the place where we experience both the passionate, exuberant joy of intense love and also the agony of the worst interpersonal discord. When stress and attachment and sex all activate together in our emotional One Ring, they call, "I am lost," to motivate us to search and search until we find ourselves in a new place: "I am home." I'll describe attachment distress–fueled sex as "sex that advances the plot," and introduce ways that we can use this dynamic to our advantage.

The goal is to help you recognize how the stress response cycle and the attachment mechanism are integrated in your sexual responsiveness, and to offer strategies for allowing them to enhance sexual pleasure, as well as to provide options when they're impairing pleasure.

We can understand women's sexual wellbeing only if we take *context* into account—and most of that context has nothing to do with sex itself. Which means we can improve our sexual wellbeing and expand our sexual pleasure without directly changing anything about our sex lives! What I've included in this chapter and the next are the contextual factors that research has shown are consistently associated with changes in women's sexual wellbeing. Improve your context, and your sexual pleasure will expand all on its own.

the stress response cycle:
fight, flight, and freeze

Let's first separate your stressors from your stress. Your *stressors* are the things that activate the stress response—bills, family, work, fretting about your sex life, all of that.

Your *stress* is the system of changes activated in your brain and body in response to those stressors. It's an evolutionarily adaptive mechanism that allows you to respond to perceived threats. Or it *was* evolutionarily adaptive, back when our stressors had claws and teeth and could run thirty miles per hour. These days we are almost never chased by lions, and yet our body's response to, say, an incompetent boss is largely the same as it would be to a lion. Your physiology doesn't differentiate much. This fact will have important implications for your sex life, as we'll soon see.

Stress is usually taught as the fight-or-flight response, but just as the "pleasure center" isn't just about pleasure, fight or flight isn't just about fight or flight. Let's call it fight/flight/freeze. Here's how it works:

When your brain perceives a threat in the environment, you experience a massive biochemical change, characterized by floods of adrenaline and cortisol to your bloodstream and a cascade of physiological events, such as increased heart rate, respiration rate, and blood pressure; suppressed immune and digestive functioning; dilation of the pupils and shifting of attention to a vigilant state, focused on the here and now. All these changes are like revving your engine before a race, or taking a deep breath before you duck underwater—preparation for the action to come.

What action that will be depends on the nature of the perceived threat—that is, it's context dependent.

Suppose the threat is a lion—the kind of threat we were dealing with in the environment where the mechanism evolved in our early ancestors. The stress response cycle notices the lion and shouts, "I'm at risk! What do I do?" A lion, your brain informs you in much less than a second, is the kind of threat that you are most likely to survive by trying to *escape*.

So what do you do when you see a lion coming after you?

You feel fear, and you run.

And then what happens?

There are only two possible outcomes, right? Either you get killed by the lion, in which case none of the rest of this matters, or you escape and live. So imagine that you successfully run back to your village and scream for help, and everyone helps you slaughter the lion, and then you all eat it for dinner, and in the morning you have a respectful burial service for the parts of the carcass you won't be using, giving reverent thanks for the lion's sacrifice.

And how do you feel now?

Relieved! Grateful to be alive! You love your friends and family!

And that is the complete stress response cycle, with beginning ("I'm at risk!"), middle (action), and end ("I'm safe!").

Or suppose the threat is a person with an angry expression on their face, who's sneaking up behind your best friend, with a little knife in their hand? Your brain may decide this is a threat you can best survive by *conquering*.

You feel anger ("I'm at risk!"—as we'll see in the attachment section, the people we love get counted as "ourselves"), and you fight.

And again, you can fight and die or you can fight and live; either way, you complete the stress response cycle by engaging in a behavior that eliminates the stressor and the stress.

These two responses, fight and flight, are both accelerator stress—the sympathetic nervous system, the "GO!" of the stress response. Fight emerges when your emotional One Ring determines that a stressor should be conquered. Flight emerges when your One Ring determines a stressor should be escaped.

But suppose the stressor is one that your brain determines you can't survive by escaping and you can't survive by conquering—you feel the teeth of the lion bite into you from behind. This is when you get the brakes stress response—the parasympathetic nervous system, the "STOP!" activated by the most extreme distress. Your body shuts down;

you may even experience "tonic immobility," where you can't move, or can move only sluggishly. Animals in the wild freeze and fall to the ground as a last-ditch effort to convince a predator they're already dead; Stephen Porges has speculated that freeze facilitates a painless death.[1]

If an animal survives such an intense threat to its life, then it does an extraordinary thing: It shakes. It trembles, paws vibrating in the air. It heaves a great big sigh. And then it gets up, shakes itself off, and trots away.

What's happening here is that freeze has interrupted the *GO!* stress response of fight or flight, leaving all that adrenaline-mediated stress to go stale inside the animal's body. When the animal shakes and shudders and sighs, its body is releasing the brakes and completing the activation process triggered by fight/flight, and purging the residue. Completing the cycle. It's called "self-paced termination."[2]

A friend offered this example of her son waking from anesthesia, after waiting in the emergency room for five hours for minor surgery on his finger:

> He came out from under the anesthesia "very distressed," said the nurses. I translate that to "bat shit crazy pants," meaning he screamed hysterically, and flailed his arms and legs wildly, and yelled that he hated me and everyone else, and cycled his legs like mad and screamed, "I just want to run, I just want to run!"

Cycling his legs and "I just want to run!" are flight. Hating everyone is fight. Anesthesia is medically induced freeze—wild animals who are anesthetized by researchers experience the same thing as my friend's son. I call it "the Feels," since it's just this thing that happens in your body without any obvious environmental cause. The kid wasn't actually in any danger, but he had a lot of Feels that needed to work themselves out. And his mom did exactly the right thing:

> I held him, remained calm, kept telling him I loved him and that I was keeping him safe, and eventually he calmed down enough to put his

clothes on (he'd literally torn them off) and leave with me. By the time we were walking into the parking garage, he was calmly telling me that he loved me very much, and when we got home, he collapsed into sleep.

He moved through the cycle and got to the relaxation at the end—affection and sleep.

Only rarely in our everyday lives does unlocking from freeze take such a dramatic form. But even in its smaller scale, that's how the stress response cycle works, beginning, middle, and end, all innately built into the nervous system and fully functional—in the right context.

stress and sex

By now it won't strike you as revelatory when I say, "To have more and better sex, reduce your stress levels." I might as well say, "Exercise is good for you" and "Sleep is important." Of course. You know this.

In fact, more than half of women report that stress, depression, and anxiety decrease their interest in sex; they also reduce sexual arousal and can interfere with orgasm.[3] Chronic stress also disrupts or suppresses the menstrual cycle, decreases fertility and lactation, and increases miscarriage, as well as reducing genital response and increasing both distractibility and pain with sex.[4]

How do the hormones and neurochemicals of stress interact with the hormones and neurochemicals of sexual response, to suppress or stimulate sexual behavior? Nobody knows precisely—but we know some things.

We know that stressed-out humans more readily interpret all stimuli as threats, just like the rats being blasted with bright lights and Iggy Pop.

We also know that the brain can handle only a limited amount of information at a time; at its simplest, we can think of stress as information overload, so when there's too much happening, the brain starts to triage, prioritizing, simplifying, and even plain old ignoring some things.

And we know that the brain prioritizes based on survival needs: breathing, escaping from predators, maintaining the right temperature, staying hydrated and nourished, and remaining with your social group are all first-order-of-business priorities—and of course these priorities sort themselves based on context. If you're starving, you'll be more willing to steal bread from your neighbor, even if it risks your membership in a social group. If you can't breathe, then it doesn't matter how long it's been since you've eaten, you will not feel hungry. And if you're generally overwhelmed by twenty-first-century life, practically everything else takes priority over sex; as far as your brain is concerned *everything* is a charging lion. And if you're being chased by a lion, is that a good time to have sex?

To sum up:

Worry, anxiety, fear, and terror are stress—"There's a lion! Run!"

Irritation, annoyance, frustration, anger, and rage are stress— "There's a lion! Kill it!"

Emotional numbness, shutdown, depression, and despair are stress— "There's a lion! Play dead!"

And none of these indicates that now is a good time to get laid.

Stress is about survival. And while sex serves a lot of purposes, personal survival is not one of them (except when it is—see the attachment section). So for most people, stress slams on the brakes, bottoming out sexual interest—except for the 10 to 20 percent or so of people like Olivia for whom stress activates the accelerator. (All the same parts, organized in different ways.) But even for those folks, stress blocks sexual *pleasure* (*liking*) even as it increases sexual *interest* (*wanting*). Stressed sex feels different from joyful sex—you know, because: context.

To reduce the impact of stress on your sexual pleasure and interest, to have more joyful, pleasurable sex, manage your stress.

Yeah, easier said than done.

When Olivia was stressed, her interest in sex increased—and it was a source of conflict in her relationship with Patrick, since when he was stressed, his interest in sex went down. And worse, sometimes the stress-driven sexual interest made Olivia feel out of control.

How can she manage that feeling?

By practicing completing the cycle.

My technical description of Olivia's out-of-control experience is "maladaptive behavior to manage negative affect"—which just means trying to cope with uncomfortable emotions (stress, depression, anxiety, loneliness, rage) by doing things that carry a high risk of unwanted consequences. Compulsive sexual behavior is one example. Other examples include:

- *using alcohol or other drugs in a risky way*
- *dysfunctional relationships—for instance, trying to deal with your own feelings by dealing with someone else's*
- *escaping into distractions, like movie binge-watching when you have other things you need to be doing*
- *disordered eating—restricting, bingeing, or purging*

Of course, many of these can be done in a healthy way. It's when we do them instead of dealing with our Feels—that is, instead of completing the cycle—that they bring the potential for unwanted consequences. Some of those consequences are fairly benign . . . and some are could-kill-you-tonight dangerous. And they're all intended to do one thing: manage the underlying feelings. We might do these things when we don't know how to complete the cycle or when the feelings just hurt too much.

As a teenager, disordered eating was Olivia's maladaptive coping strategy. She would binge-eat and then exercise, binge and exercise. As she recovered from her eating disorder, she came to realize that her behavior wasn't really about the shape of her body—"I needed something to blame for my anxiety, and cultural brainwashing made my body seem like a good target," she said. Instead, her compulsive behavior was an attempt to deal with feelings that felt too big for her to handle.

She's been symptom-free for several years. Still, she told me, "I sometimes walk through doors sideways because I think I'm too big to fit. When I catch myself doing it, I make myself go through straight, because what I learned is that it's not my body that I'm worried is too big. It's my anxiety."

Now she runs, both to manage her stress and as a productive outlet for her intensity and energy—and she limits herself to one marathon a year because, she says, "I tend to go overboard, and it helps if I set limits."

"I think you're doing something more profound than just setting limits," I said. "I think you're allowing exercise to help you complete the cycle instead of hitting the brakes. And you can do the same thing with sex."

"I can?"

"Yes."

She chewed on her lip and nodded her head. Then she said, "I don't see it."

She'll see it in chapter 5.

broken culture ⟶ broken stress response cycles

The key to managing stress effectively is to make efforts to complete the cycle—unlock from freeze, escape the predator, kill the enemy, rejoice.

But stress is more complex in modern humans than in gazelles and gorillas, for a lot of reasons. First, in modern life, we are, as I mentioned, almost never chased by lions. Our stressors are lower intensity and longer duration—"chronic stressors," they're called, in contrast to "acute stressors," like straightforward predation. Acute stressors have a clear beginning, middle, and end; completing the cycle—running, surviving, celebrating—is inherently built in. Not so with chronic stressors. If our stress is chronic and we don't take deliberate steps to complete the cycle, all that activated stress just hangs out inside us, making us sick, tired, and unable to experience pleasure with sex (or with much of anything else).

Second, our emotion-dismissing culture is uncomfortable with Feels. Our culture says that if the stressor isn't right in front of us, then we have no reason to feel stressed and so we should just cut it out already. As a result, most people's idea of "stress management" is either to eliminate all stressors or to "just relax," as if stress can be turned off like a light switch. Our culture is *so* uncomfortable with Feels that we may even sedate people who've just been in a car accident, preventing their bodies from moving through this natural process; this well-intentioned medical intervention has the unwanted consequence of holding survivors of traumatic injury in freeze, which is how PTSD gets a foothold in a survivor's brain.[5]

But third, even without medication and an emotion-dismissing culture, our ultrasocial human brains are really good at self-inhibition, stopping the stress response midcycle because, "Now is not an appropriate time for Feels." We use this self-inhibition in order to facilitate social cooperation—i.e., not freak anybody out. But unfortunately, our culture has eliminated *all* appropriate times for Feels. We've locked ourselves, culturally, into our own fear, rage, and despair. We must build time, space, and strategies for discharging our stress response cycles.

complete the cycle!

How?

Well, just as you can't grit your teeth and make a garden grow, you can't force a stress response cycle to complete. Completing the cycle requires that, instead of hitting the brakes on our stress, we gently remove our foot from both the accelerator and the brakes and allow ourselves to coast to a stop.[6] To do that, you create the right context and trust your body to do its thing.

So what's the right context?

Think about what your body recognizes as the behaviors that save you from lions. When you're being chased by a lion, what do you do?

You run.

So when you're stressed out by your job (or by your sex life), what do you do?

You run . . . or walk, or get on the elliptical machine or go out dancing or even just dance around your bedroom. Physical activity is the most efficient strategy for completing the stress response cycle and recalibrating your central nervous system into a calm state. When people say, "Exercise is good for stress," that is for realsie real.[7]

Here are some other things that science says can genuinely help us not only "feel better" but actually facilitate the completion of the stress response cycle: sleep; affection (more on that later in the chapter); any form of meditation, including mindfulness, yoga, tai chi, body scans, etc.; and allowing yourself a good old cry or primal scream—though you have to be careful with this one. Sometimes people just wallow in their stress when they cry, rather than allowing the tears to wash away the stress. If you've ever locked yourself in your room and sobbed for ten minutes, and then at the end heaved a great big sigh and felt tremendously relieved, you've felt how it can move you from "I am at risk" to "I am safe."

Art, used in the same way, can help. When mental health professionals suggest journaling or other expressive self-care, they don't mean that the construction of sentences or the task of drawing is inherently therapeutic; rather, they're encouraging you to find positive contexts to discharge your stress, through the creative process.

I'm inclined to add grooming and other body self-care to the list. Though I'm not familiar with any specific research on it, I've talked with lots of women for whom showering and the rituals, part social, part meditative, of painting their nails or doing their hair or putting on makeup—generally "getting ready" to go out (or stay in)—fully transition them from a stressed-out state of mind to a warm, social state of mind. These anecdotes aren't data, but I'm inclined to call them evidence and say: yeah. Spend time treating yourself with affection.

I have a pet theory that these rituals and behaviors are related to "self-kindness," which I'll be talking about in chapter 5, but to my knowledge no one has ever specifically measured it.[8] Anyway, our fellow apes eat insects out of each other's fur; maybe bath bombs and body glitter are the modern human equivalent.

Everybody has something that works—and everyone's strategy is different. Whatever strategy you use, take deliberate steps to complete the cycle. Allow yourself to coast to the end without hitting the brakes. Emotions are tunnels: You have to walk all the way through the darkness to get to the light at the end. I say this so often my students sometimes roll their eyes: "Not the tunnel again." Yes, the tunnel again. Because it's true.

While you're figuring out what strategies help, pay attention to your patterns of self-inhibition, and identify places and people who create space for you to have Feels. Some of those patterns of self-inhibition are important and unchangeable—for example, carefully consider any plan that involves crying at work. But some of them will be self-defeating, and everyone needs at least one place in their life where they can just Have All the Feels without worrying about being judged or freaking people out. Find that place and those people.

A final caution: Too often, we mistake dealing with the stressors for dealing with the stress. A couple years ago the leaders of the campus Peer Sex Educators sat in my office, reporting how well their Sextravaganza events had gone. They had worked for months and their efforts were rewarded with a spectacular success, but they looked exhausted and stunned and said, "Sextravaganza is over! Why do we still feel exactly as stressed out as we did the day it started?!"

"Because you've dealt with the stressor," I said, "but not the stress. Your bodies still think you're being chased by the lion."

Solution: Do things that communicate to your body, "You have escaped and survived!"

- Physical activity
- Sharing affection
- Primal scream or a good cry
- Progressive muscle relaxation or other sensorimotor meditation
- Body self-care, like grooming, massage, or doing your nails

The dance major chose physical activity, and the study of women and gender major organized a big group primal scream.

Don't Be Afraid of the Dark

Over the years, a number of people—particularly young women—have emailed me or approached me at breaks during a workshop to ask if they could talk to me in private. Without meeting my eyes, they tell me they've had anxiety since they were children. They tell me they've been in therapy since high school. And they tell me they've never been able to tell any therapists about the grotesque, disturbing, sometimes violent sexual thoughts that swamp their minds. One young woman told me the hidden thoughts had interfered with her relationships with close family members, from whom she felt she had to hide the thoughts at all costs—even if it meant never seeing beloved members of her immediate family.

People with such intrusive thoughts are hoping I can explain how these thoughts don't make them bad people. And I can!

Such intrusive thoughts are generally viewed as a kind of obsessive compulsive disorder, with anxiety manifesting not as repetitive behaviors but as repetitive thoughts. Some people have violent intrusions, some sexual, some disgusting, some religious or immoral. They don't want to do the things they think about; on the contrary, their distress comes from the very fact that they absolutely do not want to do these things, and they're worried that they might or that the thoughts mean that some hidden, awful part of them does want to.

I learned about intrusive thoughts from comedian Maria Bamford, who produced an internet show featuring a song called "Don't Be Afraid of the

Dark," a cheery little ditty that celebrates how normal it is to have dark, un-wanted things in our minds. Indeed, research has found that nearly everyone experiences some form of intrusive or unwanted thoughts sometimes, and about a third of people with OCD specifically have sexual intrusions. It's anxi-ety manifesting as all the things we've been taught to fear about sex.[9]

And effective interventions exist. A quick internet search will offer a num-ber of different approaches that generally involve gradually reducing the level of anxiety people feel in response to the thoughts, which in turn reduces the frequency, intensity, and perceived importance of those thoughts. If you have unwanted, intrusive, or obsessive sexual thoughts, know that you can disclose them to a qualified therapist and get evidence-based treatment.

when sex becomes the lion

Beyond the day-to-day stressors of life are the deep wounds that life inflicts and sometimes does not provide opportunities to heal. Given the prevalence of trauma of all kinds, especially sexual trauma—a conserva-tive estimate is that one in five women is sexually assaulted in her lifetime, and it could be more like one in three[10]—it's impossible to talk about women's sexual health without spending some time discussing trauma. From child sexual abuse to sexual assault to all forms of interpersonal violence, women are disproportionately and systematically targeted, and thus they disproportionately bring to their sexual functioning the emotional, physical, and cognitive features of a trauma survivor. In other words, if women have more "issues" than men around sex, there's good reason.

(If you're a survivor and still working through your experience, you may prefer to skip ahead to the next section.)

Trauma results when a person has control over her body taken from her, she freezes, and then she can't unlock. Whether the cause is a car accident or sexual violence, the survival mechanism kicks in: freeze, the petrified shutdown characterized by numbness and sometimes tonic immobility (paralysis) or a sense of disembodiment. Some people describe it as "going into shock." This is the life-threat stress response, activated when your brain decides you can't escape a stressor, nor can you fight it. It's reserved for the most dangerous and violent contexts.

Rape has been described by victim advocate and former police officer Tom Tremblay as "the most violent crime a person can survive."[11] Those who have not been sexually assaulted can perhaps more clearly understand the experience of a survivor by thinking of them as having survived an attempted murder that used sex as the weapon.

Sexual violence often doesn't look like "violence" as we usually imagine it—only rarely is there a gun or knife; often there isn't even "aggression" as we typically think of it. There is coercion and the removal of the targeted person's choice about what will happen next. Survivors don't "fight" because the threat is too immediate and inescapable; their bodies choose "freeze" because it's the stress response that maximizes the chances of staying alive . . . or of dying without pain.

Trauma isn't always caused by one specific incident. It can also emerge in response to persistent distress or ongoing abuse, like a relationship where sex is unwanted though it may be technically "consensual" because the targeted person says yes in order to avoid being injured, or they feel trapped in the relationship or are otherwise coerced. In that context, a survivor's body gradually learns that it can't escape and it can't fight; freeze becomes the default stress response because of the learned pattern of shutdown as the best way to guarantee survival.

Each person's experience of survival is unique, but it often includes a kind of disengaged unreality. And afterward, that illusion of unreality gradually degrades, disintegrating under the weight of physical existence and burdened memory. The tentative recognition that this thing has actually happened incrementally unlocks the panic and rage that couldn't find their way to the surface before, buried as they were under the overmastering mandate to survive.

But survival is not recovery; survival happens automatically, some-times even against the survivor's will. Recovery requires an environment of relative security and the ability to separate the physiology of freeze from the experience of fear, so that the panic and the rage can discharge, completing their cycles at last.

Neither Camilla nor Henry had a history of trauma themselves, but Henry—the nice guy, the gentleman—had a previous girlfriend who was sexually assaulted while they were dating.

We don't talk about trauma survivorship enough, and we talk even less about cosurvivorship, the emotional work of supporting a survivor. Relatively few men—the research indicates only about 5 percent— perpetrate the overwhelming majority of assaults,[12] but a lot of men have partners who have survived an assault. And yet we do almost nothing to teach men how to support survivors as intimate partners, or how to take care of themselves as cosurvivors.

Henry was barely aware of how his previous partner's trauma af-fected his approach to sex until he and Camilla developed their plan of him "chasing" her. It felt awkward for him because he loved her enthu-siastic desire more than anything else, but—remember the ticking pilot light—Camilla needed a lot of warming up before she could feel that enthusiastic desire.

How could he know she was into it? Is it really desire and consent if she "wants to want" sex, rather than plain old wanting sex?

Camilla helped him out by talking about the brakes and accelerator:

"I don't have sensitive brakes, I have a stubborn accelerator. I'm a fully loaded moving van, accelerating from a dead stop at the bottom of a hill. But moving forward slowly isn't the same as wanting to stop, right? All I need is something really awesome waiting for me at the top of the hill. And you already know I'll tell you when something feels good. Surely you trust me to tell you if something hits the brakes."

"Sure," he said.

"Well, then."

And there was one of those silences—you know, where someone's brain is turning over an idea like a puzzle piece, figuring out where it fits in the overall picture.

"Moving forward slowly isn't the same as wanting to stop," he repeated. "You have a slow hot-water heater, a ticking pilot light."

"That's right."

"And you'll tell me if you want to stop."

"Darn skippy."

Henry the gentleman, Henry the geek, nodded slowly. "I think I got it."

(He gets it slightly wrong in chapter 6, but I promise there's a happy ending.)

sex and the survivor

Sexual trauma survivorship impacts information processing for both the accelerator and the brakes. Sensations, contexts, and ideas that used to be interpreted as sex-related may instead now be interpreted by your brain as threats, so that sexy contexts actually hit the brakes. And the chronically high levels of stress activity in a recovering survivor's brain can block out sexual stimuli, categorizing them as low priority.

Sometimes, too, survivors find themselves locked in a pattern of sexual behavior. Their brains become compulsive about undoing the trauma, redoing it differently, or simply understanding it. Like biting on a cold sore or squeezing a pimple, the brain can't leave the trauma alone, even though you know you'd heal faster if you could. The result is that the survivor has multiple partners, often following a habitual pattern, without feeling perfectly in control of the decision to have those partners.

If you're a trauma survivor, chances are you've either done a bunch of emotional work to move through the trauma, or else you've got some work ahead of you. If your trauma is recent or feels unresolved (for example, if reading the previous section made your heart pound), you'll probably benefit from a more intensive level of support than this book can offer. Therapy would probably be *great*. There are excellent books about trauma and healing, the best of which, in my opinion, is *The Body Keeps the Score* by Bessel van der Kolk. Every survivor and everyone who loves a survivor will learn something important from that book. And there are books specifically about sex as a survivor, including *Healing Sex: A Mind-Body Approach to Healing Sexual Trauma* by Staci Haines and *The Sexual Healing Journey: A Guide for Survivors of Sexual Abuse* by Wendy Maltz.

If the trauma is not recent and is more or less resolved, it's normal for you to experience residual effects on your sexual functioning, even when you are largely recovered. Sexual trauma tends to wrap tendrils around so many parts of your emotional experience that you find it unexpectedly, like a persistent invasive weed that has to be pulled and pulled again.

There are three broad approaches to coping with these residual bits of trauma. We might call them "top-down," or a cognitive, thought-based approach; "bottom-up," or a somatic, body-based approach; and "sideways," a mindfulness-based approach.[13]

Top-Down: Processing the Trauma. There are several different forms of cognitive-based therapy—cognitive behavioral therapy, cognitive processing therapy, dialectical behavioral therapy, etc. They all involve some degree of recognizing the meaning that you've created around the trauma and then challenging belief patterns within that meaning, or recognizing behavioral habits that you've trained yourself into since the trauma and challenging those patterns.

They require first that you become aware of the patterns, whether of thought or behavior, and then that you develop skills to replace those patterns with new ones. Allow yourself to feel those old feelings, but now, instead of engaging in the habitual self-defensive patterns, begin practicing new patterns. In the process of changing the patterns, the residual trauma will emerge. Know that you can feel all your Feels and still be safe. Know that you did everything you could in that moment to protect yourself; grant yourself forgiveness for the things you may still blame yourself for, recognizing that the trauma is the fault of the perpetrator alone. And imagine yourself as you are now, safe and whole, sitting quietly—or imagine yourself embracing yourself as you were then, offering yourself the comfort and security you needed then, with reassurance that you survived, that your life got better. This is your new pattern: Allow the feelings to move through you.

Bottom-Up: Processing Your Body. If the idea of analyzing your patterns of thought and behavior is unappealing to you, you may prefer a body-based therapy, such as sensorimotor therapy or Somatic Experiencing (SE).[14] These approaches can stand alone as a powerful way to heal your relationship with your body and your sexuality post trauma, and they can also complement other approaches.

When I spoke with SE practitioner Kristen Chamberlin, she pointed out that body-based therapies move slowly into mainstream practice because we don't have a cultural framework for the body's natural processing of physiological stress (what I call "completing the cycle"). As a culture, we don't trust our bodies, so we override them, which makes us vulnerable to maladaptive coping strategies, as Olivia experienced.

In Chamberlin's practice, she said, the question is, "How do we work with the organic intelligence of the body to heal? Instead of managing what comes up from the body, we work with it, trusting its purpose and direction, while holding a very particular, healing framework. The result is that physiological stress can change and release." This is good news, since so many roadblocks in our sexual relationships are symptoms of unprocessed physiological stress. When we release the old, incomplete stress responses, we make space for new movement where we once felt stuck.

And when you find the stuckness, simply grant it kind, patient, gentle attention. The stuckness will change in the warmth of your attention; it will melt like snow under the sun. Let it. Emotions are physiological cascades that want to complete their cycles, and they will complete those cycles when you allow them to; they want to be travelers, not residents. They want to move on. Let them. You may tremble or shake or cry or curl up in a ball. You may notice your body doing these things without your volition. Your body knows what to do, and it will do it as long as you sit calmly with it, as you would sit calmly beside a sick or grieving child.

Sideways: Mindfulness. Perhaps the gentlest approach is the most indirect. Without ever addressing the trauma directly, you can simply begin practicing mindfulness, and gradually the trauma will work its way out, like shrapnel from an old wound. There are spectacular books on the practice of mindfulness. One of my favorites is *The Mindful Way through Depression* by Mark Williams, John Teasdale, Zindel Segal, and Jon Kabat-Zinn. Don't let the "through depression" part throw you; it's a practical guide to managing any uncomfortable emotional experience.

Here's the short version of how to practice mindfulness:

1. Start with two minutes. For two minutes a day, direct your attention to your breath: the way the air comes into your body and your chest and belly expand, and the way the breath leaves your body and your chest and belly deflate.

2. The first thing that will happen is your mind will wander to something else. That's normal. That's healthy. That's actually the point. Notice that your mind wandered, let those extraneous thoughts go—you can return to them as soon as the two minutes are up—and allow your attention to return to your breath.

Noticing that your mind wandered and then returning your attention to your breath is the real work of mindfulness. It's not so much about paying attention to your breath as it is about noticing what you're paying attention to without judgment, and making a choice about whether you want to pay attention to it. What you're "mindful" of is both your breath *and* your attention to your breath. By practicing this skill of noticing what you're paying attention to, you are teaching yourself to be in control of your brain, so that your brain is not in control of you.

This regular two-minute practice will gradually result in periodic moments throughout the day when you notice what you're paying attention to and then decide if that's what you want to pay attention to right now, or if you want to pay attention to something else. *What* you pay attention to matters less than *how* you pay attention.

This is a sideways strategy for weeding trauma out of your garden. It's a way of simply noticing a weed and then deciding if you want to water it or not, pull it or not, fertilize it or ignore it or not. The weeds of trauma will gradually disappear as long as most of the time you choose not to nurture it. And the more you choose to withdraw your protection from the trauma, the faster it will wither and die.

Mindfulness is good for everyone and everything. It is to your mind what exercise and green vegetables are to your body. If you change only one thing in your life as a result of reading this book, make it this daily two-minute practice. The practice grants the opportunity to "cultivate deep respect for emotions," differentiating their causes from their effects and granting you choice over how you manage them.[15]

origin of love

Aristophanes, in Plato's *Symposium*—and for those of you who very understandably just fell asleep, replace that with the song "The Origin of Love" from John Cameron Mitchell's *Hedwig and the Angry Inch*—offers this parable about why humans love:

Human beings used to be round, with two faces, four arms, four legs, and two sets of genitals. Some of us were two men, some were two women, and some were a man and a woman. But the gods wanted to have more control over us, so Zeus cut us in half with a bolt of lightning, and from that moment, we were susceptible to a suffering that slices, as Hedwig sings it, "a straight line/down through the heart."[16]

Love, according to the parable, is the pursuit of our own wholeness. We wander the earth in search of our lost half. And when two halves find each other, as Aristophanes says, the pair are lost in an amazement of love and friendship and intimacy, and one will not be out of the other's sight, as I may say, even for a moment: these are the people who pass their whole lives together; yet they could not explain what they desire of one another.

This isn't actually why we fall in love, but it's closer than you might think. Why we fall in love is attachment, which is sort of a biological pursuit of wholeness.

Attachment is the evolutionarily adaptive emotional mechanism that bonds infants and adult caregivers. I think human childbirth readily fits the description of pain that feels like you're being separated from a part of yourself. And then, as Christopher Hitchens put it, when you're a parent, "your heart is running around inside someone else's body." [17]

Babies attach, too, always seeking closeness with the adults who care for them. From birth, attachment is the pursuit of our own wholeness—being kept safe, and keeping safe that part of ourselves that lives in someone else's body. Attachment is love.

When we reach adolescence, our attachment mechanism gets co-opted from parental attachment to peer attachment, in romantic relationships. There are certain attachment behaviors we engage in that innately activate the attachment mechanism, whether between infant and caregiver or between two adults falling in love: eye contact, smiling, face stroking, hugging, that kind of thing. But with the shift at adolescence, sexual behavior is added to the repertoire of attachment behaviors.

Brain imaging research has found that activity in the mesolimbic systems (*wanting/liking/learning* from chapter 3) during a nondistressed experience of parental attachment is extremely similar to that during the experience of romantic attachment—and they're especially heavy on the *liking* activation, rather than *wanting* activation.[18] At the same time, attachment is why we experience "heartbreak." As infants, our lives literally depend on our adult caregivers coming when we need them. As adults, that's no longer true, but our bodies don't know it. Our bodies are pretty sure that if our attachment object doesn't come back, we'll die.

So yeah, love feels good—"I am whole."

Except when it hurts like you're dying—"I am broken."

Because: attachment.

the science of falling in love

In practice, humans build important social connections with multiple people, and our sense of wholeness emerges both from our own inner sense of wholeness and from our connection with our friends and family, as well as with our primary partner. But there is the particular experience of "falling in love" or "bonding" with one specific person that typifies what our culture has come to consider "love." If you've ever had a kid or fallen in love, you'll recognize the narrative of attachment, the series of behavioral markers that characterize the attachment process.

Proximity Seeking. You feel connected to the other person, so that it feels good to be around them (*liking*) and you desire (*wanting*) to be as close to them as possible. Most parents have experienced proximity seeking in the form of little toddler fingers under the bathroom door, while you try to have thirty seconds in a row of alone-time as you pee. In romantic relationships, proximity can take the form of social media, texting, phone calls, and email, as well as walking past their locker six times every day to see if they're there, or leaving work early to get home sooner.

Safe Haven. When things go wrong in your life, you want to tell your attachment object all about it; you seek them out for support. In adult relationships, it's the phone call to your partner after a long, hard day at work. When your stress response is activated, your attachment mechanism says, "Soothe your stress by connecting with your attachment object." This is the "tend and befriend" dynamic, which I'll talk about more later.

Separation Distress. When the person goes away, you feel pain—you miss them. For adults, it's the aching loneliness while your partner is away at a conference. It's okay for a while . . . and then it's too much, too long, too far.

Secure Base. Wherever that person is, that's your emotional home. Any adult who has come home from a business trip and fallen onto the couch next to their partner, to hold hands and make eye contact while they talk about what happened while they were away, has experienced this.

A real-life example: My sister Amelia's husband was a high school music teacher, and every other year he accompanied his choir to Europe for a week or two. And every year during that time, she sat around feeling an emotion she called "homesick," even though she was the one at home. Because he is her emotional home, her secure base. So she experienced separation distress.

Amelia's favorite book is *Jane Eyre*. Mr. Rochester, the hero of that story, expresses attachment and separation distress when he says to Jane:

> "I sometimes have a queer feeling with regard to you—especially when you are near me, as now: it is as if I had a string somewhere under my left ribs, tightly and inextricably knotted to a similar string situated in the corresponding quarter of your little frame. And if that boisterous Channel [the Irish Sea], and two hundred miles or so of land come broad between us, I am afraid that cord of communion will be snapt; and then I've a nervous notion I should take to bleeding inwardly."

attachment and sex: the dark side

Mr. Rochester's words hint at the place where attachment and stress overlap: distressed relationships.

In the previous chapter I mentioned John Gottman's stories from women in abusive relationships, who said that some of the best sex followed immediately after acts of violence, and Isabel in *What Do Women Want?*, who craved sex with a commitment-phobic ex but lacked desire for her awesome current boyfriend. Both of these puzzles make sense when we understand attachment-driven sex *when the attachment is threatened*.

Attachment is about survival; relationships are about survival. When they are threatened, we do whatever it takes to hold on to them, because there are no higher stakes than our connection with our attachment objects.

I'll illustrate this idea with some of the darkest and most disturbing science I've ever read—it's disturbing precisely because it shows us how powerfully attachment affects the emotional wellbeing of mammals like us. In Harry Harlow's series of "monster mother" studies, conducted in the middle of the twentieth century, his research team invented mechanical "mothers," to which infant rhesus monkeys attached. Once the infants were emotionally attached to the monster mothers, the mechanical devices shook the infants, spiked them, or jetted cold air onto them, to force the babies away.

And what did the infant monkeys do when their "mothers" treated them badly, shook them off, rejected them?

They ran back to their mothers.

In an episode of the radio show *This American Life*, Deborah Blum, author of a biography of Harlow, *Love at Goon Park*, puts it this way:

> The [rhesus monkey] babies came back and they did everything they could to make those mothers love them again. And they cooed, and they stroked, and they'd groom, and they'd flirt, and exactly what human babies do with their moms. And they would abandon their friends. They had to fix this relationship. It was so important to them.[19]

Of course they did. When we feel distressed, our attachment object is our safe haven. Even—or perhaps especially—if our attachment object is the source of our distress.

And just as the baby rhesus monkeys used attachment behaviors to repair their relationships with their monster mothers, women in unstable relationships may use sex as an attachment behavior to build or repair the attachment. So what Isabel "wanted," to answer Bergner's titular question, was proximity with her attachment object, in the face of separation anxiety. The hormones dopamine and oxytocin were having their wicked way with her *wanting* system, pushing her toward the attachment object who would never commit to her and who therefore chronically activated her attachment system's need for safe haven.[20]

This is the dark side of pairing stress and attachment: the "I am lost" feeling, which motivates us to stabilize our connection with our attachment object—"I am home." Therapist and author Sue Johnson calls this "solace sex," sex that's motivated by your desire to prove that you are loved.[21]

Now in a relationship with a man who is kind and attentive and committed, Isabel's "I am lost" fire is not burning—which is a good thing!—and it can't, therefore, ignite desire. Which doesn't feel so good.

Solution? Isabel needs to advance the plot.

attachment and sex: sex that advances the plot

We never get to see Jane Eyre and Mr. Rochester have sex, but I imagine it would be similar to the sex in modern romance novels, metaphorizing penile-vaginal intercourse in terms of that "pursuit of wholeness." As if Edward Rochester's penis is the key to the lock of Jane's vagina, which opens the door to her heart. Modern romance novels thrive on this kind of thing.

I am a romance reader. I do a lot of work around sexual violence, so I require "happily ever afters" in my life, and romance is a place where I can get them. It's a genre written primarily by women, primarily for women, primarily aboout women's sexual and relationship satisfaction. To that end, many twenty-first-century romance novels are not like *Jane Eyre* or *Pride and Prejudice*. They have sex in them. A lot of sex. Some of them have so much sex, they're basically Porn For The Ladies. But the best romance novels are the ones where the sex isn't just gratuitous for the sake of entertainment. In the best romances, the sex *advances the plot*, carrying the hero and heroine, against all odds and in the face of many obstacles, through one of the behavioral markers of attachment.

As just one example, the heroine of Laura Kinsale's *Flowers from the*

Storm keeps trying to leave the hero and return to her father, but as she rides away she grows "more uneasy every mile" (separation distress) "until she turn[s] her back on her father and return[s]" to the hero (proximity seeking) and reunites with him, with, ahem, "rough vigor." [22]

Romance novels are about the narrative of stressed attachment, from "I am lost" to "I am home," and sex has a starring role as an attachment behavior.

I've been discussing this idea of sex that advances the plot with my women friends, and every time, their eyes widen and they say something like, "And after you're married, the story's over. Happy ending, no more plot. Oh."

Which . . . yeah. But it makes the solution obvious. Add more plot!

So if you're thinking to yourself, "Oh, crap, that means that only in either brand-new or else dysfunctional relationships will the sex ever be exciting," there's good news—and also bad news, and then more good news.

The first good news is that sex you crave often isn't sex that feels good—remember, *liking* and *wanting* are not the same thing. This is "solace sex," which is "soothing but unerotic," in contrast to "sealed-off sex," which is "erotic but empty." [23] Solace sex can feel like a relief, because you're easing fear. But let's not mistake relief for pleasure.

Like imagine that you need to pee really, really badly, and you have to wait and wait, and then finally you pee, and it's almost pleasurable because it's such an intense relief. Sex to advance the plot in unstable relationships is like that. It doesn't feel good when you experience fear and instability in your relationship, just as it doesn't feel good to have to pee really badly. It only feels like a relief when you can finally do something about it.

And don't we want our relationships and our sex lives to be about more than just . . . relief?

So the good news is that if you're missing this kind of intense craving for sex in your relationship, it's no loss.

The bad news is that, yes, most of us will find it easier to crave sex, for what that's worth, when our relationships are unstable—either new or threatened, whether in reality or imagination. But the second good news is that there's a bunch of spectacular research on people who have great sex over multiple decades. The key is to be "just safe enough." I'll talk about that research in chapter 7, but first let's come to grips with the individual differences that influence how you manage attachment in your relationship.

When Laurie told me about her vacation fiasco and the ugly cry surprise, I asked, "What happened after the hot and dirty sex?"

She said, "I fell asleep for three hours . . . which was almost as good as the sex. I just wish I hadn't had to cry to make it happen."

"It sounds to me like crying let you discharge the accumulated stress that was hitting your brakes, which freed up your accelerator."

"Oh. Hm. So are you saying that to have more sex, I should cry even more than I already do?"

"It definitely sounds like you need more opportunities to discharge more of your stress," I said. "Especially since you don't have much leeway for getting rid of your stressors. And Johnny is your attachment object, right? He's where you turn when you're stressed, and your body totally wants to give and receive affection with him, right?"

"Right."

"So can I make a suggestion?"

"Yes, please. Anything."

"Stop. Having. Sex. Make it a rule: no sex for . . . oh, like, a month? You clearly want to give and to receive affection with your attachment object, but the stress of your life is hitting the brakes, and the bonus worry about feeling like you should be having sex just makes it worse. So until you work out more effective strategies for managing your stress, make a rule against all genital touching."

"That doesn't make sense. How am I helping our sex life by ending our sex life?"

"You're not ending it. You're changing the context."

"Which still doesn't make sense to me. We go away together and just get mad at each other; I cry all over Johnny and we get busy."

"Friend, I am not in charge of what context works for you—and neither are you. But the common denominator here is stress of all kinds, including—especially—stress about the fact that stress is hitting your brakes. So stop stressing about the fact that stress is hitting your brakes. Accept it. Welcome it. It's completely normal. You're just in a rotten context, so change the context and see what happens."

She sighed, then went home and talked to Johnny. They tried it. I'll talk about what happened in chapter 5. For now, I'll just say that one powerful way of changing the context is to take away the stress of performance anxiety that comes with feeling obligated to have sex.

attachment style

Whom we attach to as adults and how we attach—our attachment "style"—is shaped by the way we were parented.

At their broadest, we can describe attachment styles as either secure or insecure. Remember that infants' lives literally depend on their adult caregivers, so effectively managing potential abandonment is a serious issue for babies. We attach securely when our adult caregivers (usually our parents) are pretty reliably there for us when we need them. We cry, they come. We turn around, they're there. No adult caregiver is always there, unfailingly, no matter what, but when they're there reliably enough, we attach securely. Under these conditions, our brains learn that our adult caregivers will come back when they leave; they will not abandon us.

Kids who are securely attached to their adult caregivers will, as adults, most likely attach securely to their romantic partners, and kids who are insecurely attached to their adult caregivers will, as adults, mostly likely attach insecurely to their romantic partners.

But if parents are under extreme stress or have lots of other children to take care of or have an active drug or alcohol addiction or mood or personality disorder, they won't necessarily be present, physically or emotionally, when the child needs them. When our adult caregivers are less reliable, we attach insecurely. About half of people in the United States develop secure attachment styles, and half develop insecure styles.[24]

We can think of insecure attachment as fitting into two different strategies: anxious and avoidant. With an anxious attachment style, a person copes with the risk that their attachment object might abandon them by clinging desperately to them. Anxiously attached children get jealous and experience intense separation distress; so do anxiously attached adults. People with an avoidant attachment style cope with the risk that their attachment object might abandon them by not attaching seriously to any specific individual. Avoidant children don't prefer their parents to other adults; avoidant adults, according to the research, are more likely to approve of and have anonymous sex.

To give you a more specific sense of what the styles are like, here are the kinds of statements researchers use to assess attachment style in adults:[25]

Secure Attachment	Anxious Attachment	Avoidant Attachment
• I feel comfortable sharing my private thoughts and feelings with my partner.	• I'm afraid I will lose my partner's love.	• I prefer not to show a partner how I feel deep down.
• I rarely worry about my partner leaving me.	• I often worry that my partner will not want to stay with me.	• I find it difficult to allow myself to depend on romantic partners.
• I am very comfortable being close to romantic partners.	• I often worry that my partner doesn't really love me.	• I don't feel comfortable opening up to romantic partners.
• It helps to turn to my romantic partner in times of need.	• I worry that romantic partners won't care about me as much as I care about them.	• I prefer not to be too close with romantic partners.

Now, if you had to guess who has a more satisfying sex life, folks with a secure attachment style or folks with an insecure attachment style, whom would you guess?

Of course. Secure attachment folks. By a mile.

A 2012 review of the research on the relationship between sex and attachment found that secure attachment was associated with every domain of sexual wellbeing you can imagine. Secure attachers have more positive emotions during sex, more frequent sex, higher levels of arousal and orgasm, and better communication about sex.[26] They are better at giving and receiving consent and are more likely to engage in safer sex practices such as contraception use; they enjoy sex more, are more attentive to their partners' needs, feel a link between sex and love, are more likely to have sex in the context of a committed relationship, and are more sexually self-confident. Secure attachers have the healthiest, most pleasurable sex lives.

People with anxious attachment styles are the most likely to engage in anxiety-driven "solace sex"—that is, using sex as an attachment behavior—which can make sex intense without making it pleasurable. Anxious attachers worry more about sex, and yet they also equate the quality of sex with the quality of a relationship. They're more likely to experience pain with sex, particularly in low-intimacy relationships. It shows up, too, as difficulties with safer sex practices—they're less likely to use condoms, more likely to use alcohol or other drugs before sex, and, unsurprisingly, have higher rates of STIs and unwanted pregnancy. Anxious attachers experience more pain, anxiety, and health risks.

People with insecure attachment styles, anxious or avoidant, are more likely to be involved on either side of a coercive sexual relationship. People with avoidant attachment start having sex later in life, have sex less often, with fewer noncoital behaviors. They have more positive attitudes toward sex outside committed relationships, have more one-night stands, and are more likely to have sex just to fit into a social expectation rather than because they really want to. Avoidant attachers experience sex as less connected with their lives and their relationships.

In the end, insecure attachment hits the brakes. We can't understand sexual wellbeing without understanding attachment, and we can't maximize our own sexual wellbeing without learning how to manage attachment in our relationships.

managing attachment: your feels as a sleepy hedgehog

Attachment style is an inescapable factor in sexual response and relationship satisfaction—and it varies not just from person to person but also from relationship to relationship.[27] And it can change.[28] Yet these deep emotional patterns are not always very tractable and sometimes require therapy. Many people, though, can make a great deal of progress by increasing their nonjudgmental awareness of their own emotional responses and by reading excellent books on the subject. For example, *Love Sense: The Revolutionary New Science of Romantic Relationships* by Sue Johnson, who developed Emotionally Focused Couples Therapy, directly addresses attachment as it relates to sex. But couples seem to struggle with discussing sexual difficulties in specific ways. We are all so tender around this topic, so afraid both of hurting our partner's feelings and of not meeting our partner's expectations, that we need a special set of skills to help us be as gentle and kind with each other as that tenderness requires.

I've come to think of communicating about sex and love in terms of a "sleepy hedgehog" model of emotion management. It goes like this: Think of your difficult feelings about sex as sleepy hedgehogs that you discover in inconvenient places around your home. If you find a sleepy hedgehog in the chair you were about to sit in, you should:

1. *Find Out the Hedgehog's Name.* "Right now I feel . . . jealous/angry/hurt/etc." Simple, though there are usually multiple feelings involved at the same time. That's normal.

2. *Sit Peacefully with It.* Don't run away from it, don't judge it or shame it or get mad at it. Sit still with it, like it is a welcome guest.

3. *Listen to Its Needs.* The question to ask is: *What will help?* If you feel fear or anger, how could the perceived threat be managed? If you feel sadness, hurt, or grief, how can you heal the loss? There won't always be something you can actively do, apart from allowing the feeling to discharge and complete its cycle. And remember that it's not your partner's fault or obligation; their help is entirely voluntary and provides an opportunity for you to express gratitude for their support.

4. *Communicate the Feeling and the Need.* Present the feeling to your partner. "I feel x," you say, "and I think what would help is y." For example, "I feel threatened by the time you spend with your coworker, and I could use some kind of plan that will give me reassurance." Or, "I still have this hurt about that time you did x, and what I need is some time to go through that emotional tunnel so I can get to the light at the end."

Getting mad at the hedgehog or being afraid of it won't help you or the hedgehog, and you certainly can't just shove it into your partner's lap, shouting, "*SLEEPY HEDGEHOG!*" and expect them to deal with all its spiky quills. It's *your* hedgehog. The calmer you are when you handle it, the less likely you are to get hurt yourself, or to hurt someone else.

The hedgehog metaphor also illustrates the importance of making the difficulty something you and your partner share and can collaborate on, rather than a problem one of you has to "fix" on your own so the other person can be satisfied. It takes both of you turning toward that shared difficulty with kindness and compassion.

Choose to Heal

A friend of mine left a bad relationship and declared (on Facebook), "I choose to hurt no longer. [Ex-partner] can't hurt me anymore." The second sentence is 100 percent true and cause for celebration. But the first sentence doesn't make sense from an attachment/completing-the-cycle point of view. When you leave a bad relationship, you have all this pent-up hurt and rage and grief and even fear locked up inside you, which must be allowed to discharge safely.

What makes more sense is, "I choose to allow the hurt to heal." Healing always involves pain—if you break your finger, it hurts, gradually less and less until it heals. Same goes for healing emotional injury. You can't choose for your broken heart not to hurt, any more than you can choose for a broken bone not to hurt. But you can recognize the pain as part of the healing, and you can trust your heart to heal, just as you trust your bones to heal, knowing that it will gradually hurt less and less as you recover.

survival of the social

Which brings me to an additional stress response known as "tend and befriend," which we can think of as the marriage of stress and attachment.[29] As an ultrasocial species, our survival depends not just on our individual ability to fight, run, or shut down, but also on our ability to collaborate with our tribe, so that we can protect them and they can protect us. Women may be more likely than men to access this "affiliative" stress response, dealing with potential threats by connecting affectionately with people. As always, to what extent this difference is inborn and to what extent it's learned isn't clear, but the differences start early, with girls as young as eighteen months being more likely than boys to approach, rather than avoid, a parent doing scary things.[30]

Where stress and attachment overlap, the message of your emotional

One Ring is, "I am lost!" and when you escape the lion and run to your attachment object, the message is, "I am home." If you've ever found yourself checking your email obsessively when you're stressed, or scrolling endlessly through social media, or texting your partner just to say, "Hey," or calling all your friends one after the next, or, like Elle in *Legally Blonde*, running for an emergency manicure, you may have experienced the tend and befriend stress response. Both feeling taken care of and taking care of others register in your stress response as "completing the cycle."

But in modern culture, there's a contradiction built into the social remedies to stress. On the one hand, being around other people is often a core part of allowing our stress response to complete. On the other hand, we put the brakes on, self-inhibiting our stress response, in order to stay socially appropriate and not make other people uncomfortable. We hold on to our incomplete stress response in order to access the security of being with our tribe.

And, of course, this contradiction is more pronounced for women, who are the culturally sanctioned "managers of relationships." When the going gets tough in a heterosexual relationship, it often falls to the woman to rein in her own stress response, in order to create space for the man to feel his Feels. In other words, if there is stress in a relationship, cultural rules make it likely to impact the woman more than the man, and it's likely to impact her sexual interest and response. And because she has to hold on to her stress, so that her partner can let his go, she is more likely to become stuck in her stress, while he moves through his.

I blame Charles Dickens. Take Mrs. Cratchit from *A Christmas Carol*. Her son, Tiny Tim, dies, and she tells her other children that she's crying because the color of her sewing hurts her eyes, and she "wouldn't want to show weak eyes" to her husband. When I was little, I used to think, as Dickens wanted me to, *Mrs. Cratchit is so brave.* But now that I know about the stress response cycle, I want to yell, "Lady, your child died! It's not 'weak' to cry! And your other kids deserve to know that it's normal to grieve!"

Being with the tribe doesn't replace the Feels built into completing the cycle. We need to discharge the stress response, complete the cycle, before our bodies can move on. "Home" is the place—physical and emotional—where we can discharge stress without being judged or shamed or told we just need to relax or forget about it. "Home" is where we receive our partner's "loving presence." People who listen with a loving presence are calm, attentive, and warmly attuned to the other person. In the very best relationships, we're allowed to experience all forms of stress—anger, fear, shutdown—and receive the loving presence of our partner as they sit still and quietly through the storm.

Every culture has rules about how much of which kinds of emotions are appropriate in what circumstances. But our culture has constructed a social world where there is almost nowhere that we can connect with others while experiencing the full range of our emotional intensity. For a lot of us, there are times when we more readily share a loving presence through spiritual practice or with our pets than with our partners, who are mired in their own stress. God and your dog never judge or blame you for having Feels—but neither of them can make love with you.

Sex is an adult attachment behavior. When your attachment is threatened or when you and your partner share a stressor together, sex can be a powerful, pleasurable way to connect in the face of the "I'm lost" signals, so that you can find your way home. Together. But this feels pleasurable only if you can give each other time and space for Feels.

the water of life

I am at risk/I am safe.

I am broken/I am whole.

I am lost/I am home.

As you progress through these biological processes, your mental state changes, and that, in turn, changes whether and how your brain responds to contexts as sex-related or to sensations as sexually pleasurable.

Stress hits the brakes for most people, but it activates the accelerator for others—people vary. But for everyone, stress changes the context in which you experience sexual response, which changes how your perception of sexual sensations.

The key to managing stress so that it doesn't interfere with sexual pleasure is learning to complete the cycle—unlock freeze, escape the predator, conquer the enemy. Celebrate, like glitter settling in a snow globe.

Sex is an attachment behavior, reinforcing the social bond between adults. Sometimes it takes the form of passionate, joyful sex between people who are falling in love with each other. Sometimes it takes the form of desperate, grasping sex between people whose attachment is threatened. Counterintuitively, when attachment is at its most secure and stable—when your relationship is all satisfaction and no worry or "plot"—it can take a backseat in your sexual arousability.

Stress and love (in the form of attachment) can be companions to sex. Sex strengthens bonds between partners, helps each partner feel safe, cherished, and supported in a world where we are not always safe, where sometimes our only shield from chaos and terror is our chosen family.

Women tell me their stories, and I keep those stories in a mental library. One shelf in that library is overflowing: the one that holds stories of sexual violence. Like all the rest, these are awe-inspiring stories of discovery, but they are the darkest stories, revealing just how viciously indifferent the world can be to women's sexual autonomy.

Merritt's is one of those. The one-sentence version: She was a leader of the campus gay-straight alliance, out and proud, and he, she would later learn, bet his friends that he could "turn her."

It's sickening, I know. I wish no one had stories like this to tell. But it happens.

During the assault, her body went into survival mode—she froze. And until she learned about the brakes stress response, she hadn't understood why she didn't fight or run or kick the guy in the balls. She has

struggled to trust her body ever since, and her body has struggled to oper-
ate healthfully without her trust.

When a person experiences trauma, it's like someone snuck into the
garden and ripped out all the plants she had been cultivating with such
care and attention. There is rage. There is grief for the garden as it was.
And there is fear that it will never grow back.

But it will grow back. That's what gardens do.

Merritt was into the garden metaphor. She stopped me in the street
one day, phone in hand, to say, "I was thinking about the garden, and I
had to read you this thing my partner found!"

She read:

> *The water of life is here.*
> *I'm drinking it. But I had to come*
> *this long way to know it!*[31]

"'The water of life,'" she said. "It's this Rumi poem about a guy
who loses everything and goes on a quest and he's like Dorothy in The
Wizard of Oz, *he had the power all along. And you know what the*
water of life is?"

"Tell me." (This was nowhere near the weirdest thing anyone had
ever stopped me in the street to tell me.)

She quoted, "'Love is the water of life!'"[32]

I think that's right. If women's sexuality is a garden, I think of love
as the rain and stress as the sun, drawing the garden upward, nourishing
and challenging at once. It wouldn't do to have too much of either, but in
the right balance—when we are "just safe enough"—the garden thrives.

Some plants want lots of water, some want less; some gardens are
shady, while others are full of bright sun all day. Olivia, with her sensitive
accelerator, has a sunny garden full of plants that delight in the sun—
she's practically a desert, with Joshua trees and blackfoot daisies thriving
under a hot, cloudless sky. But even for her, too much of a good thing

can cause her garden to wilt and fade. Camilla, by contrast, with her rela-tively insensitive accelerator, has a montane forest of broadleaf ferns and mosses that require less light and more time to grow lush.

Meanwhile, Merritt's sensitive brakes make her garden wilt in the mildest drought, and Laurie's garden feels like it's been subjected to global warming, stripped of its native climate faster than she and her plants can adapt, and she fears the whole garden is dying. And she's afraid that if she loses her garden, she might lose her partner.

Listening to and respecting the fundamental messages that your body is trying to send you—"I am at risk," "I am broken," "I am lost"—is es-sential to creating the right context for sexual pleasure to thrive. Allowing time and space for your body to move all the way through the cycle, to discharge stress and to connect wholly with your partner, is an essential part of creating a context that grants maximum access to pleasure.

Western culture does not make this easy; it builds walls of shame and doubt between us and our essential selves, between "at risk" and "safe," between "broken" and "whole," between "lost" and "home."

In the garden metaphor, the cultural messages about women's sexual-ity are very often the weeds, encroaching in ways no one chose but that everyone has to manage.

And that's what chapter 5 is about.

tl;dr

- Stress reduces sexual *interest* in 80–90 percent of people and reduces sexual *pleasure* in everyone—even the 10–20 percent of people for whom it increases interest. The way to deal with stress is to allow your body to *complete the stress response cycle*.
- Trauma survivors' brains sometimes learn to treat "sex-related" stimuli as threats, so that whenever the accelerator is activated, the brakes are hit, too. Practicing *mindfulness* is an evidence-based strategy for decoupling the brakes and accelerator.

- In the right context, sex can attach us emotionally to new partners or reinforce emotional bonds in unstable relationships. In other words, sex and love are closely linked in our brains—but only in the right context.
- Sex that brings you closer to your partner "advances the plot," as opposed to gratuitous sex, for no reason other than that you can. To have more and better sex, give yourself a compelling *reason* to have sex, something important to move toward.

five

cultural context

A SEX-POSITIVE LIFE IN A SEX-NEGATIVE WORLD

When Johnny and Laurie took my advice and stopped having sex, something unexpected cracked open inside Laurie.

They cuddled and snuggled a few minutes at bedtime each night, without the awkward are-we-going-to-have-sex-tonight anxiety.

Into that silence one night, Laurie asked Johnny why he liked having sex with her.

He gave such a good answer. He said, "Because you're beautiful."

He didn't say, "Because you look *beautiful" or "Because you're my wife" or "Because sex is fun" or even "Because I love you." He said, "You are beautiful." It's a perfect thing to say—not least because he really, really meant it.*

Laurie being Laurie, she burst into tears. Until that moment, she had not realized how much self-criticism she was carrying with her every day, how much shame she felt about the ways her body had changed since she had the baby, as if those changes reflected some moral failing on her part—as if a truly "good person" would never allow her body to be changed by a paltry thing like having a baby.

She started listing all the things she felt uncomfortable with— her droopy boobs, her squishy tummy, her cottage-cheesy thighs, the deepening wrinkles that bracketed her mouth—a mouth that seemed to have a permanent frown now. And Johnny started touching each and every one of these "imperfect" body parts, saying, "I love that, though" and "but this is beautiful."

At last he looked into her eyes and said, "You really don't see it. You really believe this stuff makes you less beautiful. Honey, your body gets sexier every day, just by being the body of the woman I share my life with. Your belly is our belly. I've got one too. Do you love me less for it?"

"Of course not."

"Exactly, of course not."

And of course what happened next is they had totally mind-blowing sex—made all the more mind-blowing by the whispers of, "We aren't supposed to be doing this!" It turns out the pressure of what she's "supposed" to be doing works both ways.

When Laurie told me about this, she began by asking me if it was true that men weren't as bothered by body changes as women think they are.

"Yeah, I've heard that over and over from men," I told her, "especially from coparenting men. They don't notice the changes we notice, or they notice and it doesn't change how they feel, or they notice and they actively like it. We underestimate men."

And so she told me her "you're beautiful" story, emphasizing that throughout the whole encounter she never felt like he was initiating sex. It just felt like he was giving her love at a moment when she needed it.

And yes, being a sex educator is the best job ever, when people tell you stories like this.

This chapter is about the obstacles that were standing in Laurie's way, without her being fully aware of them, and how she and Johnny knocked them down.

Let's return to the garden metaphor: You're born with a little plot of rich and fertile soil, unique to yourself. Your brain and body are the soil of this garden, and individual differences in your accelerator and brakes are important characteristics of your innate garden, which is made of the same parts as everyone else's, but organized in a unique way.

Your family and your culture plant the seeds and tend the garden, and they teach you how to tend it. They plant the seeds of language and attitudes and knowledge and habits about love and safety and bodies and sex. And gradually, as you move into adolescence, you take on responsibility for tending your own garden.

As you begin to tend the garden yourself, you may find that your family and your culture have planted some beautiful, nourishing things. You may also find that your family and culture have planted some pretty toxic crap in your garden. And everyone—even those whose families planted pretty good stuff—will have to deal with the invasive weeds of a sex-negative culture full of body shaming and sex stigma. These travel not in the seeds planted by families but underground via their roots, like poison ivy, under fences and over walls, from garden to garden. No one chose that they be there, but there they are nonetheless.

So if you want to have a healthy garden, a garden *you* choose, you have to go row by row and figure out what you want to keep and nurture . . . and what you want to dig out and replace with something healthier.

It is not fair that you have to do all that extra work. After all, you didn't choose what got planted by your family and your culture. No one asked for your permission before they started planting the toxic crap. They didn't wait until you could give consent and then say, "Would it be okay with you if we planted the seeds of body self-criticism and sexual shame?" Chances are, they just planted the same things that were planted in their gardens, and it never even occurred to them to plant something different.

I was chatting about this one October evening, over poutine and beer, with Canadian sex researcher Robin Milhausen, and she said this brilliant thing: "We're raising women to be sexually dysfunctional, with all the 'no' messages we're giving them about diseases and shame and fear. And then as soon as they're eighteen they're supposed to be sexual rock stars, multiorgasmic and totally uninhibited. It doesn't make any sense. None of the things we do in our society prepares women for that."

Exactly.

Chapter 4 was about how the context in this moment—your sense of safety in your life and your sense of wholeness in your relationship—affects your sexual pleasure. This chapter is about the large-scale, long-term context—the years of "no" messages—and the deep patterns of thinking and feeling they create, patterns that are reinforced and reiterated over decades of life. These patterns are emphatically not innate, but they were learned early. You began these lessons long before you were capable of thinking critically about whether you wanted them. And just as you learned them, you can unlearn them, if you want to, and replace them with new, healthier patterns that promote confidence, joy, satisfaction, and even ecstasy.

We'll start with three core cultural messages about women's sexuality that my students grapple with as their established ideas about sex are challenged by the science: the Moral Message (you are evil), the Medical Message (you are diseased), and the Media Message (you are inadequate). Hardly anyone fully buys into any of these messages, but they are there, encroaching on our gardens, and the better we are at seeing them for what they are, the better we'll be at weeding them out.

Then I'll talk about body self-criticism. This issue is so entrenched in Western culture that most women hardly notice how ubiquitous and how toxic it is. It's so entrenched, in fact, that many women believe it's actually important and beneficial. I'll talk about the research that says otherwise. If the only change you make after reading this book is to reduce your body self-criticism, that alone will revolutionize your sexual wellbeing.

Next, I'll talk about another core emotion, like stress and attachment: disgust. Like body self-criticism, disgust is so entrenched in the sexual culture that it's difficult to know what our sexual wellbeing would be like without it. But there's growing evidence that disgust is impairing our sexual wellbeing, much as body self-criticism does, and there are things you can do to weed it out, if you want to.

And that's what I'll talk about in the last section of this chapter. I'll describe research-based strategies for creating positive change in both self-criticism and disgust: self-compassion, cognitive dissonance, and basic media literacy. The goal is to help you recognize what you've been taught, deliberately or otherwise, in order to help you choose whether to continue believing those things. You may well choose to keep a lot of what you learned—what matters is that *you* choose it, instead of letting your beliefs about your body and sex be chosen for you by the accident of the culture and family you were born into. When you take the time to notice your unchosen beliefs, and to say yes or no to those beliefs, you empower yourself to have the sexual wellbeing that fits you, custom made.

three messages

Many of my students believe that they know kind of a lot about sex, only to discover, about halfway through the first lecture, that they kind of don't.

What they do know a lot about—and they really know a *lot* about it—is not sex itself but rather what their culture believes about sex. They, we, all of us, are surrounded by messages about these beliefs, messages that are not only short on facts but are also actively self-contradictory.

I was puzzled by the false beliefs my students brought with them into the classroom, until I began reading antique sex advice manuals. And there they were in black and white, written a hundred years ago or more—the same false ideas my students believed. Students have absorbed these ideas from their families and their cultures, without any of them ever having read those books.

One day in class, I read aloud a couple of definitions of "sex." First I read from *Ideal Marriage: Its Physiology and Technique* by T. H. van de Velde, from 1926. He wrote that "normal sexual intercourse" is

that intercourse which takes place between two sexually mature individuals of opposite sexes; which excludes cruelty and the use of
artificial means for producing voluptuous sensations; which aims
directly or indirectly at the consummation of sexual satisfaction, and
which, having achieved a certain degree of stimulation, concludes
with the ejaculation—or emission—of the semen into the vagina, at
the nearly simultaneous culmination of sensation—or orgasm—of
both partners.[1]

Then I read from *The Hite Report*, published in 1976, from the chapter titled "Redefining Sex":

Sex is intimate physical contact for pleasure, to share pleasure with
another person (or just alone). You can have sex to orgasm, or not to
orgasm, genital sex, or just physical intimacy—whatever seems right
to you. There is never any reason to think the "goal" must be intercourse, and to try to make what you feel fit into that context. There is
no standard of sexual performance "out there," against which you must
measure yourself; you aren't ruled by "hormones" or "biology." You
are free to explore and discover your own sexuality, to learn or unlearn
anything you want, and to make physical relations with other people,
of either sex, anything you like.[2]

And I asked my students, "Which of these is more like what you
learned growing up?"
No contest. *Ideal Marriage.*
Many of us have absorbed ideas about sex that are at home in a
century-old sex manual, even though all the research and political change
since then has busily dismantled every single aspect of those old ideas.
Somehow the culture has not absorbed the more inclusive and evidence-
based ideas of more recent decades.
The outdated ideas consist of three interwoven cultural messages of

sexual socialization that women encounter in modern America. These are the three messages I mentioned earlier. I call them the Moral Message, the Medical Message, and the Media Message, sent by three separate but intertwined messengers. To varying degrees, each has pieces of truth and wisdom to offer, and to varying degrees each has a self-interested agenda. We've all absorbed at least a little of all of them, and they shape the story we tell about our own and others' sexualities.

The Moral Message: "You are Damaged Goods." If you want or like sex, you're a slut. Your virginity is your most valuable asset. If you've had too many partners ("too many" = more than your male partner has had), you should be ashamed. There is only one right way to behave and one right way to feel about sex—not to feel anything about it at all but to accommodate the man to whom your body belongs. Sex is not part of what makes a woman lovable; it can only be part of what makes a woman unlovable. It may make her "desirable"—and many women try to be desirable, but only as a lesser alternative to being lovable. If you are sexually desirable, you are, by definition, unlovable.

And a slut.

This is the oldest message, having changed only superficially in the last three hundred years. There are almost too many examples to choose just one, but let's take a paragraph of rhetorical questions from James Fordyce's *Sermons to Young Women*, published in 1766 and read aloud by Mr. Collins to the ladies in Jane Austen's novel *Pride and Prejudice*. The overall message of the *Sermons* is "women are appealing when they're meek and ignorant and pure." In this section, Fordyce is discussing "public diversions" involving "oaths, imprecations, double meaning, everything obscene" (he means going to the theater):

> Between the state of virgin purity and actual prostitution are there no intermediate degrees? Is it nothing to have the soul deflowered, the fancy polluted, the passions flung into a ferment? . . . Such indeed one would think were the opinion of those, who imagine there can be no harm in a passion for places of entertainment . . .

Translation: If you enjoy being entertained, you will lose your mental virginity, which makes you the same as a prostitute. Which would, it goes without saying, make you unlovable.

And a slut.

Jane Austen knew it was bogus. You know it's bogus. But it's there in the culture you were raised in, and it sneaks under the fence and invades like poison ivy.

The Medical Message: "You Are Diseased." Sex causes disease and pregnancy, which makes it dangerous. But if you're ready to take that risk, sexual functioning should happen in a particular way—desire, then arousal, then orgasm, preferably during intercourse, simultaneously with your partner—and when it doesn't, there is a medical issue that you must address. Medically. With medication. Or possibly surgery. To the extent that a woman's sexual response differs from a man's, she is diseased—except for pregnancy, which is what sex is for. One woman even told me that her (male) doctor said her low sexual desire was caused by her body shutting down her sex drive in order to prevent her from getting pregnant. She asked me if that's true. Short answer: No. Long answer: *Hell* no, and I hope that doctor reads chapter 7.

This is a newer message, dating from about the middle of the nineteenth century or later. As an example, Marie Stopes's 1918 classic, *Married Love*, has this to say on the subject of intercourse:

> Where the [man and woman] are perfectly adjusted, the woman simultaneously reaches the crisis of nervous reactions and muscular convulsions similar to his. This mutual orgasm is extremely important . . . and it is a *mutual*, not a selfish, pleasure, more calculated than anything else to draw out an unspeakable tenderness and understanding in both partakers of this sacrament.

Simultaneous orgasm can be very nice. But you know as well as I do that it is not the marker of a "perfectly adjusted" sexual experience. And yet, nearly one hundred years later, the idea of simultaneous orgasm during intercourse persists as a bogus cultural marker of "sexual excellence."

The Media Message: "You Are Inadequate." Spanking, food play, ménages à trois . . . you've done all these things, right? Well, you've at least had clitoral orgasms, vaginal orgasms, uterine orgasms, energy orgasms, extended orgasms, and multiple orgasms? And you've mastered at least thirty-five different positions for intercourse? If you don't try all these things, you're frigid. If you've had too few partners, don't watch porn, and don't have a collection of vibrators in your bedside table, you're a prude. Also: You're too fat *and* too thin; your breasts are too big *and* too small. Your body is wrong. If you're not trying to change it, you're lazy. If you're satisfied with yourself as you are, you're settling. And if you dare to actively *like* yourself, you're a conceited bitch. In short, you are doing it wrong. Do it differently. No, that's wrong, too, try something else. Forever.

This is the newest message, following close on the heels of television and the birth control pill, around the middle of the twentieth century. To see an example, just look at the checkout counter of any drugstore, where magazine racks announce in bright sans serif fonts all the exciting things you could (and, it goes without saying, *should*) be doing in bed.

You know it's just for fun. You're not really trying to live up to the standard set by characters on a TV show. But it's there, affecting your garden, whether you welcome it there or not.

> Camilla had said, "The images we see—or don't see—matter. They tell us what's possible."
>
> And it's just as true for the stories we tell as it is about the images of the people in the stories.
>
> Camilla had spent a lot of her early adolescence reading old romance novels from the 1970s and '80s. These stories stuck with her so powerfully that she even wrote her undergrad thesis on gender and race politics in ephemeral art.
>
> But now, having figured out context and the dual control model, she

revisited a collection of romance novels, examining the contexts that the narratives created for the women's sexualities.

And those contexts were bizarre.

She told Henry and me, "So here's the universal story: The heroine is a Good Girl, who has no accelerator and sensitive brakes, who has never had the slightest sexual feeling until she meets the Hero. You can tell he's the Hero because suddenly Good Girl's accelerator is going bananas. But Good Girl has to keep the brakes on because sex is inherently bad and dangerous, and so of course the Hero just has sex with her anyway—"

Henry raised an eyebrow and shook his head at this. I face-palmed.

"But gradually the purity and goodness of her squeaky-clean vagina 'tames' the Hero and they fall in love and get married."

This is both hilarious and tragic, because it is so not how women's sexuality actually works.

But here was the next-level insight:

She said, "So what I'm thinking is . . . what if the way women's sexual desire and emotions and relationships are represented in the media is just as distorted as the way women's bodies are represented? What if everything about how sex works is just as poorly drawn as the Escher Girls? What if basically everything culture says about sex is wrong, and my slow-to-heat accelerator is actually just completely normal?"

And of course it is. She's made of all the same parts as everyone else, organized in a unique way.

you are beautiful

On the day you were born, how did you feel about the chub of fat on the back of your thighs?

How did the adults around you feel about it?

Every baby needs their caregivers to hold them in their arms with affection and joy, and most of the time those caregivers are bursting with eagerness to meet that need. On the day we're born, most of us are celebrated and called beautiful.

But something happens between that joyful day when every inch, every ounce, every roll, and every bump of a girl's body is celebrated as perfect and lovable precisely as it is . . . and the day she hits puberty.

What happens is she absorbs messages about what is or is not lovable about her body. The seeds of body self-criticism are planted and nurtured, and body self-confidence and self-compassion are neglected, punished, and weeded out.

Students laugh like I made a joke when I ask, "What would happen if you met your friends at dinner and said, 'I feel so beautiful today!'?"

"Really, what would happen?" I insist.

"No one would do that," they tell me.

"But . . . how often would someone meet friends at dinner and say, 'I feel so fat today'?"

"All the time," they say.

All the time.[3]

Women have cultural permission to criticize ourselves, but we are punished if we praise ourselves, if we dare to say that we like ourselves the way we are.[4]

And it's messing with our orgasms, our pleasure, our desire, and our sexual satisfaction. There is a direct trade-off between sexual wellbeing and self-critical thoughts about your body. A 2012 review of fifty-seven studies, spanning two decades of research, found important links between body image and just about every domain of sexual behavior you can imagine: arousal, desire, orgasm, frequency of sex, number of partners, sexual self-assertiveness, sexual self-esteem, using alcohol or other drugs during sex, engaging in unprotected sex, and more.[5] The results vary somewhat among different age groups, among women of different sexual identities, and across different racial groups, but the overall result is universal: Women who feel worse about their bodies have less satisfying, riskier sex, with less pleasure, more unwanted consequences, and more pain.[6]

I don't think anyone will be surprised to hear that feeling good about your body improves your sex life. It's obvious once you think about it, right? Just imagine having sex if you feel insecure and unattractive. How would it feel to have a person you care about touching you and looking at you, when the thought of your own body makes you uncomfortable? Would you pay attention to the sensations in your body and your partner's—or would you pay attention to all the things you feel compelled to hide?

And does that activate your accelerator, or does it hit your brakes? Brakes.[7]

Now imagine having sex when you feel tremendously confident and beautiful. Imagine how it feels to have a person you care about touching your skin with their hands and gaze, when you love every inch of yourself and can feel your partner appreciating how gorgeous you are.

The *wanting* mechanism is fully on board in both cases—but in the first case the mechanism is torn between moving toward the sexual experience and moving away from your own body. In the second, when you enjoy living inside your own skin, the mechanism moves toward sex *and* toward yourself, without conflict.

So of course body self-criticism interferes with sexual wellbeing. We can't understand women's sexual satisfaction without thinking about body satisfaction, just as we can't understand women's sexual pleasure without thinking about attachment and stress. And women will not be fully, blissfully satisfied with their sex lives until they are fully, blissfully satisfied with their own bodies.

So, to have more and better sex, love your body.

Which is one of those things where you're like, "Yeah! . . . But . . . how?"

It's hard, because you never chose *not* to love your body. You didn't choose much that happened to you between the day you were born and the day you hit puberty, and that's when most of the body self-criticism was taking root. You never even got a chance to say yes or no to the self-criticism being planted in your garden.

What it comes down to is that a lot of women trust their bodies less than they trust what they've been taught, culturally, *about* their bodies.

But culture has taught you stuff that is both incorrect and just *wrong*. Hurtful. I want to address two things you've been taught that are definitely wrong, and what's right: first, that self-criticism is good for you and second, that fat is bad for you. These things are both false. Here's why:

criticizing yourself = stress = reduced sexual pleasure

Women have been trained to beat ourselves up when we fall short. We criticize ourselves—"I'm so stupid/fat/crazy," "I suck," "I'm a loser"—as a reflex when things don't go the way we want them to. And our brains process self-criticism with brain areas linked to behavioral inhibition—brakes.[8] So it's not surprising that self-criticism is directly related to depression[9]—and does depression improve your sexual well-being? It does not.

Here's how that works:

When you get right down to it, self-criticism is yet another form of stress.[10] I described stress in chapter 4 as an evolutionarily adaptive mechanism to help us escape threats—"I am at risk." When we think, "I am an inadequate person!" that's like saying, "I am the lion!" Literally, our stress hormone levels increase.[11] Your body reacts to negative self-evaluations as if you're under attack.

The solution is to practice replacing self-criticism with self-kindness.

Women tend to have a two-layered response to this idea. First, they instinctively love the idea of being more accepting of themselves and not blaming themselves when life isn't perfect. The research tells women what they already know intuitively: Self-criticism is associated with worse health outcomes, both mental and physical, and more loneliness.[12] That's right: Self-criticism is one of the best predictors of loneliness—so it's not just "I am at risk," it's also "I am lost."

But then, when women start to think concretely about it, they begin to discover a sense that they need their self-criticism in order to stay motivated. We believe it does us good to torture ourselves, at least a little bit. As in: "If I stop beating myself up for the ways I'm not perfect, that's like admitting to the world—and to myself—that I'll never be perfect, that I'm permanently inadequate! I need my self-criticism in order to maintain hope and to motivate myself to get better."

When we tell ourselves, "I can't stop criticizing myself or else I will fail forever!" that's like saying, "I can't stop running/fighting/playing dead, or the lion will eat me!" That's absolutely what our culture has taught us, so it makes sense that many of us believe it. It's so entrenched in our culture that it sounds . . . sane. Rational, even.

But it's not.

Think about it: What would *really* happen if you stopped running from yourself or beating yourself up? What would happen if you put down the whip you've been flogging yourself with for decades?

When you stop beating yourself up—when you stop *reinjuring* yourself—what happens is . . . *you start to heal*.

Self-criticism is an invasive weed in the garden, but too many of us have been taught to treat it like a treasured flower, even as it strangles the native plants of our sexuality. Far from motivating us to get better, self-criticism makes us sicker.

Later in the chapter, I'll describe three evidence-based ways for changing patterns of self-criticism, but for right now let me just point out that you can't stop criticizing yourself by beating yourself up when you criticize yourself. If you notice yourself thinking, "Ugh, I suck," and then think, "Darn it all, Emily told me to stop doing that! I *suck*!" that's not really helping, right? So when you notice yourself thinking, "Ugh, I suck," or whatever it is you say to yourself when things don't go your way, just notice that. Just notice that it's a weed. You didn't put it there—it snuck under the fence. And take that opportunity to plant a seed of something positive. For example, when you think, "Ugh, I suck," plant the thought, "I'm okay." As in, "I'm safe," "I'm whole," or "I'm home." You're okay.

And change happens—it happens all the time!

Let me tell you about my friend Ruth. We were sitting together one afternoon, talking about sex (an inevitable topic, if you talk to me long enough), and she told me, "You know, I've been through a lot of things, but my sexuality has really opened up and been so much better lately."

"Awesome!" I said. "What changed?"

"I just feel a lot more confident in myself, in my body! I know now that I'm amazing to be with and I can revel in that."

"That's *great*! How did you make it happen?"

She said, "It's like one day I just decided that it was all bullshit. Who are they to tell me I'm not amazing exactly as I am?"

Yep. That.

health at every size

Weight is just one of several things people (especially women) criticize themselves for, but it may be the most universal, with half of girls as young as three years old worrying that they might be "fat" [13]—and it's certainly among the most dangerous and needless.

People want to lose weight for two reasons: health and beauty. Whether you can measure beauty on a scale, I don't know,[14] but I do know you definitely can't measure health that way, and I'm determined to bust that myth right now, once and for all.

Here's the myth as plainly as I can state it: If I know how much you weigh, I also know something about your health.

And that's wrong. The fact is, weight alone tells us almost nothing about health. The research is painfully clear, though plenty of people have a hard time accepting it—there's been controversy about this research in the mainstream media, and even among academics, because it runs so contrary to what we've all been told, and it somehow feels dangerous to give people permission not to hate their bodies (despite the fact that the research I cited in the previous section proves that people are healthier when they don't hate themselves). But if you think about it logically for two seconds, you'll see how obviously true it is that weight is nothing more than a measure of *gravity*. Look:

- Want to lose ten pounds without diet or exercise? Cut off your leg at the knee! I guarantee, the next time you step on a scale, you'll weigh less.
- Or, hey, want to lose five pounds of fat? Have your brain removed— its mass is almost 100 percent fat!
- You know who's always thin? People who've been living in a prison camp!
- Quick and easy weight loss! Fly in a plane! Better yet, go into space! They don't call it "weightless" for nothing!

If that sounds glib, good. I think it's stupid and destructive that "experts" have been telling us that we can measure our health by measuring something we can change by removing a limb, torturing ourselves, or going on a plane and measuring it up there instead. You can achieve your medically defined "ideal weight" without improving your health at all; it might even substantially impair your health!

In case that's not compelling enough and you'd like a medical opinion, let me tell you this story. One evening during the conference where I learned about Health at Every Size (HAES), I actually went on a date with a cardiologist. I told him about the conference and asked him about this specific statistic that a speaker mentioned.

I said, "Dr. Date, is it true that it can be healthier to be seventy pounds over your medically defined 'ideal weight' than to be five pounds under it?"

And Dr. Date said, "I don't know if I'd use those precise numbers, but that's the right idea. For different reasons, being just slightly underweight carries greater risk than being obese."

The date wasn't very successful, and two years later I married a cartoonist and his two cats, but Dr. Date and I had a nice dinner and he verified that weight is not what matters, *healthy behaviors* are what matter.

My friend Kelly Coffey weighed more than three hundred pounds when she graduated from Smith College. She was completely miserable and thought her weight was to blame. So she had bariatric surgery and lost half her body weight.

And she says, "I felt happy for a few weeks, and then the depression, the self-hate, all of it came flooding back."

So when did things change for her?

"When I realized it wasn't about weight," she says. "It was about learning to respect myself and my body and treat it with love."

It's not about weight or size or fat—weight is a measure of gravity and nothing else—it's about living joyfully inside your body, as it is, today.

Which brings me to Health at Every Size. HAES is, as the name implies, an approach to living inside your body based on health rather than weight. Lindo Bacon literally wrote the book on HAES—*Health at Every Size: The Surprising Truth about Your Weight*—based on their decades of research on nutrition, exercise, and health. There are four major tenets, according to "The HAES Manifesto": (1) accept your size, (2) trust yourself, (3) adopt healthy lifestyle habits including joyful physical activity and nutritious foods, and (4) embrace size diversity.[15]

It's almost too simple: Welcome your body just as it is, listen to your own internal needs, and make healthful choices around food and physical activity. You might lose weight (you probably won't), but you'll definitely be healthier and happier.

Can it be true? Happy and healthy without losing weight?

It can.

Do you want it to be true?

That's another story.

What it comes down to is whether you're willing to try on the possibility that you *are already beautiful* and whether you're ready to prioritize real health over conforming to some cultural standard of how your body is "supposed" to look.

I know that intellectual awareness of the negative impact of self-criticism and about the lack of relationship between health and weight can't instantly undo the decades of shaming that so many women have absorbed. In my experience, women are reluctant to let go of their self-critical thoughts and the cultural thin ideal even when they believe that it's all nonsense—which it is—and they're even more hesitant to believe that they are already beautiful—which they are.

Later in the chapter I'll describe three evidence-based strategies for shifting from self-critical ways to live in your body, to compassionate and healthful ways to live in it. But in the end, it will come down to a decision to stop cultivating the weeds of self-criticism and instead nourish the flowers of confidence *today*—and then remaking that decision each day.

"dirty"

For as long as I had an office, I kept a basket of single-use bubble packs of lubricant. They were all different colors, so it looks a little like a basket of candies or lip glosses. Coming to my office for the first time, a student would poke their finger into the basket, drawn by the colors, and ask, "What's this?"

"Different kinds of lube," I say. "Feel free to take as many as you like."

About half the students say, "Cool!" and rummage around for a few they like. And the other half yank their hand away like I just told them it was bubble packs of boogers.

That's sexual disgust. It's a learned withdrawal response from things that are "gross." Everyone has something that grosses her out sexually, and everyone's "yucks" are different. And nobody ever *needs* to use packaged lube (though I recommend it; you'll see why in chapter 6)—we got along without it for a few hundred millennia—so it may not matter much if lube is on your list of yucks.

But what happens when that same sexual disgust is activated by one's own body?

"My partner wants to . . ."

I have a lot of conversations that begin this way, trailing off into embarrassed silence. In one particular case, the student continued, ". . . He wants to give me oral sex," and then she turned bright red.

"Okay," I said. And I waited.

So she said, "Well . . . I mean . . ." and she trailed off again, not making eye contact.

"Would *you* like him to give you oral sex?" I prompted.

"I . . ." she said, wincing.

"I mean . . ." she went on.

"Isn't it . . ." she finally asked, "dirty? Down there? The hair? The . . . mucus . . . ?"

I wish it were effective to respond to this question with, "Of course not, it's beautiful down there! Congratulations on having a partner who appreciates that fact!" Sometimes that is effective. But often there's a huge resistant knot of beliefs that has to be untangled before the person can get there.

Fortunately, research has provided me with a science knife designed to slice through that particular knot: Moral Foundations Theory. Jonathan Haidt and his team have found that there are six "moral foundations" in the human brain, each of which is a solution to a particular evolutionary problem our species has faced.[16] Of the six, it's the "sanctity/degradation" moral foundation I find most relevant to sex.

The sanctity foundation is about contaminant avoidance, and it's powered by *disgust*. Humans have generalized from avoidance of physical contaminants (we're innately grossed out by rotting corpses) to avoidance of *conceptual* contaminants (we can feel grossed out just by the words "rotting corpses"). You can visualize sanctity as a vertical axis, with stigmatized and taboo behaviors described as "low" and "dirty," and socially sanctioned behaviors as "high" and "pure."

We judge as wrong anything associated with lowness.

In the Judeo-Christian ethic, bodies are low and spirit is high, animal instincts are low and human reason is high, and very often women are low and men are high. Sex draws attention downward to the base, the animal, the contemptible, and it therefore triggers the disgust response.

This isn't true in all cultures or belief systems—quite the opposite.[17] And even notoriously "sex-negative" religious traditions may view sex as sacred under certain, "sanctioned" conditions. A religious fundamentalist friend in grad school surprised me after she was married with her eagerness to learn about pleasure and exploration, so that she could share it with her husband. She had to learn to think differently about her body in this new context, but once she had made the shift, her entire experience was revolutionized.

In the right context, sex and bodies are not "low" or "degrading," they can be sanctified and glorious.

But many of us were raised in cultures that say our own sexual bodies are disgusting and degrading, and so are the fluids, sounds, and smells those bodies make, as are a wide array of the things we might do with our own bodies and our partner's. "Avoid sex! Sex is gross, as well as dangerous!"

If a sexual behavior or a part of your body is considered "low," do you suppose that activates the accelerator?

Nope. Disgust hits the brakes.

Disgust is physiologically distinct from the stress response, but it's more akin to parasympathetic "freeze" than sympathetic "fight or flight." Disgust hits the brakes in the emotional One Ring—it slows your heart rate, stops your gut, and closes your throat. It doesn't matter whether it's activated by the stink of skunk or the stink of hypocrisy, the sight of blood or the sight of cruelty, the physiology is basically the same.[18]

As Merritt thought more about her brakes and her lack of trust in her own body, she came to this conclusion: "I want to learn to trust my body."

This became clear as she and Carol sat together, talking about what and how to teach their teenage daughter about sex. They made a list of all the things they wanted her to believe and experience, including

- *Recognize her own beauty of body and spirit*
- *Feel fully in control of who touches her body, and how, and when*
- *Know how to protect herself against consequences like infections and pregnancy*

When Carol (she of the feminist consciousness-raising group in the '80s) asked, "How about pleasure? I'd love her to know how to give herself pleasure and to enjoy her body," that was a tough one for Merritt. It's not that she didn't want that, it's just she . . . couldn't . . . quite . . .

Rare is the American parent who feels comfortable talking to their kid about sexual pleasure—rare but not nonexistent. My favorite story of a sex-positive parent came from a guy who told me that the first time he ejaculated (by rubbing his pelvis against his mattress), he ran to his mom, terrified that he had broken something. "Mom! Mom! All this white stuff came out of my penis while I was rubbing it!" And the mom was amazing. She calmly explained what had happened, that it was normal, and how to deal with it in the future.

When I told that story to Merritt and Carol, Carol laughed and said, "I love that mom!" but Merritt turned pale.

"If I had been that boy," she said, "I'd have burned my sheets before I would have told my mother."

Merritt, remember, didn't grow up in a sex-positive environment. But in America, each generation is rapidly overturning old ideas about social control and sex. She is the first in her family to go to college, and only the second generation to make a living doing something other than farming. And along with the social and economic revolution she represents, she's also the first out lesbian—and she's the first in her family to argue with her spouse about how to teach their kid about sexual pleasure.

"My parents taught me a lot of valuable things about commitment and loyalty and being a kind and loving person," she said. "But they also told me that if I had sex outside marriage I'd go to hell, and even

now, after almost twenty years of Carol coming home with me for Christ-mas, they still can't look her in the eye."

"It sounds like they didn't mean to teach you shame, but that's what you learned," I said.

"And when you came out," Carol said, "you were attacked."

"So no wonder you don't feel like you can fully trust your own body," I said.

Merritt closed her eyes and shook her head. "I'd never want Julia to feel like there was anything wrong with any part of her body. I am not being a role model for her."

And so, of course, she proceeded to change her entire relationship with her body and to trust herself—to relax into pleasure and swim in the water of life. I'll describe how in chapter 8.

when somebody "yucks" your "yum"

Disgust can function as a social emotion—that is, we learn about what aspects of the world (including our own bodies) are disgusting by reading the responses of the people around us. For example, infants will avoid a toy that their adult caregiver looks at with an expression of disgust.[19]

Predictably, the experience of disgust is context sensitive—we're less grossed out by sex-related things while we are sexually aroused.[20] And women tend to be more sensitive than men to learned disgust, particularly in the sexual domain,[21] though it's not yet clear why.[22]

We can see how the process of learning disgust can unfold, moment by moment, in a person's life if we imagine, for argument's sake, a pair of identical twin girls separated at birth. Let's call them Jessica and Theresa.

Imagine that both Jessica and Theresa, when they're maybe five or six years old, have a habit of masturbating in their rooms at naptime. (If you noticed a disgust-withdrawal response in yourself at the idea of a young girl masturbating, you've just experienced what I'm about to describe!)

So one day, Jessica is masturbating in her room at naptime, when her adult caregiver walks in and sees her with her hand down her pants. The parent recoils in an involuntary disgust response, and says, "Stop that!"

On that same day, in a different home, Theresa is also masturbating, and her adult caregiver also walks in and sees her with her hand down her pants. But that parent says calmly, "We're leaving for your aunt's house in a few minutes. Get your shoes on."

Jessica's brain learns to associate the shame and distress (brakes) communicated by her parent with whatever sexual arousal (accelerator) she was feeling at the moment her parent scolded her.

Theresa's brain, by contrast, learns no such association.

This one incident may not have any lasting impact. If there are no other incidents to reinforce this one, the association in Jessica's brain will be decoupled.

But imagine twenty years have passed, and Jessica and Theresa's life experiences have routinely reinforced these patterns. Jessica's brain has learned to associate sexual arousal with stress, shame, disgust, and guilt. Theresa's has learned to associate sexual arousal with pleasure, confidence, joy, and satisfaction.

Which of them has a better sex life?

Jessica will feel conflicted about her sexual sensations—they're pleasurable . . . and they're not, at the same time. And she won't have a clear idea why she feels guilty, ashamed, depressed, or even physical pain when she's sexually aroused.

If a girl has a particularly sensitive brakes system, one incident might be enough to create a tangled knot in her arousal process. For many women, though, it takes consistent reinforcement of a negative message in order for it to be embedded in sexual response, and consistent reinforcement takes a sex-negative culture.

In other words, it happens all the time.

Often disgust is reinforced in subtle ways, but sometimes we can remember a specific moment when the message is made clear. I talked to a grandmother—a badass Southern grandma sex educator, to be specific—who told me about just such a moment from when she was a teenager. She had been sitting on the front porch making out with her boyfriend, but when she went inside, her mother came up to her with disgust in every line of her face and said, "What you were just doing out there? That's *sex!*"

And this sixty-something grandmother told me, "It took me a long, long time to realize why I got so anxious about sex with my husband— and I mean *nauseated* anxious—and when I finally figured it out, I was angry for about ten seconds, and then I was just so sad for my mother."

She went on, "Now when I do health education at my church, I just say it right out loud: 'I like sex!' I want everyone to know that it's okay!"

I love this woman.

For sex educators, the rule is, "Don't yuck anybody's yum." And since we can't know what everybody else's yums are, we don't yuck anything. We know that disgust is a social emotion and that our students have already been exposed to too many people who communicate disgust around sex.

That's why sex educators and sex therapists go through an educational process of intensive exposure, deliberately designed to minimize our own judgment, shame, and disgust reactions, so that we can respond with open neutrality to whatever students or clients bring into the room. This training often takes the form of a Sexual Attitude Reassessment, a multiday training that includes values clarification exercises, guest panels and speakers, plus (in my experience) a range of porn that would surprise most people in its variety, intensity, and creativity, followed by reflection and processing of our reactions to all of it.

Unless you become a sex educator, you never need to go through a process like this. All you ever need to do is begin to recognize where your learned disgust response is interfering with your own sexual pleasure, and decide whether it's something you'd rather let go of. Your genitals and your partners', your genital fluids and your partners', your skin and sweat and the fragrances of your body, these are all healthy and beautiful—not to mention *normal*—elements of human sexual experience. You get to choose whether you feel grossed out by them.

The research tells us that disgust, as a learned response to sex, impairs women's sexual functioning and is especially associated with sexual pain disorders.[23]

In the next section, I'll describe three strategies for making your own choices about what is or isn't disgusting—they're the same strategies you use to make your own choices about self-criticism. But the first step is to begin to notice when you experience an involuntary withdrawal from sex-related things, and then try on the possibility that the sight, the smells, the sounds, the stickiness of your own sexual organism are glorious and beautiful parts of being human.

Because what if all of that actually *is* beautiful and glorious? What if your body is cause for celebration?

(P.S. It totally is.)

Sex-negative culture has trained us to be self-critical and judgmental about our bodies and our sexualities, and it's interfering with our sexual wellbeing. So let's get practical. How do we create a bubble of sex positivity for ourselves, where we can explore and celebrate and maximize our own sexual potential? How do we maximize the yum, in a world that tries to convince us we're yucky? Here are three evidence-based strategies that can genuinely create positive change.

maximizing yum . . . with science!
part 1: self-compassion

Sometimes we cling to our self-criticism. We think to ourselves: "If I stop beating myself up, I'll get complacent and lazy, and then I'll never change!"

And then we cling to our self-judgments even more tightly—after all, these are *moral* issues, involving whether you are a good, decent, worthy person or a bad, disgusting, worthless person. We think: "To accept myself as I am would be to accept that I am a flawed, bad, broken person, and to abandon all hope that I could one day be good enough to deserve love."

Remember that beating yourself up is the emotional One Ring equivalent of treating yourself as your own internal lion, experiencing yourself as a threat that needs to be escaped (which is impossible), conquered (which is literally self-destructive), or avoided through shutdown (which is counterproductive, to say the least).

And that's why we need self-compassion.

Self-compassion is the opposite of self-criticism and self-judgment. In her book *Self-Compassion: Stop Beating Yourself Up and Leave Insecurity Behind*, researcher and educator Kristin Neff describes self-compassion's three key elements:

- *Self-kindness* is our ability to treat ourselves gently and with caring. On the Self Compassion Scale (SCS), a survey used to assess self-compassion, self-kindness is described with items like "When I'm going through a very hard time, I give myself the caring and tenderness I need." In contrast, its opposite, *self-judgment*, is assessed with "I'm intolerant and impatient towards those aspects of my personality I don't like."

- *Common humanity* is viewing our suffering as something that connects us with others, rather than separates us. It's assessed on the SCS with items like "When I feel inadequate in some way, I try to remind myself that feelings of inadequacy are shared by most people." Its opposite, *isolation*, is assessed with "When I fail at something that's important to me, I tend to feel alone in my failure."

- *Mindfulness* is being nonjudgmental about whatever is happening in the present moment. I talked about mindfulness in chapter 4, and I'll be talking about it again in chapter 9. Mindfulness is important. On the SCS it's assessed with items like "When something painful happens I try to take a balanced view of the situation." Its opposite is *over-identification*, as in over-identifying with your own failures and suffering, holding fast to the pain and being unable to let it go. It's assessed with items like "When I'm feeling down I tend to obsess and fixate on everything that's wrong."

Self-judgment, isolation, and over-identification turn you into your own lion, being your own threat—"I am at risk." And they're normal—we all experience them. Self-compassion doesn't mean never feeling them, it means being kind to yourself when you do.

I like to visualize the lion of body self-criticism as a sweet little kitten that's been treated badly and needs me to give it affection and tenderness. That's what helps me to forgive my culture for teaching me such bullshit. A woman I know prefers to imagine it as an enemy, and she visualizes herself beating the crap out of it. She finds her way to forgiveness of her culture (and of herself, for having believed her culture) through a sense of conquering the enemy. Whatever works!

Both of us complete the stress response cycle with physical activity, affection, a good cry, self-care, or any other strategy that deals with the stress itself, as I described in chapter 4. We let our bodies know we have successfully escaped the lion—"I am safe. I am whole. I am home."

Self-compassion is emphatically *not* self-esteem. Self-esteem is about self-evaluation, your perceived value as a human being, which is often contingent upon your sense of personal success in comparison with others. Self-compassion, by contrast, is unconditional and non-evaluative. We can have self-compassion when we're doing well and when we're struggling—because life has treated us harshly or because we made a mistake.[24]

Nor is self-compassion the same as self-indulgence. Self-indulgence is what you do to numb emotional pain rather than allowing it to complete the cycle. Olivia's moments of compulsive sexuality are an extreme example, but for most of us self-indulgence takes the form of binge-watching Netflix or eating a pint of Ben & Jerry's in one sitting because: Feels, instead of feeling our Feels. Self-indulgence is a form of freeze, sedating the lion instead of escaping or conquering it.

Emotional pain is exhausting, and sometimes it's necessary to take a break, numb out for a while. Just remember what happens when the sedated lion comes out from under the anesthesia. The cycle has to complete, it *wants* to complete. Self-compassion is being patient with yourself through that process—and being patient with yourself when you need to take a break.

Here's an exercise to help increase self-compassion:[25]

1. Write a description of a situation that you're beating yourself up about—it can be anything from an aspect of your sexual functioning to your romantic relationship (or lack thereof) to your work to your body or anything else. Be sure to include the self-critical thoughts you're battering yourself with.
2. Then write the name of a good friend at the top of the page and imagine that that person is describing this problem. Imagine that she's asking for your help, and write down what you would tell her. Imagine that you're in your best, most empathic, calmest, most supportive state of mind, and tell her all the things she needs to hear.
3. Now reread what you wrote. It's for you.

The shorthand version of this exercise is: Never say anything to yourself that you wouldn't want to say to your best friend or your daughter.

Olivia told me this story about how she figured out how to stop hitting the accelerator when she got stressed out.

One night during finals week, Olivia tried initiating sex at bedtime. Patrick, predictably, was too tired, and said so.

In the wake of his gentle refusal, self-doubt flooded through Olivia like a fast-rising river. What if her high sex drive wasn't cool or sexy or fun or empowered? What if she was just trying desperately— pathetically—to get attention the only way she could? What if actually she was just trying to control people with her sexuality? What if— Her heart was racing and she felt like she couldn't breathe.

Into the darkness, she reached out to her partner. "Patrick?"

"Yeah."

"I'm having a meltdown."

"It's finals week. It happens. Deep breaths."

"No, I'm having a meltdown about sex."

"Babe, I'm so tired . . ."

"No, I know, I'm not saying that!" She explained in a breathless panic about the flood of self-doubt, adding her sudden recollection that her theory about testosterone and her genitals and her sexuality was wrong. "What if all *the things I've told myself about my sexuality are just an invention to mask the truth that actually I'm totally just this bully using my sexuality to manipulate you? What if I'm out of control and, like, a danger to myself and others?"*

Patrick turned on the light and looked at her. "Wow, I had no idea you had so much of this cultural brainwashing still buried in your brain. It's like the anxious part of your brain seriously believes all the women-who-like-sex-are-evil stuff, and when you're stressed out, all those beliefs come with the stress—even though the calm version of your brain totally knows how awesome you are. Keep breathing, babe, you're holding your breath."

And there it was.

When she was happy and relaxed, she had one set of opinions about herself: self-confident and self-compassionate. When she was overwhelmed, she had an entirely different set of opinions about herself: self-critical and even self-abusive.

And the negative opinions she had when she was stressed just added another level of stress and escalated the situation, which made her feel all the more self-critical, which eventually activated her least adaptive coping strategies. It was like trying to douse a fire by pouring gasoline on it.

Solution?

Stop adding fuel to the fire. Notice that you're doing it, and do something else. Let the fire burn itself out.

She had already figured out that exercise helped her complete the cycle, coasting to the end of the biological stress cycle without hitting either the brakes or the accelerator. In the next chapter, she's going to learn how to do the same thing with sex.

maximizing yum . . . with science!
part 2: cognitive dissonance

In chapter 1, I recommended that you take a good look at your genitals and notice the things you like. Now I'm suggesting that you take off all your clothes—or as many as you can bring yourself to take off—and look at your entire body in a mirror. And make a list of everything you see . . . that you like.[26]

Of course the first thing that will happen is your brain will be filled with all the self-criticism and disgust you've been holding on to for all these years. Remind yourself that the day you were born, your body was a cause for celebration, for love without condition, and that's just as true today as it was then. Let those self-critical thoughts go, let the judgments go, and notice only the things you like.

Do this over and over again—every day if you can. It will be hard at first, and there will be lots of complicated and conflicting emotions. It will be noisy in your head. Even now, as you consider doing it, you might be noticing a lot of "But Emily!" noise in your head. It's okay. It will hurt the way your hands ache when you come in from the cold—gradually they get warmer and then they feel great. Psychologist and author Christopher Germer calls this "backdraft," referencing the explosion that occurs when you add fresh air to an oxygen-deprived fire.[27] You have to allow the hurt to go through the process, let it complete its cycle.

Practice ignoring the self-critical, judgmental thoughts and focusing on the self-appreciating thoughts. And gradually it will become easier to celebrate your body as it deserves to be celebrated, to treat it with the respect and affection it deserves, and to approach sex with confidence and joy. Which is the point!

maximizing yum . . . with science!
part 3: media nutrition

Exposure to media that reinforces body self-criticism increases body dissatisfaction, negative mood, low self-esteem, and even disordered eating.[28] This is perhaps most clearly illustrated by a multiyear study of the impact of Western media—especially television—on young women in Fiji.[29] In a culture where there had been "a clear preference for a robust form,"[30] after three years of exposure to late 1990s American television (think *Melrose Place* and *Beverly Hills, 90210*), rates of disordered eating among teenage girls rose from 13 percent to 29 percent, with 74 percent reporting that they "feel too big or too fat," in sharp contrast to pre-TV culture. And this wasn't just a blip—ten years later, rates of disordered eating still hovered around 25–30 percent.[31]

If there were a food that consistently made you sick, you'd stop eating it. So if there's media that makes you feel more self-critical, stop looking at it.

As you're looking at movies or television or porn or magazines or social media, ask yourself, "After I see this, am I going to feel better about my body *as it is today*, or worse?" If the answer is "Better!" then do more of that! Increase your exposure to the media that helps you celebrate your body!

But if the answer is "worse," stop it. You don't have to get mad and write a letter to the editor or anything (though if you want to, feel free!), just pay attention to how magazines and TV shows and music videos make you feel, and stop buying anything that makes you feel worse. You don't need to be trained in media literacy and all the ways that you're being manipulated with digital alteration of images in order to know when something is making you feel better or worse about yourself.

And if it makes you feel worse, evidence suggests that it's interfering with your sexual wellbeing—even if you've been taught to believe that feeling worse about your body "motivates" you to "improve" your body. That's a psychological trap you never need to be caught in again. Stop watering the weeds.

By limiting your exposure to media that makes you feel worse about yourself, you're not just improving your own sex life, you're also voting with your eyeballs, your ears, and your cash. You're joining an audience that will pay attention only to things that make women feel better about themselves. Wouldn't it be amazing to live in a world where performers and artists and media outlets were competing to make the largest number of women feel fantastic about their bodies *right now*? On behalf of women everywhere, thank you for anything you do to make that real!

you do you

We started this chapter with three cultural messages that all of us have been exposed to in one way or another over the course of our lives: the Moral Message, the Medical Message, and the Media Message. All three messages are blended into our individual psyches; none of us lives with just one, and none of us wholly believes any of them. They've been layered over each other in our culture, each partially absorbing the others. The contradictions inherent in the three are a source of women's confusion about how sex is supposed to work.[32] Your faith community tells you one thing, the media culture tells you another, and your doctor seems to have a different attitude entirely.

So whom should you believe? What messages can you trust to promote your own sexual wellbeing?

The answer is: yourself.

Listen to your own inner voice, which hears all these messages and, somewhere deep inside you, will sound an alarm when it notices bullshit. We're all different, so what feels true and what feels like nonsense will vary from person to person. The only possible answer is: Choose what feels right for you and ignore what doesn't feel right.

Informational cherry-picking like this is a bad idea in science and in moralism. Scientific and moral systems, though different from each other in almost every other way, share the quality of developing coherent structures of meaning where one idea hangs upon the others, the way loops of metal hold chain mail armor together. When you're working in a scientific or a moral framework, an idea must take its place in the context in which it was intended.

But most of us are just trying to live our lives as best we can. When it comes to investigating and understanding your own individual sexuality, please do cherry-pick. The moral views may be sincere, the media exciting, the doctors apparently expert, but you need not buy into any system in order to create a coherent narrative of your own sexual self. You don't need to believe you'll go to hell if you have sex before marriage in order to decide whether waiting to have sex is a good choice for you. You don't need to believe you're sick or broken in order to wish you could just take a pill and want sex out of the blue. And you don't need to believe that the key to great sex is flavored lube, a giant vibrator, and the ability to deep-throat in order to want to explore, try new toys, new tricks, and new partners.

And even though I'd love you to find meaning in every page, every paragraph of this book, cherry-pick from here, too. We're all different, so what's relevant for you is definitely, absolutely not the same as what's relevant for me or for any of the many hundreds of women I've taught. Take what's relevant. Ignore what isn't; it's there for somebody else who needs it.

Treat cultural messages about sex and your body like a salad bar. Take only the things that appeal to you and ignore the rest. We'll all end up with a different collection of stuff on our plates, but that's how it's supposed to work.

It goes wrong only when you try to apply what you picked as right for your sexuality to someone else's sexuality.

"She shouldn't eat those beets; beets are disgusting."

They might be disgusting to you, but maybe she likes beets. Some people do. And you never know, maybe one day you'll try them and find you like them. Or not, that's cool, too. You do you.

"She shouldn't have taken so many fried, breaded things—she'll end up with a heart attack!"

She might and she might not, but either way it's her heart and her choice. You do you. Absorb what feels right for you and shake off what feels wrong. Let everybody else do everybody else, absorbing what feels right for them and shaking off what feels wrong.

Laurie and Johnny's story about "You're beautiful," sounds like a story about body image or disgust, but really it's about love. Laurie's body shame wasn't just about the changes to her body. She had absorbed cultural beliefs about what those changes meant about her as a person. And because she believed her body was evidence that she was somehow a lesser person, she hid behind an emotional wall, so that no one could see those parts of her she felt ashamed of. But that wall also stood between her and the love she was starving for.

We build walls for a lot of reasons. To protect vulnerable parts of ourselves. To hide things we don't want others to see. To keep people out. To keep ourselves in.

But a wall is a wall is a wall—it's an indiscriminate barrier. If you hide behind a wall to protect yourself from the pain of rejection, then you also block out joy. If you never let others see the parts you want to hide, then they'll never see the parts you want them to know.

When Laurie let the wall down, the love came flooding in.

No girl is born hating her body or feeling ashamed of her sexuality. You had to learn that. No girl is born worried that she'll be judged if someone finds out what kind of sex she enjoys. You had to learn that, too. You have to learn, as well, that it is safe to be loved, safe to be your authentic self, safe to be sexual with another person, or even safe to be on your own.

Some women learn these things in their families of origin. But even if you learned destructive things, you can learn different things now. No matter what was planted in your garden, no matter how you've been tending it, you are the gardener. You didn't get to choose your little plot of land—your accelerator and your brakes and your body—and you didn't get to choose your family or your culture, but you do choose every single other thing. You get to decide what plants stay and what plants go, which plants get attention and love and which are ignored, pruned away to nothing, or dug out and thrown on the compost heap to rot. You get to choose.

In this second part of the book, I've described how context—your external circumstances and your internal state—influence your sexual wellbeing. I've talked about stress and love and body image and sexual disgust, and I've described some evidence-based strategies for managing all of these in ways that can maximize your sexual potential.

The next part of the book focuses on debunking some old and destructive myths about how sex works. These myths are part of the context in which women's sexual wellbeing functions. In busting them, my goal is to empower you to take total control over your context and embrace your sexuality as it is, perfect and whole, right now. Even if you don't quite believe that's true yet.

tl;dr

- We all grew up hearing contradictory messages about sex, and so now many of us experience ambivalence about it. That's normal. The more aware you are of those contradictory messages, the more choice you have about whether to believe them.
- Sometimes people resist letting go of self-criticism—

"I suck!"—because it can feel like giving up hope that you could become a better person, but that's the opposite of how it works. How it really works is that when you stop beating yourself up, you begin to heal, and then you grow like never before.

- For real: Your health is not predicted by your weight. You can be healthy—and *beautiful*—no matter your size. And when you enjoy living in your body today, and treat yourself with kindness and compassion, your sex life gets better.

- Sexual disgust hits the brakes. And sexual disgust is learned, not innate, and can be unlearned. Begin to notice your "yuck" responses and ask yourself if those responses are making your sex life better or worse. Consider letting go of the yucks that are interfering with your sexual pleasure—see chapter 9 to learn how.

part 3

sex in action

six

arousal

LUBRICATION IS NOT CAUSATION

When you're a sex educator, you get phone calls like this one:

"Hey, it's Camilla. Can I ask you a sex question?"

"Sure."

"You won't be grossed out?"

"Of course not."

"Okay, so Henry and I were messing around and I said, 'I'm ready, I want you,' and he said, 'No, you're not wet, you're just humoring me.' And I said, 'No, I'm totally ready!' And he didn't believe me because I wasn't wet. So . . . should I see a doctor? Is it hormonal? What's wrong?"

"If you're having pain you should see a doctor, but otherwise you're probably fine. Sometimes bodies don't respond with genital arousal in a way that matches mental experience. Tell him to pay attention to your words, not your fluids, and also buy some lube."

"That's it? Genital response doesn't always match experience, so buy some lube?"

"Yep. It's called nonconcordance."

"But that's not what . . . I mean, is this some new scientific discovery?"

"Sorta? The earliest psychophysiological research I've read that explicitly measures sexual arousal nonconcordance is from the late seventies, early eighties, though that—"

"The eighties? Why did no one tell me this before?"

This chapter answers that question, and a whole lot more.

The idea that genital response doesn't necessarily match a person's experience of arousal runs contrary to the "standard narrative" about sex. As far as most porn, romance novels, and even sex education texts are concerned, genital response and sexual arousal are one and the same.

For a long time, I thought the standard narrative was right—of course I did, I believed what I was taught. We all do. So I had no idea what to think when, in college back in the '90s, a friend told me about her first experiences with power play in a sexual relationship:

I let him tie my wrists above my head while I was standing up, and he positioned me so that I was straddling this bar that pressed against my vulva, you know, like a broomstick. And then he went away! He just left, and it was totally boring, and when he came back I was like, "I'm not into this." He looked at the bar and he looked at me and he said, "Then why are you wet?" And I was so confused because I definitely wasn't into it, but my body was definitely responding.

Like everyone who has ever read a sexy romance novel, I was sure that wet equaled aroused. Desirous. Wanting it. "Ready" for sex. So what could it mean that my friend's genitals were responding, when she really didn't feel turned on or desirous at all?

What was going on?

Nonconcordance is what was going on.

In this chapter, I'll describe the research on nonconcordance, including answering questions like, Who experiences nonconcordance? (Everyone, actually.) How do you know your partner is turned on, if you can't use their genitals as a gauge? (Pay better attention!) And how can you help your partner understand your nonconcordance? I'll also address three wrong but beguiling myths about nonconcordance. These myths aren't just wrong, they're *dangerously* wrong.

I want everyone who reads this chapter to go on a spree of telling the whole world about nonconcordance—that it's normal, that everyone experiences it, and that you must listen to your partner's *words*, not their genitals.

measuring and defining nonconcordance

Put on your sex researcher hat again and imagine conducting an experiment like this:[1]

A guy comes to the lab. You lead him into a quiet room, sit him down in a comfortable chair, and leave him alone in front of a television. He straps a "strain gauge" (which is exactly what it sounds like) to his penis, puts a tray over his lap, and takes hold of a dial that he can tune up and down to register his arousal ("I feel a little aroused," "I feel a lot aroused," etc.). Then he starts watching a variety of porn segments. Some of it is romantic, some is violent, some matches his sexual orientation, some doesn't. Some of it isn't even humans, it's bonobos copulating. He rates his level of arousal on the dial as he watches, and the device on his penis measures his erection. Then you look at the data to see how much of a match there is between how aroused he felt—his "subjective arousal"—and how erect he got—his "genital response."

Result: There will be about a 50 percent overlap between his genital response and his subjective arousal. It's far from a perfect one-to-one correlation, but in behavioral science it's exciting to find a relationship that strong. It's highly statistically significant.

For the most part, both our research subject and his penis will respond most to the porn that matches his sexual orientation: a gay man's genitals respond most to porn featuring two men, and he'll report the highest levels of arousal in response to it; a straight man's genitals respond most to porn featuring a man and a woman or else two women, and he'll report the highest level of arousal in response to it, etc.

Now let's run the same experiment with a woman. Put her in that quiet room, in that comfortable chair, and let her insert a vaginal photoplethysmograph (essentially a tiny flashlight about the size of a tampon that measures genital blood flow), and give her the tray and the dial and the variety of porn.

Result: There will be about a 10 percent overlap between what her genitals are doing and what she dials in as her arousal.

10 percent.

It turns out that there is no predictive relationship between how aroused she feels and how much her genitals respond—statistically insignificant. Her genital response will be about the same no matter what kind of porn she's shown, and her genital response might match her sexual preferences . . . or it might not.[2]

It's called "arousal nonconcordance."[3]

This research has been in the media a lot. For example, Meredith Chivers's nonconcordance research was described in the *New York Times* and in a number of popular books.[4] Chivers's work builds on the research of, among others, Ellen Laan, whose nonconcordance studies were also covered in the *New York Times* a decade earlier.[5] Chivers replicated Laan's finding of greater arousal nonconcordance in women compared to men, with the innovation of showing research participants not only a variety of porn and nonsexual videos but also videos of nonhuman primates—bonobos, to be specific—copulating. It turns out women's genitals respond to bonobo sex, too, though not as much as to porn.

What the media coverage has failed to make clear is that women's genital response is actually very discriminating, compared to other automatic physiological responses. For example, your Achilles tendon reflex, heart rate, and skin conductance (sweating) will all increase after watching a scary segment of the movie *Cujo* and after watching porn. But your genitals have no interest in *Cujo*.[6] In fact, women's genitals don't respond to any of these videos: waves crashing on a beach, the "Ain't No Mountain High

men's arousal concordance

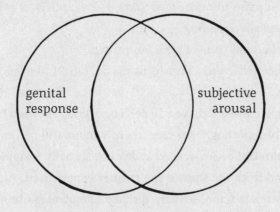

genital response

subjective arousal

women's arousal concordance

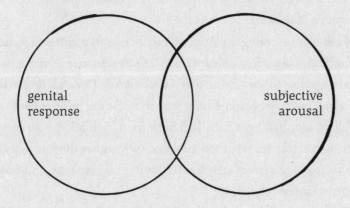

genital response

subjective arousal

There is about a 50 percent overlap between what men's genitals respond to as "sex-related" and what their brains respond to as "sexually appealing." And there is about a 10 percent overlap between what women's genitals respond to as "sex-related" and what their brains respond to as "sexually appealing." Men's genitals are relatively specific in what they respond to, and so are their brains. Women's genitals are relatively general in what they respond to, while their brains are more sensitive to context. Note that a stimulus can be "sex-related" without being appealing.

Enough" scene from the movie *Stepmom*, the telegram delivery scene in *A League of Their Own*, or a first-person view of a roller coaster.[7] Genital response is specific to sex-related stimuli—regardless of whether those stimuli are sexually *appealing*.

The *genitals* tell you, "That's sex-related."

The *person* tells you, "That turns me on," or "I like this," or "I want more, please."

For women, there's about a 10 percent overlap between "sex-related" and "sexually appealing." For men, there's about a 50 percent overlap.

A stimulus can be sex-related and yet be sexually unappealing, as my college friend from the start of the chapter experienced. A stimulus can even be sex-related and actively disliked. Remember the person from chapter 2, who emailed me that "brakes and accelerator at the same time" described her experience reading *Fifty Shades of Grey*? Her genitals responded, but she didn't feel "turned on"; the book included explicit sex, so it was sex-related, but it also hit her brakes because she disliked the characters and the story.

What we're seeing in nonconcordance is the difference between *learning* and *liking*, from chapter 3. Genital response is the automatic, trained response to something that's sex-related. Pavlov's dogs salivated when a bell rang, not because they wanted to eat the bell but because their *learning* system had linked the bell with food. Similarly, your emotional One Ring has learned what's sex-related (remember the rats in jackets?), and your *learning* system activates physiological responses to whatever it has learned is sex-related.

Women vary from each other, but different women seem fairly consistent in their level of concordance.[8] Precisely how a woman's genitals respond to sex-related stimuli seems to vary depending on the sensitivity of her brakes and accelerator. Low-sensitivity brakes and high-sensitivity accelerator leads to more blood flow, and high-sensitivity brakes and high sensitivity accelerator actually leads to less blood flow, compared with other women.[9] And women who are attracted to women tend to be more concordant than straight women . . . mostly. But it's complicated.[10] Yet again, we're all made of the same parts, organized in different ways.

What happens when a man takes erectile dysfunction medication?

It increases blood flow to the genitals during sexual stimulation.

What happens when a woman takes erectile dysfunction medication?

Same thing.

And what happens when you increase blood flow to a woman's genitals?

Not a lot. Because: nonconcordance.

Olivia and Patrick tried it. They took an ED pill together as an experiment in flipping the chasing dynamic—and also because why not? (NB: "Why not?" includes no known medical benefit and unknown medical risk. Taking a prescription medication without a doctor's supervision is always risky. But let's be real here. People do it. But don't. It doesn't do what you want it to do, as we'll see.)

Olivia's lips—the lips on her face, that is—turned dark, dark red, so that she looked like she was wearing lipstick. Other than that, she didn't notice any particular effect. For once, Olivia's experience was typical of most women's.

Patrick, on the other hand, felt like he'd taken an aphrodisiac. Olivia looked irresistibly beautiful, and his skin felt like the volume had been turned up on his nerve endings, so that every sensation was amplified, magnified. They went out for ice cream after they took the drug, for something to do while they waited for it to kick in, and they had to turn right back around because Patrick couldn't wait to get Olivia naked.

Erectile dysfunction drugs don't do any of this; all they do is increase blood flow to the genitals. Such is the power of placebo. The same thing happened occasionally when Patrick would drink at weddings and Olivia was the designated driver.

This rare experience of being the one with the lower sexual interest was revelatory for Olivia. As a woman who always felt driven forward by her sexual interest, pulling her partner along with her, being the one who was standing still and being pulled, as it were, was an inspiring experience. She allowed herself to receive Patrick's erotic attention. She allowed her arousal to build as slowly as it wanted to.

She allowed it to happen, instead of feeling like it was dragging her forward.

all the same parts, organized in different ways: "this is a restaurant"

Nonconcordance is about the relationship between the peripheral system—the genitals—and the central system—the brain: two separate but interconnected systems. And the relationship between these systems varies from person to person and from context to context.

To illustrate, imagine that a brain and a vagina are a couple of friends on vacation together, wandering down the street trying to decide where to have dinner.

The genitals notice any restaurant they pass, whether it's Thai food or pub grub, fast food or gourmet (while ignoring all the museums and shops), and say, "This is a restaurant. We could eat here." She has no strong opinion, she's just good at spotting restaurants. Meanwhile, the brain is assessing all the contextual factors I described in chapters 4 and 5 to decide whether she wants to try a place. "This place isn't delicious-smelling enough," or "This place isn't clean enough," or "I'm not in the mood for pizza." The genitals might even notice a pet store and say, "There's pet food in here, I guess . . ." and the brain rolls her eyes and keeps walking.

They pass a museum, and the brain says, "I heard about a great café in this museum," and the genitals respond, "This isn't a restaurant." But the brain has way more information than the genitals. So suppose the two friends go into the museum, and the genitals see the little café next to the gift shop. Then she says, "Oh, I see, this is a restaurant. We could eat here," and the brain says, "Yeah, this looks great." Both relevant *and* appealing!

But it's not always like that. In lesbian women, it's more like this:[11] The genitals notice only specific restaurants—diners, say—and don't notice any restaurants that aren't diners. Once they find a diner, the brain says, "A diner! I love diners," and the genitals agree, "This is a restaurant, we could eat here," unless there's some pretty compelling reason not to, like a bunch of drunks brawling outside. Even then, if our friends on vacation came across that diner with a brawl outside, the genitals might still say, "This is a restaurant," even as the brain dragged her away, shouting, "Let's get out of here! Call the cops!"

You should be able to chant this in your sleep by now: We're all made of the same parts, just organized in different ways. The relationship between the brain and genitals follows the same principle.

In other words, genitals may learn to associate certain stimuli with certain physiological responses that may have no association with desire or even pleasure. The pressure on my college friend's vulva—the bar between her legs while she was tied up—triggered an automatic genital response without triggering pleasure or desire. "This is a restaurant," said her genitals, but her brain wasn't interested.

nonconcordance in other emotions

Nonconcordance is not just a sex thing. It shows up in all kinds of emotional experiences and is a puzzle to all kinds of emotion researchers.[12]

For example, in a study of the "chills" we feel when we hear moving music, research subjects were played "My Heart Will Go On." Half of them reported experiencing chills—subjective experience—and 14 percent exhibited piloerection (their hair stood on end)—physiological response. Among those who listened to "Bittersweet Symphony," by The Verve, 60 percent experienced chills—subjective experience—and none exhibited piloerection—physiological response.[13]

From a scientific point of view, it's a gross oversimplification to say that emotions break down into "three levels," but from a regular-person point of view, it's a helpful shortcut.

First, there's the involuntary physiological response—your heart rate and blood pressure, pupil dilation, digestion, sweating, immune functioning. Genital response falls into this category, and my college friend who got wet while she was bored, tied up waiting for her partner to come back, experienced this kind of response . . . but nothing else.

Along with the physiology comes the involuntary expressive response to a feeling. Body language—or, more accurately, "paralanguage"—things like vocal inflection, posture, and facial expression—all the cues we use to infer another person's internal state. A great dinner date will be full of physiological changes and unconscious postures, gestures, and expressions, as you find yourself putting your hand on your date's arm, gazing into their eyes, and smiling. These are often influenced by culture, but have a great deal of universality, and they can be intentionally controlled to some degree, but not as much as you might think. Did you choose the expression on your face right now?

And then there's your subjective experience of a feeling. If someone asks you how you feel and you check in with yourself to find the answer, what you're noticing is subjective experience. This is subjective arousal—the conscious experience of "I want you so much I can hardly stand it"—which may or may not be accompanied by genital response or eye contact.

It might even be true that there are stable gender differences in nonconcordance between physiological response and subjective experience for emotions other than sexual arousal. For whatever reason—cultural, biological, or both (probably both)—women have more overlap between their facial expressions and their subjective experience, while men have more overlap between their skin conductance (physiology) and their subjective experience.[14] What this research suggests is that women's emotional experiences are more likely to line up with their facial expressions and vocal inflection, while men's emotional experiences are more likely to line up with their heart rates and blood flow.

Whether or not there's a gender difference, it's fair to say that what you experience as your emotional life doesn't necessarily line up neatly with what your brain and body are doing. That doesn't make you a liar, it doesn't make you crazy, and it doesn't mean you're in denial. It means you're a human being, whose emotional and motivational responses may be more complex than any other species'. Nonconcordance shows up in many kinds of emotional experiences, and men and women experience nonconcordance differently in those emotions. It's not a sex thing; it's a human thing.

> *You have to relax before you can trust. But women who are slow to trust, like Merritt, can't relax until they feel trust. It's a problem.*
>
> *The solution came when she was trying to solve a different problem.*
>
> *As a woman in her forties, entering menopause, lack of lubrication just seemed like a part of life for Merritt. Her concern was more for her partner. Carol was the birth mom of their teenage daughter, and she had struggled with intermittent genital pain ever since the birth. I recommended lube to make manual sex more comfortable.*
>
> *Merritt was into it. All I had to say was, "There are a bunch of different kinds of lube, so you might—" and she was online, browsing for a variety pack.*
>
> *The box arrived in the mail. They set a date—Friday night, with the teenager away on a camping trip—and when the night arrived, they split a half bottle of wine and got started.*
>
> *They took the importance of context seriously and started with a romantic movie and then took turns retelling each other their "Story of Us."[15] This is a trick they adapted from John Gottman's relationship research—they narrate to each other how they met and fell in love, to remind each other (and themselves) of the meaning of their shared life, their affection and admiration for each other. It works differently for each of them; it activates Carol's accelerator by making her feel in love, and it deactivates Merritt's brakes by making her feel trusting of her partner.*
>
> *But Merritt's difficulty wasn't trusting her partner, it was trusting herself. And what she learned this night is that it becomes easier to trust herself when she can see how her body brings pleasure to her partner.*
>
> *Trying out the different kinds of lube turned sex into play, instead*

*of a problem, which switched her from what she calls "noisy brain,"
where everything is perceived as a threat, to "quiet brain," where everything is perceived with curiosity and pleasure. (Remember the rat who
didn't like Iggy Pop?)*

She paid close attention to how Carol experienced each type of lube.

*As she relaxed into the pleasure of observing her partner's pleasure,
she found that when she connected with the experience of giving pleasure, her own pleasure could expand inside her, without all the brakes
and worries and fretting.*

She swam in the water.

*It happened when she moved her focus away from her own worries
and onto the task of increasing her partner's pleasure.*

*The next step, of course, was to be able to enjoy her own pleasure.
But before she could get there, she had to knock down a wall in her own
mind. She'll do that in chapter 7.*

lubrication error #1:
genital response = desire

I've noticed three errors about nonconcordance that perpetuate dangerous
cultural myths about women's sexuality. Let's do away with them, okay?

The first way to be dangerously wrong about nonconcordance is failing to recognize that it exists in the first place. Let's call this Lubrication
Error #1.

Nonconcordance isn't news—or it shouldn't be. Sex researchers have
had an increasingly clear idea that nonconcordance is a thing for a decade
or two now. It's been in the news, it's been described in mainstream sex
books . . . and yet my students and blog readers are routinely surprised
to learn about it, and both porn and mainstream culture continue to perpetuate the myth that genital response = desire and pleasure. Now that
you know about nonconcordance, you'll see people getting it wrong all
over the place.

So what gives? Why does it feel so new, when every other year a book comes out that talks about it?

When I asked this question in my class, a student raised her hand and said with comic sourness: "Patriarchy."

Totally.

For centuries, men's sexuality has been the "default" sexuality, so that where women differ from men, women get labeled "broken." Even men who differ from the standard narrative get labeled "broken." Men have, on average, a 50 percent overlap between their genital response and their subjective arousal, and therefore, the patriarchal myth goes, everyone should have a 50 percent overlap.

But women aren't broken versions of men; they're *women*.

If it weren't about men-as-default, then we'd all be just as likely to wonder, "What's up with men, that they have so much overlap?" as we are to wonder, "What's up with women, that they have so little overlap?" But no one asks about men. No student, no blog reader, no fellow sex educator, no one anywhere has ever asked me, "Why are men so concordant? Isn't that kind of . . . ?" The only people who ask that question are the sex researchers.

When we've overcome this myth of men-as-default, we'll stop mistaking "varied" for "broken." We'll remember that, like height, as I described in chapter 1, people within a particular group may vary more from each other than they do from a different group.

But in the meantime, I'm going to fight patriarchy with patriarchy. Let's make nonconcordance universally acknowledged, by understanding how it affects men.

Every guy, at some point in his life, has the experience of wanting sex, wanting an erection, and the erection just isn't there. In that moment, the erection (or lack of erection) isn't a measure of his interest—he might even wake up the very next morning with an erection, when it's nothing but an inconvenience.

Guys sometimes wake up with erections, not because they're turned on but because they're waking up out of rapid eye movement (REM) sleep, and one of the things that happens during REM is "nocturnal penile tumescence." Erections come and go throughout the sleep cycle, whether or not you're dreaming about sex. It doesn't mean anything, it's just an erection. It's nonconcordant.

Most boys, around adolescence, experienced unwanted genital response—sitting at the back of the bus, noticing a teacher's body, his own ill-fitting pants, or even just general excitement about nonsexual things (driving a car, eating a donut, really *anything*) can activate the relevant pathways and generate the physiological response in a teenage boy.

But genital response is not desire; response isn't even pleasure. It is simply response. For everyone, regardless of their genitals. Just because a penis responds to a particular idea or sight or story doesn't mean the person with the penis necessarily likes it or wants it. It just means it activated the relevant pathways—*learning*. "This is a restaurant." (Remember: Men's 50 percent overlap between genital response and arousal is highly statistically significant . . . but it's still just 50 percent, and people vary.)

Sometimes guys notice their bodies responding to something even when their brains are saying, "That's Not Okay." And they feel conflicted, because on the one hand it's clearly sexual, but on the other hand it's *Not Okay.*

I'll give you an example (and feel free to skip the next two paragraphs if you're triggered by sexual-assault-related things).

When I was in college, I was hanging out with a group of guy friends, and one of them—I'll call him Paul—told a story about a buddy of his. At the end of a party, when there were people sleeping or passed out all over the house, Paul found his buddy having sex with a girl who was passed out drunk, unresponsive, and clearly unaware of what was happening. I say "having sex with," but the technical term is "raping." And the buddy says, "Hey, you want to try this?" And my friend telling the story says, "Nah. We gotta go."

The reason that's all he said, Paul told us, rather than, "What are you doing, you douchebag? Get the hell away from her," was that he felt torn between his gut instinct that what his friend was doing was *Seriously Not Okay* and the automatic reaction of his body to the sight of sexual intercourse. He got an erection. He was horrified at himself, at the idea that any part of him might interpret this *Seriously Not Okay* situation as erotic.

Back when I heard this story, I had no idea what was going on. Genital response was desire and pleasure, I thought. It was similar to my other friend's story about being wet even though she was bored—though in this case, the guy was not bored but actively horrified!

What was going on?

What was going on was *learning* without either *wanting* or *liking*. His body recognized the sight before him as sex-related and, either because he was disinhibited by alcohol or else was just a low-brakes kind of guy, his brakes did not prevent his body from responding to the sex-related stimulation. "This is a restaurant," his penis told him, even though there was a brawl happening.

Let's imagine a different story, in a world where everyone knows about nonconcordance.

Because Paul knows that what his genitals are doing indicates only what's sex-related, not what's sexually appealing, not only does he not feel ashamed of himself or wonder if he, too, might be a rapist, but the absence of all that shame creates space in his brain for doing something more proactive to intervene! He can tell his friend to stop because what he's doing is an act of violence, a crime. Or he can call the cops and have the friend arrested, and he can take the girl to the emergency room to have evidence collected, HIV prophylaxis administered, and emergency contraception offered. Or at the very, very least he can find a friend to help her. He can be a hero.

Genital response doesn't mean anything but sex-related—*learning*, essentially a conditioned reflex—not *liking*. It doesn't indicate desire or pleasure or anything else. And by carving out space, once and for all, for nonconcordance, we're actually making the world a better place for *everyone*.

In the end, Lubrication Error #1—Genital Response = "Desire"—is actually just old-school metaphorization, like the medieval anatomists from chapter 1 ("pudendum," because shame!), though maybe without the Moral Message.

You know that the size of a person's phallus (clitoris or penis) doesn't say anything about how ashamed they are (or should be) of their genitals. At most, phallus size often—not always—predicts whether a person has ovaries or testicles. Similarly, blood flow to the genitals doesn't say anything about what the person wants or likes (or should want or like). No. At most, blood flow to the genitals often—not always—is simply information about whether a person has been exposed to something that their brain interpreted as sex-related—with no information about whether they *wanted* it.

lubrication error #2:
genital response = pleasure

A second, more science-y way to be dangerously wrong about nonconcordance is to pay attention to the science and then tell the wrong story about it, to decide that women's genitals are the "honest indicator" of what really turns them on, and the women are lying, in denial, or just repressed out of awareness of their own deep desires. Let's call this Lubrication Error #2.

This tempting—and wrong—explanation for nonconcordance lines up neatly with various cultural misconceptions about women's sexuality, like the Moral, Medical, and Media Messages that I described in chapter 5 and like the men-as-default myth. Like: Women have been socially programmed not to admit that they're actually turned on by certain things (like violent sex or lesbian porn), so when they report their perceived arousal, they're lying or in denial about their hidden desires, or possibly both. But what their genitals are doing is what's *really* true.

Daniel Bergner's *What Do Women Want? Adventures in the Science of Female Desire* begins with a description of nonconcordance research, followed immediately by a description of lie detector research. The conclusion readers are forced to draw is that women are lying—or possibly just in denial—about their arousal. Here's how Amanda Hess summarized it in her review at Slate.com: "Straight women claimed to respond to straight sex more than they really did; lesbian women claimed to respond to straight sex far less than they really did; nobody admitted a response to the bonobo sex." [16]

Note the "claimed" and the "really" and the "admitted."

Of course you know that women's genitals were just reacting automatically to a sex-related cue—"This is a restaurant"—which has only a passing acquaintance with what a woman "really" likes or wants. Readers of *What Do Women Want?* didn't get that lesson, though. They got Lubrication Error #2.

Sex-positive feminists embrace the story that women's bodies could be contradicting the outdated morality-based cultural narratives about women being "less sexual" than men: Look how much our genitals respond to stuff! Look how sexual we *really* are!

Right? That's an appealing story—as if our bodies are showing us a secret, wildly sexual self that could be into anything if we just gave ourselves the permission that our culture has been denying us for centuries!

And after all, women *have* been subjected to oppressive cultural messages that made it shameful for them to acknowledge and pay affectionate attention to their own sexuality—that's what chapter 5 was about. In fact this whole book is about paying attention to your own internal experience and trusting your body. And what could be more "trust your body" than "Your genitals are telling you what you like, even when you don't know it"?

Ah. It's that word "like" that's the problem. "Like." Like, *liking*.

But genital response isn't *liking*. It's *learning*.

Your genitals *are* telling you something, and you can trust them. They're telling you that something is sex-related, based on their experience of Pavlovian conditioning. "This a restaurant." But that's not the same as sexually *appealing*.

Do, absolutely, trust your body. And interpret its signals accurately.

We see this myth—that a woman's genitals can tell us more about how she feels than she can—everywhere. For example, as part of my research for this book, I read the bestselling novel *Fifty Shades of Grey* by E. L. James. And there it was. Arousal nonconcordance in the first spanking scene. Now, as a reader of the genre, I know what's supposed to happen in the first spanking scene in a romance novel. Our heroine should begin the scene uncertain but excited, and by the end she should be feeling like, "I know I'm not supposed to like it, but I like it *so much!*"

That is not what happens here. Our heroine, Anastasia, consents to the spanking, but she neither wants it nor likes it. During the spanking, she tries to move away, she screams in pain, and her "face hurts, it's screwed up so tight."[17] There is not one word about her enjoying the spanking as it's happening.

Afterward, hero/spanker Christian Grey puts his fingers in her vagina. Now, knowing what you know about nonconcordance, listen to what Grey tells Ana: "Feel this. See how much your body *likes this*, Anastasia. You're soaking just for me" (emphasis mine).[18]

It gets worse, though. Instead of believing her own internal experience, which she describes as "demeaned, debased, and abused," Ana believes him.[19]

The moment feels true to many readers, because so many of us were raised to believe other people's opinions about our bodies, more than we believe our own internal experiences. Certainly there are women who are turned on by being consensually debased, but the whole plot pivots on the fact that Ana isn't one of them.

So, E. L. James, if you're reading this: Lubrication means it was sex-related, which tells us nothing about whether it was sexually *appealing*. Therefore I humbly request that in the next edition, Christian says to Ana, "Feel this. See how sex-related your body considers physical contact with your buttocks and genitals, Anastasia. That gives me no information about whether or not you liked it. Did you like it? No? Double crap, let me make it up to you by reading Emily Nagoski's book about the science of women's sexual wellbeing, so that I have a clue next time."

Thank you.

If you're ever in doubt that genital response is about *learning*, without necessarily any connection to *liking* or *wanting*, just remember this:

Lubrication Error #2 wants to claim that we can know what women are truly turned on by what their genitals respond to. That would mean that women whose genitals respond to images of bonobos copulating truly are, deep down, almost as interested in watching nonhuman primates copulating as they are in watching porn.

Really? Come on.

Even in the face of such absurdities, it's an incredibly persistent myth. Alain de Botton, in *How to Think More about Sex*, goes so far as to describe lubricating vaginas and tumescent penises as "unambiguous agents of sincerity," because they are automatic rather than intentional, which means they can't be "faked."

If that's true, then when your doctor taps your knee's patellar tendon and your leg kicks out, that must mean you actually want to kick your doctor.

Or when you have an allergic reaction to pollen, you must hate flowers.

Or when your mouth waters around a mouthful of moldy, bruised peach, you must find it delicious.

Don't get me wrong—you might want to kick your doctor and you might hate flowers and you might enjoy moldy, bruised peaches. But your automatic physiological processes are not how we would know that. No. Automatic physiological processes are, ya know, *automatic*, not sincere.

And think about it from Céline Dion's perspective. Does she want an audience's hair to stand on end, or does she want them to say, "I got chills!" even if their hair stayed flat? Experience trumps physiology every time.

But it gets worse—it gets less funny and more dangerous.

If we persist in the false belief that women's genital response reflects what they "really" want or like, then we have to conclude that if their genitals respond during sexual assault, it means they "really" wanted or liked the assault.

Which isn't just nuts, it's dangerous.

"You said no but your body said yes" is an idea that shows up both in the lyrics of pop songs and in the images at Project Unbreakable, an on-line gallery of sexual assault survivors holding signs with phrases said by their rapists, their families, or even police responders.[20] But you know by now that bodies don't say yes or no, they only say, "That's sex-related," without any comment on whether it's *liked*, much less whether it's *wanted* or consented to. A penis in a vagina is sex-related, though it may be unappealing, unwanted, and unwelcome. There is no desire, pleasure, or consent necessary for genital response. It's just, "This is a restaurant," with no comment on whether it might be a good place to have dinner.

It's an ancient fallacy, this notion that physiology can prove whether someone likes something sexual. Until the 1700s, people believed that conception was the pleasurable part of sex for a woman, so if a woman got pregnant, she must have experienced pleasure, and if she experienced pleasure, then the sex could not have been unwanted.[21] Because, "She said no but her ovaries said yes."

This myth has its own degree of traction, showing up in the public discourse in the 2012 Senate race in Missouri, when Republican candidate Todd Akin said, "If it's a legitimate rape, the female body has ways to try to shut the whole thing down," which even Mormon Republican presidential candidate Mitt Romney described as, "insulting, inexcusable and, frankly, wrong."[22]

Sex researcher Meredith Chivers often says, "Genital response is not consent." Let's add to that, "And neither is pregnancy."

Genital response is no more an expression of pleasure, desire, or consent than the fertilization of an egg is. I hope that is totally obvious to you by now.

We metaphorize our bodies; we use descriptions of our physiology to stand in for descriptions of our states of mind. "I'm so wet" and "I'm so hard" are intended to say, "I'm into this." These metaphors are so entrenched that people believe they're literal. Indeed, some people actually want us to believe that women are lying—whether deliberately or because we've been culturally oppressed out of the capacity to recognize our own desires—when our genitals are responding but we say we're not turned on.

I hope that by now, six chapters into this book, you know better. You know that men's and women's sexualities are made of the same parts, just organized in different ways, and you know that no two people are alike. You know that what activates your accelerator or hits your brakes is context dependent. You know that women's sexuality is even more context sensitive than men's, that developmental, cultural, and life history factors all profoundly shape how and when our bodies respond. You know that sex-related and sexually appealing are not the same thing.

Women are not liars, in denial, or otherwise broken. They are *women*, rather than men, in a world that wants women to believe they can't understand their own internal experience.

lubrication error #3:
nonconcordance is a problem

The third way to be dangerously wrong about nonconcordance is to decide that it's a symptom of something.

Suppose you recognize that nonconcordance exists, you acknowledge that it's *learning* without necessarily indicating *liking* or *wanting*, and then you read the research that shows a correlation between nonconcordance and sexual dysfunction.[23] And so you decide that, because nonconcordance is associated with dysfunction, nonconcordance must be a problem.

Which brings me to a sentence every undergraduate who takes a research methods class will memorize: "Correlation does not imply causation." It refers to the *cum hoc ergo propter hoc* fallacy—"with this, therefore because of this"—which means that just because two things happen together doesn't mean that one thing caused the other thing.

The quintessential example in the twenty-first century is the relationship between pirates and global warming.[24] This is a joke made by Bobby Henderson, as part of the belief system of the Church of the Flying Spaghetti Monster. Henderson wanted to make a point about the difference between causation and correlation, so he drew a graph that apparently plotted increase in global temperature with the precipitous drop in the number of seafaring pirates.

Did the loss of pirates cause global climate change?

Of course not. It's absurd, right? That's the point.

Actually, we can hypothesize a third variable that influenced both the reduction in pirates and the change in global climate: the Industrial Revolution.

Like this putative correlation between pirates and global temperature, there's also a correlation between nonconcordance and sexual dysfunction. The correlation makes it easy to think that the nonconcordance is *causing* the sexual dysfunction, or that the dysfunction is *causing* the nonconcordance.

But just as pirates and global temperature can be linked together by the Industrial Revolution, nonconcordance and sexual dysfunction are linked together by a third variable: context.

How does context link sexual functioning and concordance?

Sexually functional women have brakes that are sensitive to context, turning off the offs when they're in the right context—which, remember, means both external circumstances and internal mental state. Sexually dysfunctional women's brakes stay on, even in contexts where you would expect them to turn off.

I'll illustrate this with an extraordinarily clever study published in 2010. Dutch researchers built an "ambulatory laboratory"—a take-home kit of plethysmograph, laptop computer, and handheld control unit.[25] Participants completed tests in the lab similar to other nonconcordance research—viewing erotic stimuli and measuring various automatic and conscious responses—and they took the ambulatory lab home with them and tested themselves there, too. This way researchers could measure how being in the lab influenced the results, compared to being at home. In other words, they measured the effect of *context*. They studied two groups: eight women with healthy sexual functioning (the control group) and eight women who met the diagnostic criteria for "hypoactive sexual desire disorder" (the "low-desire" group).

Result: The control group's genital response *and* subjective arousal more than doubled when tested at home, compared to in the lab. Plus they reported feeling "less inhibited" and "more at ease" at home. The low-desire group's genital response also doubled at home . . . but their subjective arousal did not, nor did they report feeling less inhibited or more at ease. Which is to say, they were less concordant because their brakes didn't turn off. Just being at home wasn't enough to turn off the low-desire women's brakes.

The sexually satisfied women were more sensitive than women with low desire to the change in context from the lab to home. To be more specific, recent research has found that sexually healthy women experience more concordance if they have *lower* sensitivity brakes.[26]

Whether it's the external circumstances or internal experience hitting the brakes, context is fundamental to most women's sexual wellbeing. Context is the crux and the key. Context is the cause.

Here's a thing that happens to me sometimes: A wife drags her husband over to me and says, "Tell him what you told me."

Laurie did that with Johnny at a lunch buffet. "Tell him what you told me. The arousal thing. Tell him, please."

"He didn't believe you?"

"He thinks I 'must have misunderstood.'"

So I told him: "Okay, Johnny. I know this is the opposite of everything you've ever learned about sex, but it's true: The state of Laurie's vagina doesn't necessarily tell you anything about her state of mind."

She thwacked him on the arm with the back of her hand and raised her eyebrows, as if to say, "See?"

He looked at me and he looked at her and he looked back at me and he opened his mouth to ask a question and then he closed it again.

Then he said to Laurie, "Go away, honey."

She did—not before giving me a knowing glance.

In a confidential whisper, he said to me, "If I can't go by her genitals, how do I know she really wants me? Because she could totally just be saying she wants me when really she's just trying to get it over with."

Johnny is a dude-bro, manly, fix-it kind of guy. I like him a lot, and often my role is to translate the science of women's sexual well-being into Manly Fix-It Dude-Speak for him. So I started by saying, "Think about it this way: Arousal is not about her genitals, it's about her brain."

Then I described the sexual response mechanism as a set of on and off switches, with each associated with a particular kind of input— genital sensations, relationship satisfaction, stress, attachment, etc.— that throws a switch on or off. Men's and women's sexual response mechanisms have the same set of dials and switches, but they tend to be tuned to different levels of sensitivity, so that just a little bit of genital stimulation throws an on switch for men, while just a little bit of stress throws an off switch for women. Laurie's life, I explained, was throwing all the off switches.

He said, "You're saying I've got this strong input from my body, but her strongest input is from her . . . life?"

"Yes!"

"So to hack the system, what I need to be paying attention to is the stuff that's hitting the brakes, because once those are off, the accelerator will take over. Is that what you're saying?"

"Yes. You've got it," I said. "I think she wrote a list of stuff that hit her brakes—"

"She did," he said. "I've seen it. I didn't know what to do with it, but now . . ." He stared at me for a moment, then shook his head and said, "This really changes everything. What this says is that the sexiest

thing I can do isn't some crazy erotic thing. The sexiest thing I can do is take away as many of the brakes as I can, which is . . . I mean, I can do that. Just . . . why did no one tell me this before?"

"honey . . . I'm nonconcordant!"

If you've got a body that doesn't always match your mind, then you've got a body that defies conventional (and wrong) wisdom, and so you might find yourself in the position of having to correct your partner's understanding. There are three things to remember, which can resolve any problem your nonconcordance may generate.

First, remember that you are healthy and functional and whole. Your body is not broken and you are not crazy. Your body is doing what bodies do, and that's a beautiful thing. Hooray! So know that you are normal. Tell your partner you are normal. Tell them calmly, joyfully, and confidently. No need to be defensive or aggressive—it's not their fault they don't know about nonconcordance. Actually, it's more my fault and the fault of all the other sex educators and researchers. We have failed to communicate this idea clearly to the world, and now you're stuck with the job of fixing our mistake. Sorry about that. So apologize for me, on behalf of all the sex educators and researchers in the world, and then give your partner the facts:

> "Emily Nagoski is sorry that you didn't already know that genital response isn't a reliable indicator of pleasure or desire. But it's true. What my genitals are doing doesn't necessarily have anything to do with how I feel. Thirty years of research confirms this. So please pay attention to my words, not my vagina."

You don't actually have to apologize for me; you can just email me and say, "Could you please email my partner an apology for the fact that

didn't know about nonconcordance?" and I'll do it myself. Seri-
, I will.

Second, offer your partner other ways to know that you're turned on.

Here are some alternative things your partner can pay attention to if
your genitals are telling them only about *learning*, not about *liking*:

- Your breath. Your respiration rate and your pulse increase with
  arousal. You begin holding your breath, too, as you get to the
  highest level of arousal and your thoracic and pelvic diaphragms
  contract.

- Muscle tension, especially in your abdomen, buttocks, and thighs,
  but also in your wrists, calves, and feet. When the tension moves in
  waves through you, your body bows and arches. For some women,
  in some contexts, this happens in an obvious way. For other
  women, or in other contexts, it is subtle.

- Most important, your *words*. Only you can tell your partner what
  you want and how you feel. Not all women feel equally comfortable talking about their desire and arousal, but you can shortcut
  with "yes" or "more."

And remember this, too: It's not about attending to any specific
physiological response, behavior, or other clue. It's about attending
with a kind of broad, receptive vigilance. Suggest that your partner
attend to you not with a magnifying glass but with the wrong end of
a telescope, or the way a chess master watches a chessboard—looking
for large-scale patterns and dynamics. Your partner should attend the
way a master chef tastes food—not just for individual flavors, but for
the way those flavors combine and create something unique and new
and delicious.

Third and finally, deal with any lack of lube-on-demand by supple-
menting with the fluid of your choice: your saliva or your partner's (when

there's no risk of infection transmission), your partner's genital fluids (ditto), store-bought lube, whatever.

What is lube for? Reducing friction, which can increase pleasure, and it always decreases the risk of tearing and pain. And *always* use lube if you're using protective barriers like condoms or dams. Lube increases their efficacy and makes them more pleasurable. Lube is your friend. Lube will make your sex life better.[27]

Sometimes people feel uncomfortable introducing outside sources of lube into their sexual connection. This hesitancy may stem from any number of life events or from simple inexperience with it or from a sense that using lube means you're somehow inadequate. Remember the sanctity moral foundation: sex-related stuff gets categorized as "dirty," even when it's a bottle filled with something you find in many hair products.

But you know now that genital blood flow has its own way of being in the world, which may or may not have anything to do with your sexual pleasure or desire. You know that lube is important because it reduces friction, which increases both health and pleasure. And you know that you get to choose which beliefs you nurture and which you weed out.

If you decide to try using lube, here are some tips for talking with your partner about it:

- *Playfulness, Curiosity, and Humor.* It is literally impossible to feel stressed and anxious about something when your approach is playful, curious, and humorous. Let it be a little silly; let it be fun. This is about pleasure, remember?
- *Make Your Partner Feel Like a Superhero.* Communicating about sex feels risky sometimes because, above all, you don't want to hurt your partner's feelings. The simplest shortcut around hurt feelings is to make the conversation about all the things your partner does well, all the ways that they can increase your pleasure beyond its already

skyrocketing heights, and all the delight you hope to add by incorporating this new element to your sexual connection.

- *Choose Your Lube Wisely.* Not all lube is created equal. Often it's a good idea to choose lube together with your partner—shop together and pick something you both feel good about, so that you are both equally invested in it.

Camilla explained nonconcordance to Henry. For her, nonconcordance was a perfect example of how the cultural narrative had failed to tell her the truth, and she was pretty pleased to find another way she was, yet again, totally normal.

It was a little more complicated for Henry, because he was still figuring out the whole desire/wanting thing. He was trying to get comfortable with the difference between the brakes version of not wanting—"I want that to stop"—versus the accelerator version of not wanting—"I like that yet feel no urge to seek out more."

He said, "I understand that genital response doesn't tell me what turns you on. You tell me what turns you on, and I believe you. But what I don't understand is how you get turned on without first wanting the thing that turns you on."

Which is maybe the most complex—and controversial—element of sexual wellbeing.

The answer to Henry's question is: Pleasure comes first—before desire, that is.

And desire is the subject of chapter 7.

tl;dr

- Blood flow to the genitals is response to sex-related stimuli (*learning*), which is not the same thing as *liking* or *wanting*, much less consent.

- Men and women seem to be different in the concordance of their genital response and subjective arousal. But, as in every other chapter, this difference between women and men doesn't mean women are broken; it's means they're *women*.
- Arousal nonconcordance is not a symptom of anything; it's just a normal part of how sex works sometimes. If you need lube, use lube!
- The best way to tell if someone is aroused is not to notice what their genitals are doing, but to *listen to their words*.

seven

desire

SPONTANEOUS, RESPONSIVE, AND MAGNIFICENT

It's a basic fact of their relationship that Olivia wants sex more often than Patrick does, so she ends up initiating most of the time. But Olivia's experience of being the target of Patrick's placebo-powered rampant lust the previous night had given her a powerful insight: It had felt good to be open *to sex, without feeling* driven *to have sex. It had felt good to* allow *sexual desire to pull her gradually and gently toward sex, rather than feeling like it was pushing her.*

So, as the next step in their experiment, they tried flipping their usual dynamic on its head. They set a "date night" and then didn't do anything to prepare; they just showed up that night in their usual states of mind—Olivia ready to go, Patrick not disinterested, but not actively interested either.

And they made Olivia follow her partner's lead, while Patrick started to explore what kinds of things he could do to shift himself into active interest. They spent a lot of time "preheating the oven": kissing and talking and massaging—and, surprisingly, a little adventure, moving from the bedroom to the kitchen to feed each other. When Patrick was in charge with full permission to do whatever occurred to him, they tried new things and played together. They learned a lot about what context worked for Patrick, because he had to create that context, had to ask for what felt right.

They learned a surprising thing about Olivia, too: When she stayed still enough to move at Patrick's pace rather than her own naturally faster pace, the gradual buildup and the sustained arousal and the necessity of holding herself back created a context that wasn't just as good as the context that worked for her. It was unbelievably better.

Olivia told me: "One of the rules we set was I had to ask for permission before I had an orgasm. And he did not always say yes when I asked. Um, we'll be doing that again."

"What was good about it?" I asked.

Olivia's expression turned serious, but with a glow. She said, "It was like . . . when we let ourselves synchronize and both of us were climbing toward orgasm at the same, deliberate pace, we, like . . . it was like I could feel his pleasure in my body. I could even feel my own pleasure inside his body. Does that sound insane?"

"Not even a little bit," I said.

Creating a great sex-positive context for the lower-desire partner resulted in a context that was mind-blowingly, almost painfully erotic for the higher-desire partner.

This chapter is about why and how that works.

Imagine a world where everyone has desert plants in their gardens—aloe plants and dragon trees and fiddlenecks and yuccas—and everyone knows how to tend them: lots of sun, very little water.

And imagine that you happen to have a tomato plant in your garden. Everybody "knows," in this desert world, that plants need very little water, so you water your tomato plant sparingly . . . and it slowly dies. You wonder, "Maybe I'm watering it too often? Maybe there's not enough sun?" And you continue to water and watch, and you wonder, "Why is it dying? I'm doing what I'm supposed to do!"

A tiny shift in knowledge—the bare fact that tomato plants are better adapted to a subtropical climate than to a desert, so they thrive on more water—can change how you tend your garden . . . which can bring your tomato plant back to life.

Now, if someone comes along and offers this fact, there will be those who say, "Plants don't need lots of water, that's part of what it means to be a healthy plant!" Others will say, "Tomato plants are crazy—broken!—to need all that water!" Some will search for a remedy for the tomato plant, to make it more like an aloe. And there will be tomato gardeners who simply can't let go of the idea that they're supposed to be able to produce abundant fruit on almost no water at all, and they will do anything to have a tomato plant that thrives in the desert.

But you try it. You give your tomato plant more water.

And you go from "Why is it dying?" to "Wow!" as you're rewarded with abundant fruit and lush, fragrant greens. All because of a tiny shift in knowledge.

This chapter is about one such tiny shift in knowledge, which can move your relationship with your sexual wellbeing from "Why is it dying?" to "Wow!"

The standard narrative of sexual desire is that it just *appears*—you're sitting at lunch or walking down the street, maybe you see a sexy person or think a sexy thought, and *pow!* you're saying to yourself, "I would like some sex!" That's Olivia's usual style. That's "spontaneous" desire.

But some people find that they begin to want sex only *after* sexy things are already happening. Rather than eagerly anticipating sex, they might have a pragmatic motivation for showing up at 7 p.m. on Saturday night, because date night is on their calendar. They put their bodies in the bed, let their skin touch their partner's skin . . . and their body wakes up and says, "Oh, right! I like this person! I enjoy this!" That's responsive desire. Where spontaneous desire appears in *anticipation* of pleasure, responsive desire emerges in *response* to pleasure.

And it's normal. People with responsive desire don't have "low" desire, they don't suffer from any ailment, they don't even long to initiate but feel like they're not allowed to. Their bodies just need some more compelling reason than, "Sex is generally fun," or "That's an attractive person right there," to crave sex. They can be sexually satisfied and in healthy relationships, and yet never crave sex out of the blue. That's Camilla. Lack of spontaneous desire for sex is not, in itself, dysfunctional or problematic! Let me repeat: Responsive desire is *normal and healthy*.

But actually? It turns out everyone's sexual desire is responsive. It just *feels* more spontaneous for some and more responsive for others, because even though we're all made of the same parts, the different organizations of those parts result in different experiences.

Research suggests about half of women might be categorizable as one or the other, spontaneous or responsive.[1] Most people's desire style is probably—drumroll, please—context dependent. That's Merritt and Laurie. And they're normal, too. These are folks who, in the hot and heavy, falling-in-love stage of a relationship, may want sex seemingly out of nowhere, but ten years and some kids later, it takes a little more deliberate effort to get them interested in sex.

So in this chapter I'll explain what desire is, how it works, how to make the most of it, and what to do if you and your partner have different desire styles.

We'll start with where desire comes from: Desire is pleasure in context.[2] We'll spend some time talking about what's unlikely to cause desire problems—hormones and monogamy—and what is much more likely to cause desire problems—sex-negative culture and the chasing dynamic. And we'll wrap up the chapter with a left turn away from mere "desire" toward what matters most: sex worth wanting.

desire = pleasure in context

Though details vary from person to person, we can experience desire in a variety of ways, depending on the context and the sensitivity of our brakes and accelerators. To illustrate, let's think through three different scenarios, each with the same stimulation, same brakes and accelerator, but different contexts.

Scenario 1. You're feeling very calm and happy and trusting, not doing anything in particular, and your partner comes over and touches your arm affectionately. The touch travels from your arm, up your spine, to your brain. In this state of mind, your central nervous system is very quiet, there's very little other traffic, and the sensation of your partner's touch says, "Hey, so, this is happening. What do you think?" And your brain says, "Affection feels nice." The stimulation continues, your beloved partner touching your arm affectionately, and the sensation travels up to your brain and says, "This is happening some more. What do you think?" And your brain says, "Affection feels *really* nice," and tunes its attention more to that sensation. Then your partner starts kissing your throat, and that sensation makes its way to your emotional brain and says, "Now this is happening, too. What do you think?" And by then the brain says, "That is fantastic! Go get more of that!" In that context, sexual desire feels *responsive*.

   Scenario 2. You're stressed, exhausted, or overwhelmed, it's very noisy in your brain, there's heavy traffic, lots of yelling and horns honking about all the stuff that's stressing you out. Your partner's affectionate touch travels from your arm, up your spine, to your brain, and it says, "This is happening. What do you think?" And your brain says, "WHAT? I CAN'T HEAR YOU OVER ALL THIS NOISE!" And by then the sensation is over. (Sensations are a little bit like Snapchat.) If your partner keeps touching you, the sensation keeps asking your brain, "This is still happening. What do you think?" And eventually it might get your brain's attention, and your brain might say, "ARE YOU KIDDING ME? I'VE GOT ALL THIS OTHER NOISE TO CONTEND WITH!" And if the sensation ever gets noticed enough to expand out of your brain's emotional One Ring, it comes out in the form of, "Not now, honey."

   Scenario 3. Your sexy, sexy partner has been away for two weeks, but you've been sending each other frequent texts, which started out flirty but have been gradually escalating in explicitness and intensity as you get more and more into teasing and tormenting each other. By the end of the two weeks, just the sound of your phone receiving a text makes you gasp and tremble. There's noise in your brain, but all of it is chanting, "Sexy,

sexy partner!" By the time your partner gets home and touches your arm affectionately, you're set to go off like a rocket. In that context, sexual desire feels *spontaneous*.[3]

In all three scenarios, stimulation comes first, whether it's your partner's touch or just the idea of your partner's touch. If the context is right, the stimulation feels good and leads to desire. All three scenarios are normal, healthy sexuality.

Sometimes the stimulation may not feel good but can still lead to desire—wanting without pleasure. This can also be normal, healthy sexuality, but as we'll see toward the end of the chapter, desire without pleasure is not the sexuality of people who have great or even good sex.

What all of this means is that if you want to expand your access to spontaneous desire, all you have to do is look for the contexts that facilitate it. Go back to the worksheets in chapter 3 and consider what partner characteristics, relationship characteristics, setting, ludic factors, and other life circumstances create pleasure that leads to urgent longing. Then see which of those you can alter in your life to create spontaneous desire. And if your life doesn't currently allow for the context that facilitates spontaneous desire, you know you're normal. You can enjoy responsive desire until you find your way to a day-to-day life that allows for spontaneous desire.

So sexual desire emerges in response to pleasure.

When it works.

Which sometimes it doesn't.

What causes desire to misbehave, and what do you do when it does? Women's own reports of why their desire diminishes will probably sound familiar to you: exhaustion, issues with mental and physical health, changes in body image, feeling overwhelmed by their many roles and obligations, and feeling anxious and worried about sex itself—worries ranging from unwanted pregnancy to "taking too long" to get aroused to not meeting partner expectations.[4]

In the next sections, I'll talk about the unlikely culprits for desire issues (hormones and monogamy) and the most likely culprits:

brakes-hitting cultural messages and the relationship issue that I call "the chasing dynamic." And then I'll talk about paradigm-shifting research on people who have *extraordinary* sex lives, sustaining sexual connections over many years.

> *Camilla and Henry had embraced her erotic "slow heater" and were collaborating to find contexts that activated her accelerator. But Henry was left with a lingering discomfort that it felt forced to do things to turn Camilla on when she wasn't already "in the mood." It felt somehow unnatural.*
>
> *Sometimes you can watch a fact drop into a person's brain like ink into water. I saw it happen when I explained to Camilla and Henry that, in fact, her desire style was totally normal.*
>
> *"Pleasure comes first, before desire—for everyone, not just Camilla," I said.*
>
> *"Pleasure comes first?" Henry said.*
>
> *"Yup. Desire emerges when pleasure crosses the person's individual threshold. Camilla, you happen to have a high threshold, but it's the same basic process for everyone."*
>
> *"You are kidding me," Camilla said. "Seriously, has pop culture gotten anything right about sex?"*
>
> *Henry didn't give me a chance to answer—this was important for him, the solution to his turn-Camilla-on-when-she-doesn't-yet-"want"-sex conundrum. "You're saying we just have different thresholds, is that right?"*
>
> *"Right."*
>
> *For Henry, sometimes just seeing Camilla walking around after a shower was all the pleasure it took to activate desire. He said, "And I like that! I like seeing her walking around all damp and naked. I wouldn't want her to stop doing it just because I wasn't turned on before I saw her. So . . . if the equivalent is true for you"—he turned to Camilla—"I don't have to feel uncomfortable creating equivalent contexts for you, right?"*

"I want you to!" said Camilla. "Tease my ticking pilot light! Build up the water pressure!"

So that's what they decided to do. Henry turned everything into low-key, no-pressure, zero-expectation foreplay, the way her walking around after a shower was a kind of low-level foreplay for him. Cuddling and touching. Slow kisses. Flowers. Affectionate attention. Like when they were first falling in love—a constant, steady stream of reminders that, "This guy is amazing!"

Henry loves Camilla's enthusiastic desire, and all it takes to get her there is enough pleasure, built up gradually.

This is not a story we see very much in pop culture because it's not about tension and ambivalence. But it turns out this is how it works for many couples who sustain a strong sexual connection over the long term.

good news! it's probably not your hormones

If you're experiencing pain with sex, talk to a medical provider—there may well be hormonal issues involved, along with a variety of neurological and physiological factors. But if you're experiencing low desire, hormones are the least likely culprits.[5] Lori Brotto and her colleagues tested six hormonal factors to determine which predicted more or less dysfunction in women with low desire, and not one of them was significantly predictive of low desire.[6]

So if it's not your hormones, what has the research found to be predictive of low desire? According to Brotto, "developmental history, psychiatric history, and psychosexual history." In other words, all that stuff from chapters 4 and 5—stress, depression, anxiety, trauma, attachment, etc.

People sometimes feel more comfortable with the idea that their sexual desire has everything to do with their chemistry and nothing to do with their life. After all, these days it's easy to change your chemistry! But hormones are a small—often negligible—part of the context that shapes a woman's sexual wellbeing, so changing them can make only a small—often negligible—impact. Stress, self-compassion, trauma history, relationship satisfaction, and other emotional factors have far more influence on a woman's sexual desire than any hormone.

If you sometimes experience low desire, unless there's some medical issue interfering, chances are you don't have to fix *you*—you're not broken—you only have to change your context.

It's Not a Drive

Most of us are used to thinking about sexual desire as a drive, like hunger. A drive is an uncomfortable internal experience that pushes you to go fix a problem. And what's the consequence if you don't solve the problem? Ultimately, you will die. Hunger is a drive. So is thirst. Thermoregulation. Sleep—you can literally die of sleep deprivation.

For centuries, scientists thought sex was a drive. It's probably how you think about it, too. It's how I thought about it for a long time.

Turns out, no.

It's easy to prove that sex is not a drive: As animal behaviorist Frank Beach put it in 1956, "No one has ever suffered tissue damage for lack of sex."[7] Put more colloquially, nobody ever died because they couldn't get laid. Maybe they wanted to, but that's frustration, and people don't literally die of frustration.[8]

If it's not a drive, what is it? It's an "incentive motivation system."[9]

Most people associate the word "incentive" with the idea of a prize, something worth working for. The biological meaning is similar. Where drives are about being pushed by an uncomfortable internal sensation, incentive motivation systems are all about being pulled by an attractive external stimulus. Curiosity is the quintessential example of an incentive motivation system, as natural to us as hunger, but without the threat of actual death.[10]

When you hear "drive," think "survive."

When you hear "incentive motivation," think "thrive."

This matters for at least two reasons:

First, if sex were a drive, like hunger, then people who rarely or never experience spontaneous desire for sex would be . . . well, what would we call a person who never experienced spontaneous hunger for food, even when they hadn't eaten in days or weeks or months? That person is definitely sick! And when you believe you're sick, your stress response kicks in. And we know how great stress is for sexual pleasure and desire, right?

The myth that sex is a drive is bad for people's sex lives.

But there's a more important reason that it matters that sex is like curiosity and not like hunger: If someone steals a loaf of bread because they're starving, on some level we can have sympathy and mercy; even when stealing is wrong, we acknowledge that people do what they have to do to survive. But if someone steals a loaf of bread simply because they're curious what someone else's bread tastes like . . . do we have the same sympathy, the same mercy?

Because sex is not a drive, it is not a biological "need," and no one is entitled to it, and no one ever has permission to steal it from anyone, under any circumstances.

more good news! it's not monogamy, either

Much has been made recently of the "unnaturalness" of monogamy and the death of erotic connection when people commit to a long-term, sexually exclusive relationship. By now you can probably anticipate my view of the subject: It's the context that matters, and no two people are alike. Some monogamous couples create a context that sustains and enlivens desire, and some couples . . . don't. The same is true for people in open relationships. It's not that either monogamy or polyamory is inherently good or bad for desire, it's the way people *do* monogamy or polyamory that can kill desire. If monogamy is your preferred relationship structure, this section is for you.

There are currently two general schools of thought on strategies for sustaining desire in long-term monogamous relationships. I'm going to frame them as the Esther Perel school and the John Gottman school, though that's just a shorthand for a much richer and more complex issue.

In *Mating in Captivity*, Esther Perel presents a contradiction at the core of modern relationships: the antithetical pull between the familiar versus the novel, the stable versus the mysterious. We want love, which is about security and safety and stability, but we also want passion, which is about adventure and risk and novelty. Love is having, desire is wanting, and you can want only what you don't already have, goes the reasoning.

If the problem is that long-term love is antithetical to long-term passion, then the solution, says Perel, is to maintain autonomy, a space of eroticism inside yourself, as a way to maintain the distance necessary to allow *wanting* to emerge. As Perel puts it, "In desire, we want a bridge to cross."[11] This means intentionally adding distance that creates an edgy instability or uncertainty, a slight and enjoyable dissatisfaction.

By way of contrast, John Gottman, in *The Science of Trust*, says that the problem is not lack of distance and mystery but lack of deepening intimacy. From this point of view, intimate conversation, affection, and friendship are central to the erotic life of a long-term relationship. Gottman reports the findings of a study of one hundred couples, all age forty-five or older, half with good sex lives and half with poor sex lives. Those who reported that they had good sex lives, he writes, "consistently mentioned: (1) maintaining a close, connected, and trusting friendship; and (2) making sex a priority in their lives."[12] In other words, sustaining desire isn't about having a bridge to cross but about building a bridge together.

"Turn toward each other's desires," says Gottman.

"Keep a comfortable distance," says Perel.

Are you wondering who's right?

They both are—depending, I think, on how you conceptualize "desire." Remember back in chapter 3, the distinction between *wanting* and *liking*? For Perel, desire is *wanting*. Longing. Seeking. Craving. The discrepancy-reducing pursuit of a goal, to put it in romantic terms.[13]

And for Gottman and the couples in the research he cites, "desire" has more to do with *liking*. Holding. Savoring. Allowing. Exploring this moment together, noticing what it is like, and *liking* it. The *Mating in Captivity* style of desire is higher adrenaline; it's inherently exciting. We relish this kind of perpetual itch-scratch-relief-itch cycle. We *like* to *want*, so much that we can't always separate the experience of *wanting* from the experience of *liking*. It's a good fit for the existing narrative that says spontaneous desire is the right way to experience desire. The *Science of Trust* style of desire is lower adrenaline, more a celebration of sensation in context, a celebration of togetherness.

Perel's style is about hunger as the secret sauce that makes a meal delicious. Gottman's is about arriving home from work and cooking dinner with your partner, having a glass of wine while you cook, feeding each other all the strawberries you meant to keep for dessert, then sitting down together and savoring every mouthful. In the Perel style, you come to your partner with your fire already stoked. In the Gottman style, you stoke each other's fire.

My personal inclination is more toward Gottman's style, while my twin sister said, "Why would closeness ever make anyone want more closeness? *Space!*" I know people who swear by one or the other. I know people who are too exhausted to try either. I know people who are convinced that one is the True Way to desire, even though I think they'd benefit from trying the other. It's a matter of fit. And I think that in the end, both are strategies for accomplishing the same overall goal: increasing activation of the accelerator and decreasing the brakes.

The two approaches are more alike than they sound on the surface, and their similarities are where we find the deepest truth: Both are clear that passion doesn't happen automatically in a long-term, monogamous relationship. But they're also both clear that passion *does* happen—as long as the couple takes deliberate control of the context. For some couples that context feels like creating closeness. For others, it feels like creating space.

Following Johnny's revelation about the dials and switches and what Laurie is sensitive to, they decided to try one of those box subscriptions. Every few months, a box would come in the mail—like a Fruit of the Month thing, only instead of fruit they got kits with a sort of prefabricated sexy fantasy. They both feared it would be kind of cheesy, but they also figured it was worth a try. They were paying attention to context, and even though Johnny's context was, "Give me two minutes to brush my teeth," Laurie's was, "Get me the heck out of mommy mode or I'll never get to hey-sexy-lady mode."

So the box arrived and they opened it together.

Their first impression was . . . well, disappointment.

"That was a lot of money for some arts-and-crafts supplies," was how Laurie put it.

"We already have a vibrator," was how Johnny put it.

But they thought, What the hell. We paid for these arts-and-crafts supplies. We got your mother to babysit. We made a hotel reservation. Let's just go, and whatever happens (or not), happens (or not).

The box included instructions, laying out their evening and some rules, but they didn't follow the rules. They talked about it all in the car on the way to the hotel, laughing the whole time.

They had a pizza delivered and they kept talking about it, and talking about other things, too—work, kid, family. They just talked about stuff and remembered how much they like each other. Then Laurie had a bubble bath, taking a book of erotic stories with her into the tub.

I'll fast-forward through the rest of the evening by suggesting you hum "Can You Feel the Love Tonight?" to yourself for a few minutes.

At what point in the evening did Laurie start experiencing something she would describe as actual "desire"? About halfway through the massage Johnny gave her when she got out of the tub and strolled to the bed wearing nothing but a lacy bra and perfumed body lotion.

At what point did Johnny start experiencing desire? In the car on the way there.

But it worked out just fine.

It was an expensive night, and it required a significant amount of planning ahead, but it got Laurie all the way out of the parenting-bosslady-student-OMG-life state of mind and into a Johnny-and-me-sexytime state of mind that allowed her stressors to slip into the shadows of her attention for a while, while hey-sexy-lady stood in the spotlight.

And all they changed was the context.

"why can't I just take a pill?"

When you believe there's something wrong with you, your stress response kicks in. And when your stress response kicks in, your interest in sex evaporates (for most people). Insisting that spontaneous desire is the only "normal" desire is insisting that a healthy person with responsive desire is sick. Say it often enough and eventually they'll believe you. And when they believe you, suddenly it's true. The myth makes people sick.

This is exactly what I saw during the FDA approval of the drug Flibanserin, a drug to treat "low desire." It's a pill you take every day. For what benefit? According to the FDA analysis of the data, women on the drug had less than one additional "satisfying sexual event" per month, compared to those on the placebo; overall, approximately 12 percent of study participants were "at least minimally improved" above placebo, which means that about 88 percent of participants experienced *not even minimal benefit* above placebo.[14] (Unsurprisingly, it was not a bonanza.)

A second drug, approved in 2019, is an abdominal injection you give yourself an hour or so before sex. In clinical trials, it did not increase sexual frequency, nor did it increase participants' reported sexual satisfaction. It *did* increase participants' scores on a general survey of sexual functioning—a survey developed by the pharmaceutical industry.[15] (This drug, too, was not a bonanza. Unsurprisingly.)

But the real story behind these drugs isn't simply that they don't "work"—that is, they don't increase spontaneous desire or sexual frequency, except perhaps in a small minority of women. The real story is that even the women for whom the drugs "work" were never broken in the first place.

One woman who had a great experience on Flibanserin during the trial phase told *Cosmo* what her sex life was like before she started the drug.[16] She said, "Once I started, it wasn't an issue. It was getting me started."

Sound familiar? That's responsive desire. Healthy and normal.

Another participant said something similar: "I miss really wanting to have sex. I hate having to 'wind myself up' to do it. It makes me feel broken. It takes a really dedicated effort for me to be there physically and mentally." [17]

Again and again in mainstream media coverage, research participants were describing intact *responsive* desire.[18] Which is healthy and normal! Their relationships were strong and their health was good—both things had to be true for women to qualify to participate in the drug trial— yet they believed their responsive desire was a disease. And so they felt broken.

Of course they felt broken. They were taught the same thing that the rest of us were taught, the same thing even their doctors were taught, about sexual desire: that it "should" be spontaneous. That a person who doesn't spontaneously just crave sex is diseased.

Does feeling diseased and broken activate the accelerator?

Are we starting to get the picture, that telling women they're broken is a great way to break women?

The starkest example of this, to me, came during the FDA hearing for Flibanserin. FDA panel member and urologist Dr. Phil Hanno asked why women in the study were having, on average, two to three "satisfying sexual events" (SSEs) per month *before the drug trial began*.[19] If they lacked desire, why were they having any sex?

Which . . . okay, Dr. Hanno. Can I call you Phil? Phil. Sometimes women have sex because they're bored. Sometimes they have sex because their partners want to have sex and they love their partners, so sure honey, let's do it. Sometimes it's to end a fight. Sometimes it's because they feel so loving they want to express that love, and maybe sex is a way to do that.[20]

But here is what a presenter from the drugmaker said in response:

"Once they engage in activity, it's pleasurable."

Jaw drop. What the drugmaker was saying—explicitly! Right to the FDA's face!—is that they were attempting to "treat" *healthy women*. Because if you experience pleasure in the context of a mutually consenting "sexual event," that is a normal, healthy sex life. Period.

No wonder the drugs are ineffective. They're trying to fix something that isn't broken. The only thing that's broken is the culture that tells women they have an illness.

Let me say this categorically: Drug companies would very much like you to believe that responsive desire is a disease. It is not. When they want to medicate someone who says, "Once we get started, everything is great; it's just getting started that's a lot of work," they are trying to medicate someone who is normal and healthy.

Unfortunately only three of the twenty-four FDA panelists were sex researchers, therapists, or educators, so the panel believed the same old myth most of us were raised with—that desire must be "spontaneous."

They are wrong.

I am working to help therapists, educators, and medical providers of all kinds to stop believing desire must be spontaneous. If your medical provider or therapist thinks desire should be spontaneous, feel free to suggest they read this book; a lot of clinicians actually refer their patients and clients to the book once they, too, learn that desire needn't be spontaneous. Some medical schools even assign *Come As You Are* as a text, and I hope you get one of those doctors. But in the meantime, you are likely to encounter helping professionals who have not integrated responsive desire into their understanding of normal, healthy desire.[21] (Drug companies have a much bigger PR budget than sex researchers, therapists, and educators do.)

Please tell everyone you know: If you have responsive desire, you are already normal. No one needs to "crave" sex out of the blue to be a fully healthy person.

If you want to experience more spontaneous desire, just for the fun of it, you don't need to change *you*, you can just change your context, which you learned how to do way back in chapter 3. But you don't need to experience spontaneous desire in order to be healthy and normal.

it might be the chasing dynamic

Remember the tomatoes and the aloes: Our expectation that people are supposed to be all one way will only make some people "right" and other people "wrong," when there's nothing wrong that a different context wouldn't fix—and nothing right that the wrong context couldn't break.

That brings us to the most common issue for which couples seek sex therapy: low desire. Low desire is, by definition, a relationship issue. The partner with "low" desire is the one who wants sex too infrequently for the other partner's satisfaction. It's not that one person's desire for sex is somehow inherently "too low" or the other's is "too high." They're just different—at least in the current context.

But it's not the differential itself that causes the issue; it's how the couple manages it. Problematic dynamics emerge when partners have different levels of desire *and* they believe that one person's level of desire is "better" than the other person's. For example, let's say Partner A has more spontaneous desire and Partner B is more responsive. In this scenario, Partner A may feel rejected and undesirable because they almost always do the initiating, and then Partner B may start to feel pushed and judged and so will resist more. Partner A asks and asks and asks and feels rejected and hurt and resentful because Partner B keeps saying no, no, no; and Partner B feels defensive but also guilty and hurt because just being asked makes Partner B feel like there must be something *wrong* with them. Meanwhile Partner A may even start to wonder, "Am I broken? Do I want sex too much? Am I sexually obsessed or compulsive?" It's a mess.

I call it "the chasing dynamic."

And how do you "fix" the chasing dynamic?

We know the answer by now: The problem isn't the desire itself, it's the context. You need more sex-related stimuli activating the accelerator and fewer things hitting the brakes. The chasing dynamic hits the brakes.

To disrupt it, take away the chase. Take sex entirely off the table. No sex—whatever "sex" means in your relationship, but generally no genital contact and no orgasms with the other person present.

The purpose is to remove every trace of expectation or demand that sex will result from any physical contact between you. There might be other things you put off-limits, too—anything the lower-desire Partner B resists because of feeling pushed. Without the dread of "Ugh, what if this perfectly pleasant kiss turns into an expectation of sex that I still don't want?" both of you can relax and enjoy the physical intimacy you do share.

For how long? A month. Or two weeks, or three months. Long enough to feel like there's a substantial barrier.

When you take sex off the table in order to break down the chasing dynamic, both partners must agree fully and equally that they are creating the dynamic together. Neither partner is the problem; the dynamic they're stuck in is the problem.

After your phase of no sex, you can gently increase the intimacy of your physical contact, but ultimately the solution is attitudinal rather than behavioral. Feeling like there's something wrong with you (or with your partner) or feeling like your partner feels there's something wrong with you—these are desire-killing contexts, every time.

So look, I've got a message for Partner B, the one who feels chased. I'm going to say something, and you're going to believe me because all the scientific evidence is on my side. Actually, you'll believe me because what I'm about to say is *true*. Because in the patient corners of your heart, you've always known it's true. It's this:

You're not broken. You are whole. And there is hope.

You might feel stuck. You might be exhausted. You feel depressed, anxious, worn out by the demands of taking care of everyone else, and in desperate, dire need of renewal. You might be tired of feeling like you need to defend yourself and tired of wishing your body would do something different. You might wish that for a little while, someone else would defend you so you could lower your guard and just be. Just for a while.

Those are circumstances; they're not *you*. You are okay. You are whole. There exists inside you a sexuality that protects you by withdrawing until times are propitious.

I completely get how terribly frustrating it can be that your partner's body feels like times are propitious *right now*, while your body is still wary. And it's even worse because the more ready your partner's body seems, the more wary your body becomes. It sucks, for both of you.

But it's in there, your sexuality. It's part of you, as much as your skin and your heartbeat and your vocabulary. It's there. It's waiting. Just because you've had no call to use the words "calefacient" or "perfervid" lately doesn't mean they're no longer available to you. If the opportunity arises, there they will be, ready, waiting. Like your best friend, your sexual desire is waiting for your life to allow it to come out and play. Let it, whenever it feels safe enough.

And a brief message to Partner A—the one who wants sex and keeps asking for it: I know that it can feel like Partner B is withholding and I know that that can feel *deeply awful*. Your role in untangling your relationship knots is very difficult because it requires you to put down your hurts and be loving to the person who, it sometimes seems, is the source of those hurts. Boy, is that hard.

I know, too, that sometimes you might worry that you want sex too often, that you're making unreasonable demands, or that you're sick to want sex as much as you do. No, you just have a higher level of sexual interest than your partner does—your parts are organized in a different way. It's normal. Neither of you is broken, you just need to collaborate to find a context that works for both of you.

Give Partner B space and time away from sex. Let sex drop away from your relationship—for a little while—and be there, fully present, emotionally and physically. Lavish your partner with affection, on the un-derstanding that affection is not a preamble to sex. Be warm and generous with your love. You won't run out.

Put simply, the best way to deal with differential desire is: *Be kind to each other.*

Remember the sleepy hedgehog. Untangling the knots of sexual dy-namics in a relationship takes time, patience, and practice.

Because desire difficulties are the most common sexual problem, I devote many worksheets to it in the *Come As You Are Workbook*, which you can explore on your own, with a partner, or with a therapist. But per-haps the most powerful tool you can use during your sexual hiatus is to ask each other—and yourself—the question, "What kind of sex is worth wanting?"

Brakes are Merritt's big challenge, so she tried out a trick she learned in her political organizing days: Connect a behavior to your identity.

"Don't just run, be a runner," she told me. "If you run because you have to or you feel like you're supposed to, rather than because it's part of who you are, you won't run very far or very often, and you probably won't enjoy it much when you do. Ditto if I have sex because I feel like I'm supposed to. So how about I try on the identity of a woman who loves sex?"

"Worth a shot!" I replied.

So she tried it. And the first thing that happened is she got really angry.

"Why should I have to love sex?" she stormed to Carol. "Why can't I just be a woman who doesn't want sex? I'm tired of all the pres-sure to want sex more than I do and be a person I'm not!"

So she did a remarkable thing. She made that her identity: "I'm a woman who doesn't want sex." For while, she made her identity out of saying no. Angrily.

You'll remember from chapter 4 that anger is a "fight" stress response, and that stress responses are cycles that want to complete.

Merritt's life had afforded plenty of opportunities to start these cycles, but not nearly enough opportunities to complete them. She would just get angry and then shut herself down, get angry and shut herself down, hitting the brakes in the middle of the cycle. So she had a big backlog of incomplete stress response cycles.

Gloria Steinem said, "The truth will set you free. But first it will piss you off." What she didn't say is how to get from being pissed off to being free. They way to do it is to complete the cycle, walk through the tunnel.

So Merritt let herself experience her anger, because for the first time she was less afraid of the anger itself than of what might happen to her if she kept the anger locked up inside her forever. She let it all out.

And she made a fantastic choice about where to put all that non-specific anger: She channeled it into her writing, allowing her main character to brutally kill an enemy—and she shook and cried, teeth gritted, while she wrote. She could equally have channeled it into her morning walk, letting herself get aggressive with the big hills . . . or she could have channeled it inappropriately toward her family, taking her nonspecific anger and trying to make it specifically about them, using her anger as a weapon against others. But she's smarter than that. She made writing her outlet.

And the anger did what anger does when you allow it to blow through you like a strong wind: It blew itself out. It took some time, and it was uncomfortable. She had multiple decades of accumulated stuff to finish, and even a couple of weeks of No! was just a beginning. But what mattered most was that she had given herself permission to feel the anger and was learning the skill of allowing it to move through her, rather than holding on to it. She didn't do anything with it, she didn't direct it toward anyone, she just released it into the world; she just allowed it. Merritt trusted her body to release all that pent-up rage. She visualized it settling into the hole in the ozone layer.

Then one day, her anger blew itself into quietness, and into that silence she could ask, "So if I don't want sex, what do I want?"

She remembered the lube night, how good it felt to give pleasure, and the answers came fast and furious. She wanted to give pleasure, to connect, to receive pleasure and share it with the love of her life. To experience pleasure—all kinds of pleasure, but the pleasures of her own body especially—without the defenses that had kept her safe in an unsafe world.

It wasn't that she had never before had pleasure in her life, but it was so walled up by her self-protection that it couldn't expand beyond a small imprisoned domain within her.

When she focused on her partner's pleasure, her brakes weren't activated. She knew that much. How was she going to let go and experience pleasure for herself?

Orgasm.

But that's chapter 8.

"sex worth wanting"

When I teach about responsive desire, many students feel suddenly relieved and optimistic. They stop beating themselves up for not "craving" sex and instead get busy creating contexts that allow their brain to access enough pleasure for desire to emerge in response.

But one time I was out with friends and they asked, super casually, "So, hey, Emily . . . how do couples sustain a strong connection over the long term?" They were a young couple with two small children, and both of them worked full time.

I said what I always say. I explained responsive desire and concluded, "So you show up. You put your bodies in the bed, you let your skin touch your partner's skin, and—"

But when I said that, the lower-desire partner leaned away from the table with a cringe of disgust on her face.

"Okay, wow," I said gently. "So the problem isn't that you don't desire sex. The problem is you don't *like* the sex. Tell me what you don't you like about the sex."

And she talked about feeling ignored for years.

Ignored!

For *years*!

Of course she didn't like the sex! And if she didn't like it, of course she didn't desire it! In my all years of reading the research on sexual desire and talking with couples, therapists, scientists, and medical providers, I have seen no more powerful key to treating "problems" with desire than to understand that *it is normal not to want sex you don't like*.

As Peggy Kleinplatz and her team write, "[P]erhaps much of what is currently diagnosed as sexual desire disorders can be best understood as a healthy response to dismal and disappointing sex." [22]

When couples with low desire see Kleinplatz, a sex therapist and researcher, she asks them, "What kind of sex is worth wanting?"

Remember from chapter 4, "Sex That Advances the Plot"? It's sex that moves you toward a larger goal, powered by more than just the sexual response cycle. That's the kind of sex Kleinplatz's clients describe as "worth wanting." People don't just want orgasm, they want *more*.

And she helps them find their way to more.

She leads a team of researchers who have spent years studying people who self-identify as having extraordinary sex lives. These people come from every background imaginable, every sexual orientation, and every gender identity; some are kinky, some are vanilla, some are monogamous, some are not. They are many different ages, with different health statuses and different bodies. What they share is an inspiring capacity to access a sense of connection and pleasure through sexuality. The results of the research are described in *Magnificent Sex*, coauthored by Peggy Kleinplatz and Dana Ménard. They report that people who have these "Optimal Sexual Experiences" describe it with these eight major components:

- *Being present, focused, and embodied.* This is the experience of slowing down, letting go of distractions and inhibitions, and paying attention to what's happening right now, to the exclusion of everything else.

- *Connection, alignment, merger, being in sync.* Feeling aligned with your partner was described by many participants as essential to extraordinary sex.
- *Deep sexual and erotic intimacy.* Not just during sex, but in the whole relationship, these folks felt deep mutual respect, genuine acceptance and caring, and a deep and penetrating trust with their partners.
- *Extraordinary communication, heightened empathy.* Extraordinary lovers are also, necessarily, extraordinary communicators, which means they are extraordinarily empathic, tuned in to their partners' inner worlds.
- *Authenticity, being genuine, uninhibited, transparency.* Extraordinary sex involves emotional nakedness and a shame-free expression of sexual pleasures and desires, which usually requires going through a process of rejecting the sexual scripts and "shoulds" we're raised with.
- *Transcendence, bliss, peace, transformation, healing.* Yes, extraordinary sex can include feeling like you're melting into the universe and connecting with the divine in a way that changes you, heals you, and truly makes your life and relationship better. When our daily lives require a lot of boundary setting, our sex lives are transformed when we are willing and able to dissolve our boundaries with a trusted partner.
- *Exploration, interpersonal risk-taking, fun.* This is much like the "ludic factors" from chapter 3—the context of play, curious investigation, discovery, experimentation, creativity, and laughter.
- *Vulnerability and surrender.* Extraordinary sex is also characterized by profound trust, with nothing held back from partners, where your authentic self is received by someone else as a cherished gift.

These participants' experiences show us that great sex is not about what you do with your partner, nor about which body parts go where or how often, or for how long, but about how you share sensation in the context of profound trust and connection. Which sounds astonishing, right? But this research isn't about setting an impossibly high bar for the rest of us to reach for, it's about recognizing the difference between what great sex is really like and what most of us expect great sex to be like.

For example, notice anything missing from that list?

How about desire?

Turns out, desire is not a big part of extraordinary sex. It was not mentioned by the majority of participants, and was only rarely emphasized as a necessary aspect of great sex. "Lust, desire, chemistry, attraction" was, at most, a minor component of optimal sex. Even among people who have extraordinary sex, responsive desire is normal.

And they're not alone. "Optimal" sex is remarkably similar to the "good sex" described by survivors of child sexual violence, including qualities researchers identified as "communication," "openness, vulnerability," being "present in the moment," and being an "active, assertive participant."[23] In another study that asked twenty women to describe "good sex," only three participants mentioned being "in the mood" or "wanting it" as hallmarks of "happy and joyful" sex.[24] More common in these women's narratives of good, happy sex were comfort and naturalness, basic pleasure, and, above all, emotional connection.

But magnificent sex goes further and deeper. As Kleinplatz and Ménard put it, "Magnificent sex requires growing beyond the conventional scripts most people learn in their youth. Disappointing sex lives can change. The goal here is not merely to discard sex guilt, shame, and inhibition. Rather it is to jettison the entire aspirational package of paint-by-numbers sex."[25] People who have magnificent sex don't just show up and put their bodies in the bed—e.g., good sex. They deliberately cultivate a context that's "just safe enough" to dare the leaps of faith they take into the wild places in their souls. That's magnificent sex. And out-of-the-blue desire has almost nothing to do with it. When people who have magnificent sex want sex, they don't just want the sex we see performed in the mainstream media or porn. They want to know themselves and their partners more fully, and they want to be seen and known more fully, felt more deeply, held more closely. This is what I call "magnificent desire."

As Gottman and his colleagues found, couples who sustain a strong sexual connection over the long term prioritize sex—but. It's also normal for there to be times when sex drops off the list of priorities. When you have a new baby, when you're caring for a dying parent, when you're both overwhelmed with work, sometimes there truly isn't time or energy to pause and turn toward each other with erotic intention. You can allow that to be true, knowing that it's a phase of life you'll pass through together, and you'll find your way back to each other on the other side.

And it's worth considering what you will each find there, on the other side of your shared dry spell. Is it play or connection or exploration or peace? Or is it more like a chore or an obligation or drudgery? If you dread the idea of showing up and putting your body in the bed, lack of desire is not the problem. Lack of pleasure is the problem.

To want sex may be to want the routine pleasures of the body and of play. Sometimes, though, it is to want something *more*. Precisely what that "more" is varies from person to person and changes across our lifespans, but people who have magnificent sex describe sex that gives them far more than pleasure. It tunes them in to their partner at a deep, physiological level. It reveals their own desires to themselves, and it dares them to reveal those desires to a partner. It takes them deeper into their own personhood, even into their own divinity, and it takes them deeper into their partner's internal world.

Ask yourself: What kind of sex is worth wanting? And how far would you go to create that in your life?

sharing your garden

Just as women are often taught to trust cultural messages about their body more than their own internal sense of what's healthy, we often trust our partner's opinions and ideas about our sexuality more than we trust our own. Especially if our partner's sexuality is a better match with the standard narrative about how sex is "supposed" to work, we're ready to believe that we're broken.

But you know better now, and you know how to make the most of any desire style. Embrace responsive desire. Adore it. It asks that your partner help you in creating good reasons for you to be turned on.

Couples who sustain a strong sexual connection over multiple decades have two things in common: They are friends who prioritize sex. Let's be clear that it is normal for there to be times in your relationship when sex is not a priority, and in some relationships it is never a priority.

But when the context is right, you long to welcome someone into your garden. When you do, remember that they are used to working in their own garden, and their garden is different from yours. Their body, their brakes and accelerator, the seeds that their family and culture planted, the way they were taught to tend the garden, may be similar to yours, or they may be totally different. If you and your partner are different from each other, remember that *neither of you is better or worse*—even if one of you conforms more to the cultural standard. A potato farmer would be plain old wrong to suggest that your roses should be growing underground. What works for aloe won't work for tomatoes.

I hope that anyone you like and respect enough to invite into your garden likes and respects you, too. Just as you'd want to help their garden thrive, so they should want to help your garden thrive. They just might not know how to do it.

So you have to teach your partner about responsive desire. You're not broken, you're a tomato plant in a world that expects you to be an aloe. If you thrive on more water, tell your partner, and celebrate it together. Tell each other what contexts activate your accelerators and what contexts hit your brakes. Talk about the sexiest sex you've had together and what you can do to make it happen again.

Good things happen when you create space in your relationship for responsive desire. When Olivia and Patrick flipped their desire styles on their heads by making Patrick, with his context-sensitive desire style, the initiator, he had to figure out what exciting things would propel him from idling to interested. Olivia patiently allowed Patrick space and time to explore his desire, and she was rewarded with an intensity of erotic experience that her own spontaneous style rarely allowed for.

This level of mutual acceptance and self-acceptance is itself a specific and vital characteristic of the most exuberantly sex-positive context. It requires not simply being aware of how each person's sexuality works, but also accepting and welcoming those sexualities, just as they are. It's not how your sexuality works that matters; it's how you feel about your sexuality. How your partner feels about theirs. And how you both feel about each other's.

That right there is the ultimate sex-positive context. And it's what chapter 9 is about.

But before we get there, we need to talk about orgasm.

tl;dr

- Some people have a spontaneous desire style—they want sex out of the blue. Some have a responsive desire style—they want sex only when something pretty pleasurable is already happening. The rest, about half of women, experience some combination of the two, depending on context.
- If partners have different levels of sexual desire, the higher desire partner doesn't have the "right" amount of desire and the lower desire partner doesn't have the "wrong" amount of desire, and vice versa. People vary.

- If spontaneous desire goes away, it's because the context changed, not because someone is "broken." To bring spontaneous desire back, change the context.
- The most important thing to know about desire is that it's not what matters. *Pleasure* is what matters. If you create a context that allows your brain to interpret the world as a safe, fun, sexy, pleasurable place, you'll create *sex worth wanting*.

part 4

ecstasy for everybody

eight

orgasm

PLEASURE IS THE MEASURE

Spectatoring is the art of worrying about your body and your sexual functioning while you're having sex, and Merritt was a master practitioner. Rather than paying attention to the pleasant, tingly things going on in her body, her head would fill with anxious thoughts about how her breasts were moving or how she didn't have an orgasm the last time they had sex or what her inability to focus on pleasure meant about her as a sexual person. She worried about the sex she was having, instead of liking the sex she was having. And worry is the opposite of pleasure. Worry hit the brakes.

And when the brakes are on, orgasm doesn't happen.

Which is why she could easily count the number of orgasms she had had with Carol in their two decades together.

And which also is why she decided that orgasm was the perfect way to practice the pleasure—and the trust in herself that pleasure required—that she wanted to build in her life.

"Okay so tell me how," she said to me. "How do I make orgasm happen?"

"Ah, you don't make orgasm happen. You allow it," I said.

She nodded—then shook her head. "I don't know what that means."

I recommended she read Becoming Orgasmic *by Julia Heiman and Joseph LoPiccolo. Although it's written for women who've never had an orgasm, it's really the quintessential guide for all women who struggle with it. Merritt got the book, read it, and did some exercises . . . and then she did another remarkable thing. She decided not to try to have orgasms with Carol after all.*

"For me, having sex until I have an orgasm would be like running until I lose weight. It just doesn't work that way, and it's not even the point. So I'm going to stop trying."

Once a week, she and Carol traded massages and kisses and oral sex. They just played, and they paid attention to how it felt, and they weren't goal directed at all.

And guess what happened.

Yup.

This chapter is about orgasm, the full range of orgasmic experience available to women and the barriers that stand between women and ecstatic pleasure. Merritt's sensitive brakes made orgasm—especially orgasm with another person—elusive. She used the science I describe in this chapter to turn off the offs and find her way to a more profound experience of orgasm than she thought she would ever experience.

Several years ago I supported a friend as she began her first sexual relationship, having never so much as masturbated in her life, much less had an orgasm. She asked me questions from time to time, and one of them was, "How do I know when I've had an orgasm?"

I told her that orgasms feel different to everyone and that orgasms can vary from each other, depending on the mode of stimulation, whether you have a partner with you, maybe even where you are on your menstrual cycle—any number of factors. Sometimes you feel a rhythmic pulsing of the muscle around your vagina, sometimes not. The main thing most women describe most of the time is a sense of "doneness," a sense that you've crossed a threshold and something has completed. There's often a peak of tension where your muscles tighten and your heart pounds. Orgasms are like art, I told her. You know it when you see it. It may not be what you expect, but it will be different from everything else.

She nodded eagerly and said, "I think I had that!"

And then one day she walked up to me, grinning from ear to ear, and said, "It wasn't what I expected, but you were right. It was unmistakable."

This great variety and variability makes orgasm almost impossible to define—though scientists spend thousands of words puzzling over it. But when you strip it down to the universal essentials, here's what you get: Orgasm is the sudden, involuntary release of sexual tension.[1]

Notice how much is missing from that definition: genitals, muscle contractions, sexual behavior, pleasure, or indeed anything that specifies what it feels like or how it happened. Orgasms vary—from person to person, and from context to context. They happen while you're making love—and sometimes they don't. They happen while you're masturbating—and sometimes they don't. They can happen from clitoral stimulation, vaginal stimulation, thigh stimulation, anal stimulation, breast stimulation, earlobe stimulation, or mental stimulation with no physical contact at all—or not during any of these. They can happen while you're asleep, while you're exercising, or while you're in a variety of other completely nonsexual situations. They can be delightful, humdrum, spiritual, annoying, ecstatic, fun, or frustrating. Sometimes they're awesome. Sometimes they're not. Sometimes you want them. Sometimes you don't.

In this chapter, we're on a quest to explore the entire landscape of orgasmic experience, so that we can find our way to the secret garden at the center of it all. To begin, I'll tell you what orgasm is not: It is not a genital response, "pleasure," or hierarchical. I'll roll out a red carpet of statistics and a cheering crowd of women's stories, to normalize your experience (or lack thereof) of orgasm. Then I'll describe what it takes to overcome difficulty with orgasm, whether it's learning to have that first orgasm or learning to orgasm in different contexts. And I'll tell you how to find inside yourself the kind of orgasm that makes the stars explode into rainbows.

I want to prove to you that whatever your orgasms are (or aren't) like is normal, and I want to empower you to have the most profound and intense orgasms you're capable of, orgasms that turn the universe inside out. It's possible for everyone, I believe, but only when you let go of all the things orgasm isn't.

What to Do if You Find Yourself Spectatoring

Humans, unlike all other species, can be in control of their brains, rather than their brains being in control of them. We can notice what we're thinking or feeling, and we can do something about it. That's the key to managing any form of performance anxiety, including spectatoring: Notice what you're paying attention to, and then shift your attention to the thing you want to pay attention to.

This is easier said than done at first, but with practice it becomes easier done than said. Here's how:

Suppose you're standing in line at the grocery store or sitting on the bus. Let yourself notice your breathing. In. Pause. Out. Pause. In. Pause. Out. Pause. Two breaths, just like that. Notice, and smile. Notice five to ten times a day.

And notice, above all, when your attention wanders during those two breaths—which it will, that's normal. When you notice your mind wandering, smile at those other thoughts, let them go, and gently return your attention to where you want it to be. That skill right there? That's mindfulness. Noticing when your attention wanders from the thing you're trying to notice is the skill that will help you stop spectatoring, because you'll learn to notice the spectatoring and to redirect your attention to the sensations in your body.

nonconcordance—now with orgasms!

The first thing orgasm *isn't* is a "genital response."

In chapter 2, I described Masters and Johnson's research measuring the physiology of the sexual response cycle. There were certain cues that the research used to mark when orgasm happened, particularly contractions of the pelvic floor muscle at the entrance of the vagina.

Yeah, it's not that simple.

Remember nonconcordance from chapter 6—what your genitals are doing doesn't necessarily match what you're experiencing? There's evidence that this is true for orgasm as well—at least among women who are able to orgasm in a laboratory while their genital response is being measured.

For example, in one study, research participants were asked to masturbate to orgasm in the lab and then "grade" their orgasm on a scale of 1 ("weak or poor") to 5 ("most powerful or excellent").[2] Result? There was no relationship between the grades women gave their orgasms and the genital responses traditionally treated as "markers" of orgasm, such as number of contractions of the pelvic floor muscle.

Those rhythmic, involuntary contractions are perhaps the most nearly universal physiological marker of orgasm—but even that can't be relied on all the time. In one study, two out of eleven women exhibited no vaginal muscle contractions at orgasm.[3] And in another study, some women exhibited the muscle contractions without orgasm.[4]

In other words, genital physiological markers of orgasm are not always predictive of a woman's subjective experience of orgasm. Which makes perfect sense if you recognize that orgasm—like pleasure—isn't about what happens in your genitals, it's about what happens in your brain.[5]

no two alike

Which brings us to the second thing orgasm isn't: "a pinnacle of pleasure."

Orgasm is a lot like being tickled. Sometimes it can be fun, other times it's annoying, and sometimes it feels like almost nothing. Pleasure is a *perception* of a sensation, and perception is context dependent. That's just as true for orgasm as it is for tickling. But no one ever asks me, "Why is it that a lot of the time when my partner tickles me it feels fun and pleasurable, but then other times it really doesn't?" We all know intuitively that the perception of tickling sensations is context dependent. There's a time and a place for tickling.

And yet people ask me all the time, "How come sometimes my orgasms are great and other times they're really not?" It's as if we believe that orgasms are somehow different from other sensations, that they should feel a certain way, no matter the context.

All orgasms are the sudden release of sexual tension. How that release *feels* depends on context. Which is why some orgasms feel amazing and others . . . really, really don't. A handful of examples:

- A woman told me, red faced, that she had an orgasm during her exercise class. She was too embarrassed to feel any pleasure, and she was confused both by the orgasm and the lack of pleasure.[6]
- A friend with major depression said she could have orgasms but she didn't experience pleasure with them. I told her that was normal, that pleasure comes from context, and her context was gray and flat. Normal for a person with depression.
- An undergrad was turning paler and paler during my guest lecture about sexual assault. I had mentioned in passing that sometimes women have orgasms during rape and that that's basically just a reflex, it doesn't mean pleasure or consent. She came up to me afterward and said I'd changed her life with that one sentence.[7]
- A woman periodically orgasmed in her sleep and would wake up midorgasm, sometimes from a dream, sometimes not, but always puzzled by the warmth and pulsing that were not necessarily accompanied by any particular enjoyment.[8]

Orgasms differ from each other because the context for those orgasms differs. The quality of an orgasm is a function not of orgasm itself but of the context in which it happens.

all the same parts . . .

The third thing orgasm isn't: hierarchical. All orgasms are different, and there is no "right" kind or "better" kind of orgasm. It's even hard to say that there are different kinds of orgasm—because they're all made of the same basic parts (sudden release of sexual tension) organized in different ways.

Instead of thinking about "kinds" of orgasm, we can think about different *ways* to have an orgasm. Here's a small sample of the highly pleasurable orgasms women have described to me:

- Orgasm from clitoral stimulation.
- Orgasm from vaginal stimulation.
- Orgasm just from breast stimulation.
- Orgasm from having her toes sucked.
- Orgasm when her partner penetrated her (well-lubricated) anus with a finger, while pinning her to the bed by her hair. The most erotic sensation, she specified, was his warm palm resting gently on her butt cheeks.
- Orgasm when her partner slowly and gently stroked fingertips upward along her outer labia . . . again . . . and again . . . and again. She said, "What started out as an appetizer turned into the main course."
- Orgasm without any genital stimulation, while she was giving her partner oral sex. She was so closely tuned to his arousal that when he came, she did, too.

Are these clitoral orgasms, vaginal orgasms, breast orgasms, toe orgasms, butt cheek orgasms, labia orgasms, and oral orgasms?

Nope. Despite the painstaking efforts of women's magazines and even researchers to identify and label the various kinds of orgasms we could be having—G-spot orgasms, blended orgasms, uterine orgasms, vulval, and all the rest[9]—there can be only one. (Like *The Highlander*.) There's just the sudden release of sexual tension, generated in different ways. Anatomically, physiologically, even evolutionarily, it doesn't make much sense to talk about kinds of orgasms based on what body parts are stimulated.[10]

It's true that orgasms generated through clitoral stimulation often *feel* different from orgasms generated through vaginal stimulation. But it's also true that vaginally stimulated orgasms feel different from each other, and clitorally stimulated orgasms feel different from each other. Orgasms with a partner may feel different from orgasms without a partner, and orgasms with one particular partner may feel different from orgasms with a different partner, and orgasms with one partner may feel different from sexual encounter to sexual encounter. If we were going to categorize orgasms by how they feel, we'd need a new category for every orgasm a woman has.

Just as all vulvas are normal and healthy just as they are, so all orgasms are normal and healthy, regardless of what kind of stimulation generated them or how they feel. An orgasm's value comes not from how it came to be or whether it meets some arbitrary criteria but from whether you liked it and wanted it.

It comes to this: *Pleasure is the measure*. Pleasure is the measure of your orgasm—not what kind of stimulation created it, not how long it takes to get there, not how long it lasts or how strongly your pelvic floor muscle contracts. The only measure of your orgasm is how much you enjoy it.

Orgasms were not Laurie's problem. Once she got going, she found orgasm pretty reliable. No, Laurie's problem was that the stress in her life built a stone wall between her and sexual pleasure of any kind. She and Johnny were learning how to break down that wall by changing the

context . . . but following their "Can You Feel the Love Tonight?" suc-
cess, Johnny got cocky. He pushed his luck. He started asking and press-
ing and chasing, which made Laurie feel more and more pressured, and
soon she started to resent that he was asking, especially since he knew—
he knew—that when she felt pressured, her interest evaporated. It was
like he was trying to ruin it.

A perfectly normal and very tempting way for Laurie to think about
this situation would have been to say, "Look, my life is out of whack,
therefore my sexual interest is out of whack. So be it. No sex for me."
Plenty of women think the same thing every day and are rightly satisfied
to wait until their lives improve before they try to get their sex lives back
into whack. It's a matter of priorities. And in fact, the main reason Lau-
rie kept trying to want sex more was not that she really wanted to want
sex, but that Johnny wanted her to want it.

In frustration, she booted him out of the house for the day, sent him
with Trevor to the library so that she could have the luxury of the house
to herself, to do laundry, get some work done, and maybe, if she was
really lucky, take a nap.

And once they were gone . . . she missed them.

Often the best part of her day was her son's bath time—far from
being an exhausting chore or a hassle, she loved to splash and play
with him. And now she found herself looking forward to their return,
because . . . bath time!

And then she compared her feeling about sexy-pleasure to her feel-
ing about mommy-pleasure. She thought, "It's not selfish of me to enjoy
being with my kid—enjoying it makes me a better parent! So how come
I can give myself permission to have that pleasure, but I can't give my-
self permission to enjoy other kinds of pleasure?"

Something clicked. She had all kinds of insights about having
been taught that being a mom was the best thing about being a woman
but having sex wasn't okay, that the pleasure of delicious food was
blocked by guilt about her body . . . lots of things. But in the end,
something just clicked, and she let go of a bunch of stuff. She started

wondering if maybe sex could be for her pleasure, too, rather than something "for Johnny."

Laurie remembered Johnny saying, "Maybe it's about what it feels like, not about where we are or what we're doing." Maybe she could try that, try paying attention to what it feels like, regardless of what's going on.

your vagina's okay, either way

I get asked a lot about orgasm during penile-vaginal intercourse, so let's spend a little time with that. As we saw in chapter 1, the clitoris is your Grand Central Station for erotic sensation. The dominance of the clitoris in women's orgasms explains why 80–90 percent of women who mastur-bate typically do so with little or no vaginal penetration, including when they use vibrators.[11]

But ya know, there's this old saying: "It ain't the size of the boat, it's the motion of the ocean."

The wisdom this attempts to convey is that it's not the size of the penis penetrating the vagina, it is the collaborative stimulation between partners (or possibly the skill of one or the other of the "sailors") that creates pleasure and orgasm for a woman during intercourse.

The fact is, it's not the size of the boat, and it's not the motion of the ocean either. Women just vary. Despite what you've learned from movies, romance novels, or porn, in reality less than a third of women are reliably orgasmic with vaginal penetration alone, while the remaining two-thirds or more are sometimes, rarely, or never orgasmic with penetration alone.[12]

Yet women ask me all the time, "Why can't I have an orgasm during intercourse?" The reason they can't is very likely the same reason most women can't: Intercourse is not a very effective way to stimulate the cli-toris, and clitoral stimulation is the most common way to make an orgasm happen. In fact, research has found that one reason why women vary in how reliably they orgasm with penetration is the distance between the cli-toris and the urethra.[13] It's essentially a matter of anatomical engineering.

So the question is not so much why some women aren't orgasmic from vaginal penetration as it is why *are* some women? There are several hypotheses, but probably the two best contenders are: (a) stimulation through the front wall of the vagina of the urethral sponge (the female homologue of the prostate and the original hypothesized source of the "G-spot"); or (b) the vestibular bulbs, extending down to the mouth of the vagina from the head of the clitoris. But in the end, the answer is: People vary.[14] People vary in the layout of their genitals and the sensitivity of the tissue. My guess is that both of these hypotheses have merit, but you can imagine how challenging it is to get funding to do research on women's orgasm, so it may be a while before we know for sure.

Now, if penetrative orgasms are comparatively uncommon, why do women ask about it so often? Why is it so often viewed as "the right way to orgasm"?

And the answer is, of course, "Ugh, patriarchy." Men-as-default again. Centuries of male doctors and scientists—Freud is often pointed to as a key offender here, and rightly so—claimed that orgasms from vaginal stimulation are the right, good, normal kind, and clitoral orgasms are "immature."

But it's men-as-default in a different way from how it worked with arousal and desire. Culture sanctions spontaneous desire as the "expected" kind of desire because that's how men experience desire (though not all of them do, of course), and culture sanctions concordant arousal as the expected kind of arousal because that's how men experience arousal (though, again, not all of them do) . . . but if women's expected kind of orgasm is whatever men experience, then that should be orgasms from clitoral stimulation, since anatomically the clitoris is the homologue of the penis. To say that women should have orgasms from vaginal penetration is anatomically equivalent to saying that men should have orgasms from prostate or perineal stimulation. Certainly many men *can* orgasm from that kind of stimulation, but we don't judge them if they don't, and they don't usually wonder if they're broken if they don't.

So apparently, according to cultural myth, women should be just like men—with concordant arousal and spontaneous desire—right up until we actually start having intercourse, and then we're supposed to function in an exclusively female way, orgasming from a behavior that also happens to get men off very reliably. Men's pleasure is the default pleasure.

Camilla, with her relatively insensitive sexual accelerator, had always been slow to orgasm and wasn't all that interested in having more of them. They were a lot of work most of the time, and not rewarding enough to bother. She had masturbated very rarely in her life, and then more out of curiosity than desire. And she often wasn't too interested in having an orgasm when she had sex with Henry.

Henry, gentleman that he was, had a hard time with this.

"If you don't have an orgasm, how can I tell that I satisfied you?" he would ask.

"You can tell because I say that I'm satisfied! If I eat less pizza than you and say that I'm full, do you doubt me? If I have two glasses of wine and feel as tipsy as I want to feel, am I supposed to try to increase my tolerance? If I read a novel but don't feel compelled to read the sequel, is there something wrong with that?"

"Of course not," was the answer to all three questions.

"So why," Camilla said, "do you need me to experience some physiological reflex in order to feel like I've had an awesome time?"

"Because that reflex is how I know you were satisfied!"

It was one of those disagreements where each person's point of view is so obvious to each person but so foreign to the other person that they didn't even know where to start. Their solution was the kind of problemsolving that shows me they'll be together for decades. They literally switched places—they swapped seats—and took on the other person's point of view. Camilla argued for Henry, and he argued for her.

Camilla said, "If you don't have an orgasm, then I can't feel certain that you really liked and wanted the sex we had."

Henry said, "If I don't have an orgasm, all that means is I had as much pizza as I wanted, it was great, and now I'm all set."

And then he said, "Oh."

Camilla continued, "But pizza isn't the same as sex. Sex has a destination, a goal, a 'Final Real Ultimate It,' and if you don't have that, then I've failed you!"

And then she said, "Oh."

Henry said, "The only way you fail me is if you can't accept me the way I am."

Camilla said, "Your orgasm tells me you accept me the way I am."

And they both said, "Oh."

And then she moved from Henry's chair to sit next to him with her head on his shoulder. "Does my orgasm really mean that much to you?" she asked.

Henry answered, "If I make you a special pizza and you only eat one slice, how can I not wonder if you didn't like it?"

"Hm. We'll have to see if we can think of a logical solution," Camilla said.

They do, in chapter 9.

difficulty with orgasm

Very early on in grad school, two classmates and I sat together before class one fall afternoon, talking about—what else?—sex. One of them was recently married but had yet to have an orgasm with her new husband.

"I can orgasm on my own, but somehow when he's with me, I can't get there," she said, her eyebrows sad and her mouth quirked in confusion. "I know he feels rejected and takes it personally, but I love him, I *want* to have an orgasm with him. I just can't."

She blamed herself. Her husband blamed himself. Both felt ashamed and broken and anxious that they would never experience "normal" sex.

At the time, I had no idea what was going on, but not long after that I began a clinical internship where I learned that such challenges are both common and eminently solvable.

Distress about orgasm is the second most common reason people seek treatment for sexual problems (after desire), occurring in about 5 to 15 percent of women.[15] Difficulty with or absence of orgasm in certain contexts is very common. For example, only 11 percent of college women report having an orgasm the first time they "hook up" with a new partner, compared with 67 percent of college women having sex in the context of a relationship of more than six months' duration.[16] Around 12 percent of women have not had an orgasm, or are unsure whether they've had an orgasm, by age twenty-eight.[17] And there probably are some women who never experience orgasm—the research indicates something like 5–10 percent.[18] I met a woman in Boston who told me she had her first orgasm of her life in her seventies, so I'm convinced that anyone can have an orgasm, though for some people it really requires just the right context to make it happen.

Orgasm is, in some ways, like riding a bicycle—it comes more naturally to some people than others, and if you're not motivated enough to keep trying until you figure it out, you'll never learn. And it's a rare person who genuinely needs to learn to ride a bicycle.

Most problems with orgasm are due to too much stimulation to the brakes—too many worries, too much stress, anxiety, shame, or depression, including stress, anxiety, shame, or depression *about* orgasm.[19] If you're interested enough to want to have an orgasm, chances are you can, given the right stimulation and a context that lets you turn off the offs. And if you can orgasm now in an *ideal* context, chances are you can orgasm in a new and different positive context—like with your partner.

Never Had an Orgasm . . . as Far as She Knows

Students laugh when I add "as far as she knows," but several times I've talked about what childhood masturbation to orgasm is like—squeezing your legs around a swing set pole or rocking your vulva against a stuffed animal, as well as touching your genitals with your hands or pressing your pelvis into the mattress—and people have said, "Oh! So that's what I was doing!" Memories of childhood orgasm are often more like sleep orgasms or exercise orgasms; they're not particularly erotic. You're not having sexual fantasies to fuel your accelerator, but nor do you have a decade or more of cultural shaming to hit your brakes.

The most common word women used to describe their struggle with orgasm is "frustrated."[20]

So how does frustration work?

Imagine a little monitor, like a referee, sitting next to your brain's emotional One Ring.[21] She's got two jobs, this monitor:

1. She watches to make sure the world is behaving according to her expectations (expectations set by all her previous experience with the world).
2. She directs the investigation when there is any discrepancy between the world and her expectations.

When the world is meeting her expectations, the monitor feels satisfied. Nothing is lacking. But sometimes there is a gap between the world and the expectations—some ambiguity needs to be resolved, some novelty needs to be explored to see where it fits in the expected order of things, or some very appealing stimulus needs to be approached and obtained.[22] When this happens, she goes into command mode. She makes *reducing the discrepancy* her purpose in life. Her entire world is made up of these three things:

- The goal of closing the gap—which might mean resolve the ambiguity, explore the new thing, approach the incentive, or simply complete the task.
- The effort you're investing in the pursuit of that goal—the attention, resources, and time you're allocating to it.
- The progress you're making toward that goal.

So the little monitor keeps track of how much progress you're making in relation to how much effort you're investing. She tallies your effort-to-progress ratio, and she has a strong opinion about what that ratio should be. This opinion is called "criterion velocity."[23] And this is where it gets really interesting.

When the monitor feels that you're making good progress—when you're matching or exceeding the criterion velocity—she is satisfied, motivated, eager. But when the monitor feels that you're not making enough progress, she becomes frustrated, and she prompts you to increase your efforts to get closer to your goal. If you still aren't making enough progress to satisfy the little monitor, she begins to get angry . . . and then enraged! And eventually, if you continue to fall short, at a certain point the little monitor gives up and pushes you off an emotional cliff into the "pit of despair," as the monitor becomes convinced that the goal is unattainable. You give up in hopeless desolation.

When you're continually "failing" to reach orgasm, your little monitor grows frustrated and then angered and eventually despairing.

When I teach about the little monitor, my students' eyes widen and their jaws drop. The little monitor is a crucial part of your sexual wellbeing, but she shows up in nearly every domain of life. If you've felt the thrill of winning a race or a game, that's your little monitor having her criterion velocity satisfied—effort-to-progress ratio met or exceeded! If you've experienced road rage, that's your little monitor's how-long-this-trip-should-be-taking criterion velocity going unmet—effort-to-progress ratio much too large! If you've ever collapsed in a hopeless heap in the face of failure, that's your little monitor reassessing a goal as unattainable, uncontrollable. The little monitor and her opinions about how effortful things should be is the foundation of a wide range of frustrations and satisfactions, orgasm not least among them.

impatient little monitors

Our culture absolutely teaches us to have impatient little monitors, with criterion velocities set as small as they can be, which means many of us are easily frustrated, enraged, and eventually despairing when we can't easily achieve our goals—including orgasm. If you feel like you should have had an orgasm already, but you haven't, you'll begin to get frustrated . . . and will that frustration make it easier for the brakes to release?

Quite the opposite.

The little monitor is a gremlin of irony.

Unlike the One Ring and the brakes and accelerator, we *can* create intentional change in the little monitor. Actually, humans may be the only species that can do something deliberate about this kind of frustration, and I bet if you think critically about it for a minute you can work out how to do it. There are three potential targets of change, right? [24]

- Is this the right *goal* for me?
- Am I putting in the right kind of *effort*, as well as the right amount?
- Am I realistic in my *expectation* about how effortful this goal should be?

Suppose the goal is orgasm in ten minutes or orgasm from vaginal intercourse. If orgasm doesn't happen that quickly or from that kind of stimulation—which it doesn't for most women—your monitor will begin to get frustrated.

And does frustration fuel your accelerator . . . or does it hit the brakes?

Yeah. Brakes.

The central approach to orgasm difficulties is to change the goal by making *pleasure* the goal, not orgasm. When you begin to feel frustrated, remember that's your little monitor feeling like you're not making progress toward the goal of orgasm. That's the time to remind yourself that you are already at the goal as long as you are experiencing pleasure.

Orgasm isn't the goal. Pleasure is the goal.

For women who sometimes (or always) struggle with orgasm, I've included step-by-step instructions for practicing the skills of paying attention to pleasure and letting go of the goal, including ways to adapt the skill to having orgasm with your partner (see appendix 1).

Vibrators

At least half of women in the United States have used a vibrator, and these women are more likely to report better arousal, desire, and orgasm.[25] Eighty to ninety percent of those women report experiencing no side effects, and of those who did report side effects like numbness or irritation, nearly all of them said it lasted for less than a day.

A small study of women using vibrators as part of sex therapy found that women varied a great deal in their response to the vibrator and had a wide range of feelings about the experience.[26] Initial resistance ("I should be able to orgasm without having to use a 'tool'") and concerns about whether vibrator use somehow disrupts sexual connection with a partner ("Am I cheating on him with it?") often gave way to a sense of freedom and exploration. While there was a great deal of variety, even in a sample of only seventeen women, the overall experience was a new kind of pleasure and opening up their perspective on the idea of sexual autonomy.

You'll recognize the worry that it's not "natural" as the "sanctity" moral foundation that I described in chapter 5. The idea that there's a pure, good, natural way to have an orgasm and a wrong, bad, unnatural way to have an orgasm is a cultural pigeonholing of experience shaped by those three messages—Moral, Medical, and Media—from chapter 5.

The concern people most often bring to me about vibrators is that they'll get "addicted" to them, but it doesn't happen. Here's what does happen: Orgasm with vibrators occurs relatively quickly for many women because a vibrator provides such a high intensity of stimulation. And some women get very comfortable with how quickly they orgasm with their vibrator, which leads them to forget how long it took without the vibrator. And when they get frustrated by how long that takes, the frustration makes it take even longer. But by this point in the chapter, you probably know the answer to this problem: frustration = impatient little monitor. So change the goal, change the effort, change the criterion velocity. Pleasure, not orgasm, is the goal. If it takes five minutes, that's five minutes of pleasure. Hooray! If it takes thirty minutes, that's thirty minutes of pleasure! Also hooray!

ecstatic orgasm: you're a flock!

Orgasms can certainly happen in subideal or even adverse contexts—but the brain-melting, toe-curling, turn-the-stars-into-rainbows type of orgasm happens only in a spectacularly good context.

And what exactly is that context?

The answer to that question is the same as the answer to this question: Why would wearing socks make it easier to have an orgasm?

Some students asked me this while I was eating lunch and chatting with them. Brittany and Tiffany and I were talking about sex science, as usual.

"Huh?" I said through a mouthful of salad.

"I read about it on the internet. Socks make it easier to orgasm," Brittany said.

"Oh! Well, if you read it on the internet, it must be true," I joked.

"No, I read it, too!" said Tiffany. "I think it was a real thing. I'll find it and send you the link."

She did, and it was true . . . kind of. It turns out putting on socks made it easier for research participants to orgasm while masturbating in a brain imaging machine.

You have to wonder why. Are all brain imaging sex research participants secret foot fetishists? Does it have something to do with redirecting blood flow?

Nothing so arcane. Gert Holstege, the researcher leading the study, said the research participants "were uncomfortable, because they had cold feet."[27]

Put on socks, have warmer feet, and have easier orgasms. Even in the unerotic setting of a research laboratory, such a small shift can make a difference.

And that type of shift is the key to moving from very nice orgasms to award-winning orgasms. Here's the science that tells you how.

All your internal states—your physical comfort, hunger, thirst, sleepiness, loneliness, frustration, etc.—interact deep in the emotional

One Ring of your brain, and they influence each other in a process called "integration."[28] When one state—like cold feet—interferes with another state—like sexual arousal—that's "subtractive integration."

And when one state actively reinforces another state, that's "additive integration." That's what Laurie and Johnny experienced when they were trying not to have sex and Johnny also told her the reasons he loved making love with her. The proximity seeking of their attachment mechanism mixed with their sexual motivation, and both were intensified.

Additive integration can be an unmitigated good in your sexual experience . . . and sometimes additive integration can draw you into unhealthy dynamics, too. Olivia's tendency to feel "driven" toward orgasm when she's stressed is one example. The stress adds to her sexual motivation in an unhealthful way. And the women in John Gottman's research who experienced intense sex after their partners were physically abusive were experiencing additive integration: The threat to their attachment made it important that they bond with their partner. Sex is a crucial attachment behavior for human adults, so the two states—separation anxiety plus sexual stimulation—reinforced each other, to give rise to a sexual experience that was intense but ultimately unsafe and unhealthy.

You can visualize the effect of integration if you think of your brain as a flock of birds.

Do you know how a flock works? There is no leader, no individual who controls the group and says, "Hey, everybody, let's fly this way!" Instead, each bird is individually following a set of rules, along the lines of, "Avoid predators, fly toward the magnetic pole, and also stay by your neighbors." When all the birds are following these rules, flocking emerges without anyone having to be in charge.

If you think of your brain as a flock, then each "bird" is a different drive or incentive motivation system—stress, attachment and social belonging, food appetite, curiosity and exploration, thirst, sleep, plans for the future, emotional baggage from the past—all your competing roles and identities in life are there in the flock. You can think of your sexual accelerator and brakes as birds in the flock, too.

Ultimately, the "you" that is consciously aware of being a "self," an individual distinct from other individuals, is a composite self, a hologram built of these multiple motivational and cognitive processes all engaging with the environment and with each other, in a noisy, messy, multidirectional tug-of-war. As a person capable of desiring multiple things at once—food, sleep, sex, warmth, to be left alone, etc.—you are a *collective of motivations*. A flock.

Complex things can happen in a flock because there's no leader. If one bird notices a predator, it will fly away (following the "avoid predators" rule), and then all the birds around it will follow, pulled as if by a magnetic force, not because of the predator but because they're following the "stay by your neighbors" rule.

And if your brain is a flock, then orgasm is a destination the flock can fly toward—a magnetic pole—and sexual pleasure is *the flock itself*. Sexual pleasure emerges, like flocking behavior, from the interaction of all these different birds.

The more birds you have flying toward orgasm, the greater the pleasure you experience. If some of the birds are flying toward orgasm but others are trying to accomplish some other goal—as in, you're trying to masturbate to orgasm, but your feet are cold—the "flock" that is your brain will not move simultaneously in the same direction. Some of the birds may arrive at orgasm, but the experience won't be the same as if *all* the birds got there.

"Subtractive integration" happens when the birds flying toward foot warmth actively tug at the birds who would otherwise fly toward orgasm. Put on socks, and those birds are freed up and can move toward orgasm. "Additive integration" happens when the birds flying toward an attachment object (your sex partner) tug their neighbors to fly faster and more enthusiastically. Fall wildly in love, and your flock may rush to orgasm at the littlest prompting.

The technical language for what I'm describing here is that sexual pleasure is an emergent property of a complex dynamical system. But all you need to remember is that peak sexual pleasure happens when the whole collective works together, when all the birds are flying in the same direction, when all of your motivation systems are coordinated and attuned to the environment in a way that gives rise to every system moving collectively toward orgasm. Turn on all the ons and turn off all the offs. Get rid of all the predators and pile on different kinds of incentives at the magnetic pole: attachment, curiosity, expansive pleasure—all the motivations orgasm can fulfill. The more the whole system is moving in the same direction, the more the orgasm takes over your whole awareness, with every cell of your body focused on the same thing: pleasure. Peak sexual pleasure requires *all of you*.

The most pleasurable orgasms happen when every part of you is present and collaborating in pursuit of one shared goal: ecstasy.

If you haven't figured it out by now, Olivia—the marathon runner, the intense, driven, sensitive accelerator woman—is a perfectionist. So here's what she said when she learned about the little monitor:

"Well that explains . . . you know, my whole life."

Perfectionists set goals that are impossible—and if they somehow manage to achieve a goal, they assume that goal must be worthless and they set another, even more impossible goal. Which puts them in a state of perpetual dissatisfaction.

"And then I'm my own lion, like, all the time," Olivia said. "And when you add the cultural brainwashing, that puts me in that out-of-control place with sex.

"Jesus," she added.

Her experience moving at Patrick's slower pace showed her the potential in slowing down and allowing more of herself to align with the goal of experiencing sexual pleasure—to take control of the little monitor, so that it didn't take control of her.

As an experiment one Saturday afternoon, Olivia tried meditating while she gave Patrick an erotic massage. She practiced keeping her mind quiet and focused on the present. Any time a stray thought entered her mind, she acknowledged it fleetingly and then let it go, returning her attention to the sensation of her partner's skin under her hands. She found herself becoming aroused, and she noticed that her thoughts were increasingly turning toward orgasm, as her little internal monitor got impatient to reach her goal. But each time she felt pulled toward orgasm, she took a deep slow breath and returned her attention to Patrick.

She didn't hit the brakes, she just took her foot off the accelerator.

After Patrick's orgasm, they switched, and Olivia kept her attention tuned to the sensations of her body. As her arousal grew, she continued to breathe deeply and slowly, not allowing her abdominal muscles to tense too much.

The result was an orgasm that lasted several minutes as her body shuddered and rolled, and Patrick stayed with her, holding and kissing her, fingers pressed against her vulva. It ended with joyful tears and a kind of bubbly chattiness quite unlike Olivia's usual postorgasmic self. She felt open and raw and tender.

She told me later, "It was like being way out in the center of the ocean, when I usually just surf on the shore. Bigger and slower . . . and scarier, too, in some ways. I was all the way open. I had to let go of all control. I had thought I was an erotic powerhouse because I could have a lot of orgasms and because I wanted sex often. But it turns out my greatest erotic power only emerged when I stopped pushing toward orgasm and just allowed pleasure to be still inside me."

Not every woman wants to experience this kind of radical vulnerability with her sexuality. Not every woman trusts her partner enough to allow herself to let go so thoroughly. Not every woman has a life that allows the time—an hour, generally, for most people—and relaxation necessary to get there.

But given the right context, I believe every woman is capable of it, and, in my opinion, every woman deserves the opportunity to try it. Even if you don't experience minutes of oceanic ecstasy, it will still be an hour well spent!

how do you medicate a flock?

The kitschy 1968 cult movie *Barbarella* imagines a forty-first century in which people take "exaltation transference pellets" to have orgasms, to save on the mess and bother of having sex. You take the pill, sit palm to palm with your partner, and within a minute your body pulses and your hair curls. Boom. Done.

You can see the appeal. I want ecstasy to be easy and instantaneous, too, like taking a pill. Many of us live lives of constant tension, doubt, obligation, and effort. Couldn't pleasure, of all things, just happen, without our having to work at it?

The closest we can come to that in the twenty-first century is a vibrator. The right vibrator provides an intensity of stimulation for your accelerator that you just can't replicate with any nonmechanical stimulation. Even if your brakes are still on—you're stressed out, anxious, sad, or frustrated—a vibrator is often intense enough to generate an orgasm much faster than manual stimulation.

A vibrator won't necessarily persuade all the birds to fly in the same direction. It provides high-intensity stimulation for the parts of your brain that respond to sex-related stimuli; it can turn on the ons like nobody's business, but it doesn't turn off the offs.

The idea of pleasure as an emergent property of the interactions of a collective of desires (aka a flock) is what makes medicating pleasure, arousal, desire, and/or orgasm so difficult. A drug would have to twiddle not just the accelerator and brakes but also the stress and the love and the body image and trauma history and the relationship trust and the other things that are known to impact women's sexual wellbeing. Tugging one bird toward orgasm won't help you if the rest of the birds are busy avoiding predators.

Pleasure is an emergent property of the interaction of multiple systems—it's a *process*, not a state, an *interaction*, not a specific area of the brain or the body. Pleasure is the whole flock. Pleasure is all of you.

flying toward ecstasy

What the science gives us is this: To have more and better orgasms, turn off all the offs and slow down how you turn on the ons. Give your whole brain time to get on the orgasm train.

But what science can't give you is *permission* to experience ecstatic pleasure. In the end, that's the key to spectacular orgasms. And only you can give you that. Science can't tell you how to feel about your orgasms. Science can tell you only that how you feel about your orgasms changes your orgasms. Science can tell you that feeling shame, judgment, frustration, and fear about orgasm will diminish your orgasmic experience, while acceptance, welcoming, confidence, and joy will expand your orgasmic experience. Science can tell you that your brain is like a collective of desires, and the more the collective collaborates, the more of you can move toward ecstasy.

But not one word of that science makes you more or less entitled to the pleasure of your own skin and mind and heart. Your orgasms belong to you, and all the science in the world can't make you more delighted with them or more afraid of them or more curious about them. The science can't do that. Only you can do that.

You were born entitled to all the pleasure your body can feel. You were born entitled to pleasure in whatever way your body receives it, in whatever contexts afford it, and in whatever quantities you want it. Your pleasure belongs to you, to share or keep as you choose, to explore or not as you choose, to embrace or avoid as you choose.

So, if you wanted to, how would you find your way to ecstasy? How would you get all the birds flying together in the same direction?

Patience, practice, and a sex-positive context.

You already know how to create a sex-positive context. And you understand how to build patience—by training your little monitor to make sure you've got the right goal, the right kind and quantity of effort, and the right criterion velocity.

Which leaves us with the "practice" part.

Practice what?

Practice turning off the offs. Here's how:

The brain states that are dragging parts of your flock away from orgasm—stress, worry, spectatoring, chronically wondering if your kid is going to knock on the door, or even just literal cold feet or other physical discomfort—need to be taken seriously and have their needs met. They need to be respected and treated like the sleepy hedgehog from chapter 4.

Be kind and gentle with each of the offs, listen to what they need in order to feel satisfied, and then satisfy them. Go back to your context worksheets: What hits your brakes? Consider the things in your environment and also your own thoughts and feelings. What context do you need in order to turn off those offs?

Most of the offs women experience have *nothing to do with sex*, and many of them have straightforward, pragmatic solutions. Chronically stressed? Complete the cycle with a good cry, a brisk walk, a primal scream, or other physical release, as described in chapter 4. Give yourself a solid twenty to sixty minutes to allow the stress of the day to wind down with whatever rituals or practices help. Baths, walks, exercise, cooking, meditation, yoga, a glass of wine, whatever works.

Constantly monitoring for footsteps in the hallway? Arrange for a time when no one else is home.

Tired? Take a nap, or even just rest for twenty minutes. Squicked out by grit on the sheets? Change them! Cold feet? Put on socks! Sometimes it really is this simple.

Other offs are more complex and require longer-term solutions, such as those I addressed earlier: self-critical thoughts or other body image challenges, lack of trust in your relationship, trauma history, sexual disgust. It took decades of planting and cultivation to create the garden you currently have. It won't change overnight. Give yourself permission to make progress gradually, and celebrate all the incremental steps between where you are now and where you'd like to be.

And the most important turn-off-the-offs practice of all: self-kindness. Too often women get stuck in their sexual growth because they can't get past their belief that something "shouldn't" hit their brakes. It shouldn't turn them off to have the lights on, they shouldn't be so hung up about their bodies. "Should" is all about what you're "doing wrong."

Pop quiz: Does a belief that you're Doing Something Wrong with sex hit the accelerator . . . or the brakes?

Yeah.

So when something hits the brakes, what do you do? You take it seriously. Listen to it. Be gentle with it, like a sleepy hedgehog. Even if you wish something like having the lights on didn't hit your brakes, the fact is it might, and that's okay. It's also okay to wish it didn't. But believing it "shouldn't" only hits the brakes more. Recognizing that frees you up to do something about it—something like having sex with unlit candles in the room for a week or two, then with one lit tea light candle, then two, then three . . .

You see, sex is not context dependent—sex can happen more or less anywhere. *Pleasure* is context dependent. Create a context where you can experience pleasure, and sexual ecstasy will follow, given time, practice, and genuine solutions to turn off the offs.

Appendix 2 offers instructions for achieving ecstasy. Try it! Remember: Each member of the flock has its own needs and motivations. Turn off all the offs, and turn on all the ons.

Merritt had believed all her life that orgasm was supposed to be easy, and that her struggle with it made her a freak. She believed that it was supposed to feel a certain way and have a certain effect. But she wanted to learn to trust herself, so that she could open the door wide to pleasure. So she stopped comparing her experience with her expectations and simply allowed her experience to be what it is. She just enjoyed the sex she was having instead of worrying about whether it was the sex she "should" be having. She created an environment of acceptance, where the parts of her mind that needed to worry, that needed to avoid something bad happening, could instead move toward something good. It took time. And practice. And positive nonjudging.

Did it work? For her, it did.

Merritt is a writer and she was raised religious, which might explain the email she sent me near the end of her don't-have-an-orgasm-with-Carol experience. Or it might not. Lots of people start talking about God and spiritual experiences when they find their way to ecstasy. The language of mundane human experience, anatomy, physiology, even relationship doesn't feel large enough to contain it.

Anyway, this is what she wrote:

> *No storm can shake my inmost calm*
> *While to that rock I'm clinging.*
> *Since Love is lord of heaven and Earth,*
> *How can I keep from singing?*

It's from a hymn called "How Can I Keep from Singing?" Pete Seeger and Enya and many others have recorded it. It's about what happens when you make contact with the peace at the center and core of yourself, which is the same peace at the center and core of the universe, and it resonates through you, like you're a bell that's ringing.

That is what happens when you turn off all the offs and allow all the ons to focus on one shared goal: pleasure.

tl;dr

- Orgasms happen in your brain, not your genitals.
- Less than a third of women are reliably orgasmic from vaginal penetration alone. The remaining 70+ percent are sometimes, rarely, or never orgasmic from penetration alone. The most common way for women to orgasm is from clitoral stimulation. And we are all normal.

- All orgasms are created equal. It doesn't matter what stimulation generates them, the quality of an orgasm can only be determined by how much you enjoy it.
- To have bigger, better orgasms, turn off more of the offs, and turn on the ons more gradually.

nine

love what's true

THE ULTIMATE SEX-POSITIVE CONTEXT

Laurie and Johnny had tried all the tricks. But in the end, what made the difference was when Laurie chose pleasure—for herself.

Armed with the decision to start paying attention just to what it feels like, Laurie went to a weekend mindfulness retreat called something like Awakening the Feminine Divine. She practiced yoga and slept nine hours a night. She ate mindfully. She breathed mindfully. She shared her feelings with strangers, made new friends, and found a renewed sense that she was not alone in her struggles. And, let me just emphasize this, because Laurie would want me to: She slept nine hours a night.

She focused for twenty-one hours (the time she wasn't sleeping) on really noticing what it felt like to be alive and move through the world.

And she came back a new woman.

"I can't be a source of joy in the lives of the people I love if I can't even be a source of joy for myself," she announced. "And what I want, more than anything, is to be a source of joy in the lives of the people I love."

"Wait a second, Johnny and I and everyone else who loves you, we've all been saying that for months," I said. "What did they do to you at that retreat?"

"I stood in the Divine Gaze of Lakshmi, the Goddess of Auspicious-ness, and I felt my own power and beauty," she recited seriously. Then she cracked a grin and said, "You'll probably tell me that's just a meta-phor for activating something or other in my mesolimbic whatever, but I don't give a damn about the science. It frickin' worked."

This chapter is about the science Laurie doesn't give a damn about.

It frickin' works.

Here we are in the final chapter. So far we've learned that in some impor-tant ways your sexual response may not follow the "standard narrative" of sexual functioning:

- You may have more or less sensitive brakes and a more or less sen-sitive accelerator.
- Your genital response may not predict your subjective experience of being "turned on."
- Your sexual desire may emerge in response to pleasure, rather than in anticipation of pleasure.

All of which may come as a surprise if you're among the 10–20 per-cent of women whose sexual response is similar to the "standard narra-tive." (We also learned that people, especially women, vary widely from each other and change substantially across their life spans.)

Which brings me to confidence and joy.

"Confidence and joy" is a phrase I've used a lot for many years, but it didn't become the core of my work until, one semester, a student raised her hand in the middle of a lecture and said, "Wait, Emily. Could you please define those terms? What are confidence and joy?"

"Uh . . ." I said. "Let me get back to you."

And I went home and thought about it for a week. I read a lot of sci-ence. I reread a lot of my own blog posts. I watched my dogs romp in the yard. And when I got to class the following week, this is what I told my students:

fidence is *knowing what is true* about your body, mind, sexuality, life. Knowing that your genitals are made of the same parts as everyone else's, organized in a unique way. Knowing about the brakes and accelerator. Knowing about context and about the difference between liking, wanting, and learning. Knowing about arousal nonconcordance and responsive desire. Knowing what's really true, even when it's not what you were taught "should" be true. Knowing what's true, even when it's not what you wish were true.

Joy is *loving what is true* about your body, mind, sexuality, and life. Loving your genitals, your brakes and accelerator, and the way your brain responds to context. Loving the context itself. Loving arousal nonconcordance and responsive desire. Loving what's true, even when it's not what you were taught "should" be true. Loving what's true, even when it's not what you wish were true.

I said all this to my class, and the student who had originally asked me to define my terms raised her hand again.

She said, "Joy is the hard part."

In the years since, students and workshop attendees have agreed: Joy *is* the hard part.

Fortunately, the research shows us a practice that can teach us, well . . . how to joy. This chapter is about that practice. We'll begin with why confidence alone is not enough, then describe the process of "reality checking," to bridge from confidence to joy. We'll conclude with an exploration of "nonjudging," the key skill that bridges from joy . . . to long-lasting, sustainable access to ecstasy.

why confidence is not enough

Consider "Ms. B.," whose story opens a *New York Times* article about women's sexual medicine. The article begins:

Since Ms. B. entered her mid-40s, she says, sex has been more about smoke and mirrors than thunder and lightning. She is rarely if ever interested enough to initiate it with her partner of 10 years, and she does not reach climax during the act.

She wishes it were otherwise.[1]

Having gotten this far in the book, you'll recognize that Ms. B.'s desire style may be responsive rather than spontaneous, and it sounds like she's not reliably orgasmic with intercourse. Both of these put her squarely in the majority.

And she wishes it were otherwise.

Which is perfectly understandable. I imagine she learned (as most of us do) that spontaneous desire and orgasms with penetration are normal, and since that's not what she's experiencing, she believes she's abnormal. Broken. If I believed I were broken, I would wish it were otherwise, too.

But she's not broken, she's normal—in fact, she's typical. And what effect does wishing her normal sexuality were otherwise have on her sexual wellbeing? Does it activate the accelerator or hit the brakes?

The result is that she herself describes herself as "sexually dead."

And it doesn't get much worse than that.

For someone who feels this bad about her normal sexuality, knowledge alone (and the confidence that comes with it) often falls short.

I've seen confidence fall short at least three different ways. First, you may know something is true, but still believe it's a failing. A reader of my blog learned about responsive desire but commented, "I think you're glossing over the fact that 'responsive desire' is a lesser desire than [spontaneous] desire."

Most women have "a lesser desire?" Yeowch.

The construction of responsive desire as "lesser" is not a "fact," of course; it's a value judgment, an opinion. "I shouldn't have to put all this effort in," you think. "Desire should just *happen*." And beneath that thought is the feeling, "I shouldn't be like this. I'm inadequate."

And is the feeling "I'm inadequate" going to activate the accelerator, or hit the brakes?

Right.

A second way confidence alone falls short: Sometimes sexual confidence is like body acceptance. You welcome it enthusiastically as you learn about it, and then you try to put it into practice. You look at your body in the mirror and write down everything you see that you like . . . but then you go out into the world and some misogynist asshat sneers at you and whispers something foul. No matter how much you practice turning toward your body with kindness and compassion, some part of the world will still tell you you're broken. And maybe that part of the world is your partner or your friends or your family or even your medical providers. It's hard to hold on to what you know when everyone around you is saying you're wrong.

And a third way confidence falls short: It isn't just outside voices protesting that you're still broken. You spent decades *internalizing* messages—Moral, Media, and Medical—about the ways you are damaged, inadequate, and diseased. Part of you might have become convinced that you're a disgusting failure who can never show her true sexual self to anyone. You may "know" it's not true, but that small part of you, cowering in a corner of your psyche, cannot be persuaded by any amount of science.

If you know something is true, but you resent it or judge it or hate it or feel ashamed, it can't expand your sexual wellbeing. If you know it's true, but important people in your life disagree, confidence can slip out of your hands like soap in the bath. And if you know something is true, but part of you has been so wounded that knowledge alone can't heal it, then confidence per se can't be the gateway to ecstasy. You need joy, too. You need to love what's true.

The first step to move from knowing what's true to loving what's true is expanding what it means to "know what's true."

step 1: your feelings are always true

Beyond the facts of your sexuality are the facts of your feelings about your sexuality.

Notice how you feel.

When simply knowing something is true isn't enough to release you from the myths and lies, you can return to the little monitor in charge of your frustration or satisfaction. When you experience your sexuality in the way your monitor expects, she feels good. When you experience your sexuality in a way that creates a discrepancy between your experience and the monitor's expectations, the monitor gradually becomes frustrated . . . and then angry. Eventually she pushes you off an emotional cliff into the pit of despair, as she gives up and decides you can't achieve your goal.

We saw in chapter 8 that there are three ways you can address the gap between where you are and where you expect to be. You can ask yourself, "Is this the right *goal* for me?" or, "Am I putting in the right amount of the right kind of *effort*?" or, "Are my *expectations* of how much effort this particular goal requires realistic?" All three of these are different kinds of *reality checks*.

We've seen these reality checks in action throughout the book: in chapter 5, when Laurie decided to stop trying to want sex with Johnny and just allowed herself not to, she closed the gap between where she was and where she wanted to be, which opened the door to affection without performance demand. In chapter 8, when Olivia meditated her way to an extended orgasm, she was practicing being present as she was, rather than pushing forward to some goal. She kept the same goal—ecstasy—but she changed the kind of effort she was investing. And in chapter 7, when Merritt, instead of trying on the aspirational identity of a woman who loves sex, embraced the identity of a woman who did *not* want sex, she was changing the kind of effort she invested, to attain her goal of trusting herself. The result was not sinking down forever into a state of not wanting sex—on the contrary! Allowing herself to be where she was opened the door to where she wanted to go.

By contrast, Ms. B.'s little monitor is deeply dissatisfied, convinced that there is a wide gulf between where she is and where she ought to be—and furthermore, she feels utterly helpless to do anything about it. She's in the pit of despair. She has collapsed into the hopeless grief that comes when the little monitor is convinced that a particular goal is unattainable. Did she try to create change and fail and try again and fail again, or, when her sexuality fell short of the mark (a mark set by cultural standards that have nothing to do with reality), did her body go right to shutdown? I don't know. But I do know that her little monitor can learn, and Ms. B. can teach it—if she chooses to. She can change her goal, her effort, or her expectations.

For example, suppose you're not reliably orgasmic from intercourse. Because you've read chapter 8, you know you're normal and you've learned about other ways to have orgasms, especially from clitoral stimulation. Knowledge! But what if you still feel frustrated about your lack of orgasms with intercourse? Or ashamed? Or sad? Or judgmental? Will that make it easier or more difficult to try out new ways to access pleasure and orgasm? Yeah. This is when it's time for a reality check. What is your goal? What effort are you investing? What are your expectations for how much effort it will take to attain this goal?

For many of us, the goals we have in mind—such as spontaneous desire or orgasm with intercourse—are not goals we have chosen consciously for ourselves. We absorbed them from our culture in the form of sexual scripts. These scripts provide the structure for the beliefs through which we interpret the sexual world. These scripts, too often, are barriers between us and joy.

Over the last few decades, research has followed how sexual scripts have changed in Western culture. Recent cultural scenario scripts may include, "Men's sexuality is simple and women's sexuality is complex," or, "Women don't have as strong a sex drive as men," or, "Orgasm is central to a positive sexual encounter."[2]

The scripts are written into your brain early, by your family and culture—remember the Moral Message, the Medical Message, and the Media Message from chapter 5?

But scripts aren't about what we intellectually believe is true. They act as a template for our emotional One Ring and for our little monitor to filter and organize information. You can disagree with a script and still find yourself behaving according to it and interpreting your experience in terms of it.

The technical term for this process of organizing your experience according to a preexisting template is "probabilistic generative model." It means that information—anything you see, hear, smell, touch, or taste—goes first to your emotional brain, where prior learning (possibly about lemons or little rat jackets, possibly about body image or sexual disgust) plus your present brain state (stress, love, self-criticism, disgust, etc.) combine to shape the initial decisions your brain makes about whether to move toward or away from that information. That initial decision sets off a series of expectations about what else might be true and what might happen next.

A simpler way to understand it, I think, is in terms of maps versus terrains.

the map and the terrain: a tool
for reality checking

A map is an abstract representation of something that exists in reality. It's a simplified picture of an actual place that exists. A place that does not look like the map. If we think of our sexual scripts as a "map," we can begin to compare it to the terrain—the real thing that actually exists, which the map is supposed to represent. You try to navigate the sexual world by following the map.

If the map doesn't match the terrain, is the terrain wrong?

No. The map is the problem. The mapmakers made a mistake or based the map on another map they saw instead of on the terrain itself, or might even have wanted to mislead you deliberately. Maps can be wrong, and that leaves you looking from the map to the terrain to the map again, feeling lost.

Sadly, most people's sexual maps are hugely out of date. We're like

Brendan Fraser's character in the movie *Blast from the Past*. His parents raise him in a bomb shelter, mistakenly believing that there was a nuclear attack in 1962, and when he finally goes out into the world thirty-five years later, he is navigating through a landscape that has almost nothing to do with what he has been taught. Like him, we've got this map in our heads and we step into the terrain expecting to find a path in one place, and instead we're instantly lost.

As we saw in chapter 5, our maps may have places that are way more than thirty-five years out of date.

But perhaps the biggest challenge is that when the map and the terrain don't match, our brains try to make the map true, forcing our experience into the shape of the map. "No, no, this is the trail," we say as we stumble through the thicket. "It says so on the map."

A couple years ago, I talked to a young woman who had learned most of what she knew—or rather, what she thought she knew—about sex by watching porn. She was genuinely surprised when nothing in her first sexual encounters happened the way she expected. She thought orgasms would come easily and often. She thought direct clitoral stimulation would always make her see stars. She thought wrong. But she kept trying to make her experience match the map. She kept behaving the way people in the videos behave, assuring herself that because she was doing what she was supposed to be doing, the feeling she was having must be pleasure.

It was months before the dissonance between what she expected to experience and what she was actually experiencing became clear to her. That's when she came to me, convinced that she must be broken.

When I told her that women are more likely to have orgasms later in a relationship than the first time they have sex with a new partner, she truly didn't believe me, so convinced was she that the map was right and the terrain—her body—was wrong.

I also told her that pleasure is context dependent, so that even clitoral stimulation doesn't feel good unless it's in the right context. "Like tickling," I said. "If it doesn't feel good, that just means you haven't got the right context yet. When clitoral stimulation doesn't feel good it's not because your clitoris doesn't work, it's usually because you're not turned on enough yet."

The first step toward joy is recognizing a mismatch between the map and the terrain, with the knowledge that the terrain is always right.

Olivia is One Big Yes when it comes to sex, which has the potential to create profound ecstasy . . . or profound self-doubt and anxiety, not to mention the chasing dynamic. And it all depends on how she feels about her capacity for Yes.

Way back at the beginning of the first chapter, Olivia found out that her "map" wasn't true—the story she told herself about wanting sex because of her hormones was a metaphorization that shielded her against the cultural messages that would tell her she's a bully.

But she drew a new map—grounded in the science and in nonjudgmental attention to her own internal experience. She realized that her sensitive accelerator could team up with her little monitor to create that out-of-control feeling, and they could also team up to create joyful pleasure. She got the out-of-control feeling when she allowed the spiral of stress/self-criticism/stress to escalate. She got the joyful pleasure when she learned to deescalate by allowing the stress to run its course, without hitting either the brakes or the accelerator.

"Slow down. Stay still." That's Olivia's advice for all higher-desire partners. "Don't chase, don't push or pull. Be like the person with the broom on a curling team. Clear the path to sex."

When there's no pressure to perform, Patrick is creative, curious, playful, and unabashedly experimental. He knows what a gift Olivia's sensitive accelerator can be, and he's aware of the challenges it presents.

So. When Olivia finished her master's degree, he set up a kind of sensual treasure hunt for her, involving most of her collection of toys, two kinds of lube, at least one instance of being carried, naked, handcuffed,

and blindfolded, down the hallway to another apartment in their build-
ing, and several of their very good friends. (Which may be the best "sci-
ence made my sex life better" story I've ever heard.)

At the end of it, over a giant meal, Olivia, swimming in endorphins
and oxytocin, asked Patrick to marry her—mostly kidding.

Mostly.

Some people don't believe me when I tell this story, which I share
with permission. Oddly, it's the only story they don't believe, as if an un-
conventional, wide-open celebration of pleasure is the only real cause for
skepticism around women's sexuality. But it's out there, pleasure and un-
ruly exploration and partners who adore a woman's whole sexual being,
from the wounds of her past to the wilds of her imagination. Stories like
this give me hope that more and more women will heal from shame and
find love that embraces their whole selves, eroticism and all.

Olivia is One Big Yes. It's a gift. It's a challenge. She maximizes
her sexual potential when she allows her sexual response to grow to ca-
pacity, without pushing in any specific direction.

Slow down. Stay still. Don't push or pull. Allow sensation to take
over.

Your best source of knowledge about your sexuality is your own
internal experience. When you notice disagreement between your experience and your expectations about what you "should" be experiencing—
and everyone does, at some point—always assume your experience is
right.

You can also assume everyone's experience is different from
yours—as are everyone's ideas about what their experiences "should"
be. Everyone's terrain and everyone's map are different from everyone
else's. When the map doesn't fit the terrain, the map is wrong, not the
terrain.

I've used hypothetical twins a few times throughout the book, but
this time I can use real-life twins to illustrate my point. My sister Amelia and I are identical twins. We have the same DNA, were born within

minutes of each other, grew up in the same house, went to the same schools, watched the same TV shows, and read many of the same books. And yet by the time we started our sexual lives, we had very different maps in our heads.

I had my own unique version of the Media Message in my head. I believed that the Ideal Sexual Woman was an adventurous, noisy female whom men lusted after for her skill and her enthusiasm. She was—of course!—easily orgasmic from penetration, she experienced spontaneous desire, and her vagina got *so wet*. Any woman who didn't want to try new things was a prude, hopelessly hung up and neurotic.

Notice that the Ideal Sexual Woman does not necessarily enjoy a great deal of pleasure; she just appears to experience pleasure. That's what a sexual woman should be, as far as my culture had taught me, and so that's what I performed. By the time I started my first sexual relationship, I was a sexual product, processed and packaged for the pleasure of others.

This map was so potent and persuasive that I couldn't separate what I believed I should be experiencing from what I actually was experiencing. At eighteen, in my first sexual relationship—with a man who would later become my stalker and threaten to kill me—I would dream that my partner was hurting me, and in my dream I would laugh. I would laugh until even I didn't know if I liked being hurt.

At the time, I had no idea how screwed up that was.

It was toward the end of that relationship (which ended when I called the police) that I first looked at my vulva and wept.

I had the improbable good fortune of beginning my training as a sex educator in the same semester that I got into that abusive relationship. At the same time that I was marketing myself as a sexual product, in accordance with my instruction by women's magazines, romance novels, and porn, I was learning the truth about sexual wellbeing. Over the next decade, I gained a vast store of knowledge, but more importantly I gained a radically more healthful attitude: that a woman's body and her pleasure belong to her and no one else; that it's possible to say no to intercourse without saying no to all the other things that come with it—the love and the affection and the pleasure and the play; and that my own internal experience was a legitimate guide for whether or not I wanted to try something.

Perhaps most compelling of all, I recognized that it is normal for my internal experience sometimes to be self-contradictory (I'm a flock!), and the more gently and patiently I pay attention to the full depth of my own internal experience—especially if I am gentle and patient with the uncomfortable feelings—the more I experience confidence and joy.

Amelia, by contrast, had her own unique version of the Moral Message in her head by the time we got to adolescence. Smart women didn't want sex, she believed. Smart girls were interested in minds, not bodies; only stupid girls were ruled by their "base animal instincts." This is a classic middle-class Victorian attitude. She believed the Ideal Sexual Woman was more or less asexual, and she took her own lack of interest in sex as evidence that she was intelligent.

And then she started having sex, and eventually even liking it! So she opened up a new area on the map, explored new territory. She created space for the idea of sex as recreation, a fun thing to do on a Friday night, as long as X-Files wasn't on. She redrew the map to allow for both being smart and enjoying sex as a source of pleasure, but still she was navigating through a fairly narrow band of terrain.

It was only when she met the man she would eventually marry that she began experiencing sex as something through which she could discover human connection and a deeper pleasure than mere entertainment, a pleasure connected to her personhood.[3] This was a whole new map, which included terrain she had never known existed—though it had been there the whole time, unexplored.

She's been with the same partner for decades and has had many of the same pleasures and struggles that so many women experience in long-term relationships. And while I had the great good fortune of becoming a sex educator, she had the good fortune of having a sex educator for a sister, so she could be among the women who called me or emailed me to say, "Is this normal?" She's like a lot of women—context-sensitive desire and nonconcordant arousal. And so, like a lot of women, she sent my blog posts to her husband and said, "This! See?"

We're an example of how even genetically identical gardens, planted with very similar seeds, may still grow into very different terrains. It turns out she's got slightly more sensitive brakes than I do, and I've got a slightly more sensitive accelerator. So perhaps the Media Message was a slightly better fit for my native sexuality and the Moral Message a slightly better fit for Amelia's, and so different ideas took root and grew.

For both of us, by the time we began having sex with partners, we had some set ideas about what that experience was supposed to be like. And both us of, like nearly all women, went through a time of realizing how poorly prepared we were and then relearning what it meant to be a sexual woman.

For both of us, education about the science of sexual wellbeing helped us draw maps that better represent our sexual terrains, which in turn allowed us to communicate about our sexual wellbeing more effectively with our partners. It also helped us let go of judging other women for having experiences that contradicted our own—because it turns out everyone really is just different. But it was our willingness to believe our own internal experience, even when it didn't match what we thought we "should" be experiencing, that empowered us to embrace that science—the science in this book.

But learning what's true, redrawing the map, was not the hard part—not for either of us, not for the woman who learned about sex from porn, and not for most of the women I talk with.

Upon learning that they are normal, many women instantly feel liberated and satisfied with their sexuality in a way they never have before. The light goes on and they say, "My map was wrong all along and I'm actually normal!" But some women, even though they can accept that their responsive desire or nonpenetrative orgasms are normal, can't accept that this new kind of normal is something worth being. Knowing how your sexuality works is important. But welcoming your sexuality as

Emily Nagoski, Ph.D.

it is, without judgment or shame, is more important. And that's the hard part for a lot of women.

And when it is, that's where nonjudging comes in.

step 2: the hard part (or, how to "nonjudging")

If you're anxious about your sexuality, or you're angry with yourself for feeling (or not feeling) a certain way, or you're ashamed, what you will often do is put it that feeling about your sexuality in a box and hide it somewhere deep inside you. And the feeling sits in that box, waiting to complete its cycle. You haven't gotten rid of it, you've just put it on hold. But eventually it has to complete it cycle.

Suppose that instead of putting it in a box, you're aware of your feelings about your sexuality and are curious about them, or you're gently affectionate toward them, as you would be toward a tearful newborn or a sad, shy kitten. Or suppose you're simply neutrally observing from the sidelines of your own internal experience. These kinds of compassionate self-awareness create a context that doesn't hit the brakes and instead allows your internal state to complete its cycle.

I used to think that it was the *awareness* of your internal state that mattered, but in study after study, "observation" of internal state is not a significant predictor of wellbeing. Instead, the most important variable is "nonjudging."[4]

People who score low on mindfulness assessments that measure nonjudging agree with statements like, "I tell myself that I shouldn't be thinking the way I'm thinking" and "When I have distressing thoughts or images, I judge myself as good or bad, depending on what the thought/ image is about." People who are high on nonjudging say the opposite: When they have distressing thoughts, they simply recognize that that's what's happening, without judging it as good or bad, right or wrong. In other words, nonjudging allows you to feel what you feel, whether or not it makes sense to you, whether or not it's comfortable, whether or not it's what you believe you should be feeling. Nonjudging is neutrally noticing your own internal states. With nonjudging, it doesn't matter how you feel; what matters is how you feel about how you feel. And the most wellness-promoting way to feel is . . . neutral.

I'll illustrate this with my favorite research paper on the subject, a small study that looked at the role of mindfulness in people's experiences with generalized anxiety disorder.[5] The researchers measured, among other things, participants' anxiety symptoms and the degree of interference with daily life these symptoms caused, along with participants' responses on the Five Facet Mindfulness Questionnaire (FFMQ). Two of the five facets are "observe"—noticing your internal experience—and "nonjudge"—not categorizing your internal experience as either good or bad.

So dig this: Research participants who were less affected by their symptoms did not experience lower frequency or severity of symptoms, nor were they more aware of their internal state—the "observe" factor. Nope. The people who were less impacted by their symptoms were those who were more nonjudging! In other words, it isn't the symptoms that predict how much anxiety disrupts a person's life, it's how a person feels about those symptoms. It's not how you feel—it's not even being aware of how you feel. It's how you feel about how you feel. And people who feel nonjudging about their feelings do better.

The body of research specifically measuring nonjudging in relation to sexual functioning is steadily growing. In an early, tiny study of sensorimotor sex therapy, women in the treatment group reported that the therapy helped them to feel less like they "should" be experiencing something in particular and more able to be gentle and forgiving with themselves.[6] (Sound like anything from, oh, say, chapter 5? Remember self-compassion?)

But the real win in recent research on nonjudgment and sex is the development of the Sexual Mindfulness Measure, based on the FFMQ. This development found that sexual mindfulness—nonjudgmental awareness—predicted sexual satisfaction, especially in women.[7] Notice, though, it's not awareness per se that makes the differences. For example, overall body awareness doesn't affect arousal nonconcordance—it's not that people are "unaware" that their bodies are doing stuff.[8] It's that people can be aware and nonjudging, or they can be aware and judging, afraid, ashamed, frustrated, resentful, or despairing. It's the nonjudgment that makes the difference.[9]

Let's look at five situations where nonjudging can help: feelings that happen for "no good reason," healing trauma, resolving pain, increasing pleasure, and mourning the "shoulds."

What says, "You are awesome in bed!" more clearly than your partner's orgasm?

Your partner not being able to stop themselves from having an orgasm—especially if that partner has a slightly stubborn accelerator.

Camilla thought through the "If I make you a pizza and you only eat one slice, how does that make me feel?" problem logically and came to a smart conclusion:

They made a rule against her having orgasm.

They could do anything else they wanted, but Camilla wasn't allowed to have any orgasms. It's a reverse psychology trick that you'd never expect to work in real life—"You don't want to have an orgasm? Fine. You're not allowed to have an orgasm!"—but it actually does.

The rule did two things. First, it genuinely took away performance pressure from Camilla and frustrated expectations from Henry. They could both relax and forget about it, which made them both feel better.

It had another impact, too. Henry had already shifted the way he thought about foreplay and was thinking of their entire relationship as an opportunity to tease Camilla's ticking pilot light. The new rule took that to another level.

See, taking orgasm off the table put Camilla's little monitor in a puzzling situation. If Henry was, say, going down on her, and she felt so aroused that she thought she might have an orgasm, she'd remember that she wasn't supposed to have an orgasm, and then the little monitor would keep checking her arousal level and comparing it with her goal state of not having an orgasm, which means her monitor would keep thinking about orgasm and how close she was to it.

Embedded in the thought "Don't have an orgasm" is ". . . have an orgasm." And if I say to you, "Don't think about a bear," what's the first thing that happens?

Orgasms aren't as automatic as thoughts, but in the right, sex-positive context, if you make orgasm against the rules and then give the person a lot of time to try not to have an orgasm . . . I'll just say it's a fun game and you might want to try it sometime.

Which brings me to the orgasm your partner can't stop themselves from having.

Henry is just about as smart as Camilla. I know this because one day she called me and said that he had stuck to their agreement better than she had—he was using a vibrator on her and she had been close and actually wanted *to have an orgasm, but he stopped before she got there.*

She was frustrated. And even a little pissed. But hey, the rule was her idea. He was being a gentleman.

He did this two more times—got her close, then backed off.

Because he is such a gentleman.

And eventually he got her so close that she genuinely couldn't stop herself from having an orgasm. Which is a neat trick—women don't have a "point of no return" for orgasm the way men do for ejaculation. To get a woman to be unable to stop herself from coming takes a high level of persistent arousal.

And yes, again, being a sex educator is the best job in the world when people tell you stories like this.

nonjudging 1: "no good reason"

Here's something I hear a lot: "If there is no solution to an uncomfortable feeling, there's no point feeling it."

Sure there is!

The point of feeling a feeling you can't do anything about is to let it discharge, complete the cycle, so that it can end.

I was talking about the nonjudgment research with my colleague Jan, and she told me she'd had a relevant experience over the weekend. She had noticed herself getting disproportionately enraged about a small thing—losing a stamp when she was trying to mail a letter—and she later made the connection that her anger wasn't really about the stamp. The anger had been activated the night before, when she watched a movie about a misogynist jerk, which triggered her own history with a misogynist jerk from two decades ago.

"So what did you do with the anger?" I asked.

"I told myself I didn't need to feel angry, because the jerk is gone from my life now."

"You judged? You hit the brakes?"

"What else was I supposed to do? Be mad at a guy I haven't seen in twenty years?"

The threat—the misogynist jerk—wasn't around anymore to fight against or run away from . . . and yet she had these feelings. So what could she do with them?

She could complete the cycle. The Feels exist in her body, without reference to the jerk whom she successfully left behind.

But this is not the habit most of us learn early in our lives, and it takes practice. When we have feelings we can't really do anything about and we don't know how to let ourselves simply feel without doing anything, our brains will look for some situation it *can* do something about, and it will try to impose the feelings on that situation.

So don't be mad at the guy who's long gone. Just allow the anger to move through you. It doesn't matter what it's about, it's just random Feels, left over from the past, that have to work themselves out. Don't hit the accelerator, but don't hit the brakes either. Notice the anger and allow it. Be still, and it will blow through you like a hot desert wind or a typhoon.

nonjudging 2: healing trauma

When a person experiences trauma, it's like someone snuck into their garden and ripped out all the plants they had been cultivating with such care and attention. This is particularly awful when the person who tears up the garden is not a stranger but someone the person trusted. There is rage and betrayal, there is grief for the garden as it was, and there is fear that it will never grow back.

But it will grow back. That's what gardens do.

And you facilitate that growth by allowing the garden to be what it is, in process, rather than what it was or what you wish it were. How? Self-compassion: self-kindness, common humanity, and mindfulness. Patience. Feeling okay with feeling not-okay.

Healing hurts. If you break your leg, there is no stage in the healing process when your leg feels better than it does after it has healed. There is pain and itching and loss of strength. From the moment your leg is broken, it continues to feel bad . . . until, gradually, it starts to feel less bad. It's appropriate that it hurts.

If you numb physical pain, healing can still happen. Alas, if we try to "numb" emotional pain, we get a break from the pain . . . but the healing is put on pause, too. People who are more evolved than I am can go through emotions like grief and panic without suffering, but for most of us, heart healing doesn't happen without suffering. Sorry.

I worked with a survivor of sexual violence who was early in her healing process. She was by turns angry and despairing and frozen—and she was afraid all the time. Though she had been practicing meditation for a long time, the intensity of her emotions felt too big for her to allow them to move through her; they bottlenecked inside her. She felt panicked and stuck in the pain. She wanted to know what to do with all the feelings, how to fix them. She wanted to know how to stop hurting and how soon the pain would end.

"All I can tell you," I said, "is that everything you're experiencing, all the contradictory feelings and all the pain, is a normal part of the healing process. Everyone goes through it differently, and there's no way to know how long it will last. It sucks for a while, and then gradually it gets better. But I can tell you this for sure: Every single survivor I've ever known has found their way through it."

We sat in silence while she absorbed the idea of not knowing when the pain would end and having to simply trust her body and her heart to heal in their own time. At last she said, "It's like . . . I'm sitting with a stunned bird in the palm of my hand. If I get tense and try to hurry it, it will just stay frozen. But if I'm still and patient long enough, the bird will wake up and fly away."

Yes. That.

nonjudging 3: pain

There are only two sexual experiences I'm willing to call "abnormal": lack of consent and unwanted pain. If everyone involved is glad to be there and free to leave whenever they choose, then anything they do is normal. And if everyone is experiencing sensations they want and like, then anything they do is normal. But unwanted pain with sex—pain with penetration, pain with genital contact, any unwanted pain—is not normal.

And a key to treating such pain is nonjudgmental awareness of those sensations.

This is a tricky one because, on the one hand, nonjudgmental awareness is a key to healing from sexual pain, but on the other hand, many women have been told all their lives that pain with sex is normal, it's just part of life, have a glass of wine, why are you complaining, get over it. Can we be nonjudgmentally aware of our pain and also take it more seriously than our culture has taught us to believe we "should"?

I had a chance to talk with Caroline Pukall, coauthor of *When Sex Hurts: A Woman's Guide to Banishing Sexual Pain*. She pointed out that some women tolerate pain with sex "just because they have this belief that, 'I guess some pain is to be expected.'"

She went on, "There's something about women bearing pain longer than they need to," perhaps in other domains of their life, as well as in sex. They tolerate pain because they think that is their only option, that effective treatments aren't available (they are!), or that the hassle of seeking treatment isn't worth the potential benefit (it is!). And medical professionals sometimes reinforce this tendency by not taking pain seriously or assuming that if there is no infection or injury, the pain is "all in her head."

If women (and our medical providers) had the same criterion velocity about our genital pain that men have about their own genital pain, women would never hesitate to seek treatment. Our willingness to tolerate greater effort—in this case, pain—is learned. And it can be changed, simply by becoming aware of it and allowing the possibility that it could be different.

This is the kind of story that fills me with righteous anger: A woman in a wheelchair approached me after a public talk and told me that my presentation was the first time she had ever heard that there are effective treatments for vaginismus, chronic tension of the pelvic floor muscle, which makes penetration of the vagina either impossible or very painful. Her doctors had never mentioned that her vaginismus might be treatable.

Why didn't they tell her? Was it because the doctors didn't know? Was it because they didn't feel comfortable talking about sex with any twentysomething woman? Was it because it didn't occur to them that a woman in a wheelchair has just as much right to a satisfying sex life as any other woman? I don't know. But I can't help wondering if those doctors would have ignored complaints of sexual dysfunction and pain from a twentysomething man in a wheelchair.

Here is an ultrashort primer on the nature of pain:

All pain is created in the brain, in response to the body's signals that there is some kind of threat.[10]

Pain is a signal that your brain perceives a threat, and you might need help. If you use your own internal experience, rather than culturally imposed criterion velocities, as your most accurate source of knowledge about sex, you'll be able to hear your brain's signal that you need help, and you'll take it seriously.

Part of what complicates our understanding of women's sexual pain is that there are so many different potential "threats," from well-understood tissue damage, such as tearing during childbirth or allergic contact dermatitis, to less understood hormonal changes with menopause that lead to dryness and atrophy, to newer domains of study, such as hypersensitivity of the central nervous system in response to childhood abuse or neglect.[11]

This is as literal as it gets: It's not how you feel (pain). It's how you feel (tolerant or not) about how you feel. Nonjudging doesn't mean resignation. It means turning toward what's true with kindness, without self-criticism. With nonjudging, you can ask for help.

nonjudging 4: pleasure

We've talked about practicing nonjudging with experiences like frustration, pain, and trauma. But for some of us, the most difficult experience to accept is pleasure—and the bigger the pleasure, the more we shut it down with "shoulds."

Remember the salad bar metaphor from chapter 5? That you can take what you like and leave the rest, and everybody will come to the table with a different plate? Too many women make their choices based not on what they like, but on what they believe their partner likes or what they've been told they "should" like. You're supposed to want kale and fat-free dressing, but not the candied pecans, and if you bring a plateful of taboo foods to the table, you'll be judged. So you preemptively deny yourself the things that bring you pleasure. And if you suffer as a consequence, well . . . raise your hand if your family or culture taught you that suffering is somehow a virtue.

Suffering is not a virtue and pleasure is not a sin. We've been lied to all our lives.

In my experience, women struggle with nonjudging pleasure more than they struggle with nonjudging discomfort. We shut down pleasure so intuitively we don't even notice we've done it. I had a student many years ago who was coming out from under several months of depression, beginning to access moments of pleasure in sunshine and friends and school.

"It feels wrong," she said. "It doesn't seem right to feel good when so much of the world is such a mess."

I reminded her of the conversations we had had about nonjudging as a way to cope with her depression. "That skill applies to pleasure, too. Don't judge it. It's not right or wrong, it's just what's happening in your body right now. You don't have to be ashamed of it, you don't have to worry that when it passes it will never come back, you don't have to do anything but say hi to it and let it be what it is."

She looked at me skeptically, and when we talked again a few weeks later, she said, "So I tried that nonjudging pleasure and joy thing and, uh . . ."

She bit her lip and tears filled her eyes.

I waited.

After a long silence, she sniffed and said, "If you don't judge it, it grows."

This is a strange truth about nonjudgment. When you turn toward suffering with nonjudgment, the suffering diminishes as wounds heal. When you turn toward pleasure with nonjudgment, it expands to fill the space judgment once filled. I don't know why this is true, but it's an essential fact about nonjudgment.

"You didn't warn me about that," she accused.

"If I had warned you, would you have tried it?"

"Oh, hell no," she agreed. "But . . . I also like it."

"And how do you feel about the fact that you like pleasure?" I prompted.

She rolled her eyes—at herself or at me, I still don't know—and she said, "Well when you put it that way, it seems pretty normal."

It is normal. But that doesn't mean it's easy or simple. Many of us have been taught that pleasure is selfish, sinful, a waste of time, or something to be ashamed of. How dare we attend to what feels good, when we ought to be attending to other people's needs or our partner or making sure we meet other people's expectations?

But here is the truth: Pleasure is a gateway to accessing your fullest, truest personhood. Pleasure is where you find a no-holds-barred connection with yourself and with those you love most. Why? Because pleasure only happens in a context where your brain feels safe enough to be completely and entirely *you*, without shame or social performance or "shoulds." Ecstasy comes to us when we leave behind everything that doesn't delight us or spark our curiosity. Ecstasy comes when we surrender to pleasure without reservation. You are allowed to like pleasure. And the first step toward that is simply to notice it with nonjudgment.

Merritt is the queen of not doing it the way you expect her to. She began to trust herself not when she could give herself pleasure, but when she could give her partner pleasure. She embraced herself as a sexual woman . . . when she allowed herself not to be sexual. She sank down in the light of intense pleasure . . . when she let go of trying to experience pleasure.

"It's like how your fingers feel when you come in from the cold. It hurts for a while, but then they're warm." That's how she described the experience of letting go of the sexuality she thought she was supposed to have and opening up space for the sexuality she did have. "You'd think a middle-aged lesbian would know better than to accept what the world says about how women's sexuality works. But letting go of all that is hard."

"You've got sensitive brakes," I said, "and you've probably had those brakes a lot longer than you've had feminist politics."

One last story:

Merritt and Carol got married not long after their daughter graduated from high school. That kid—a peer sex educator in her high school, of course—organized a bridal shower for her moms that included, among the more pragmatic gifts of garden store gift cards and new towels, a kit from their daughter containing sparkling cider, scented candles, and massage oil, in a pretty basket with a bow.

"I can't believe my child is giving her parents date night parapher-nalia," Merritt said.

"Oh, puh-lease. It's not like I'm giving you a dildo and a whip!"

At this Merritt and Carol, both red faced and laughing, tried to send her to the kitchen to do the dishes.

But their daughter continued, "I mean, come on, it's the twenty-first century. You're here, you're queer, you get naked together sometimes because you're in love with each other. Get used to it."

Which is exactly what she's been doing ever since, side by side with Carol.

nonjudging 5: mourning the "shoulds"

For some people, knowing what's true is enough to set them free from the old, oppressive myths. Other people need to know what's true and also notice their judgmental feelings about what's true. When they notice they've been harboring judgment about themselves, they can release those attitudes and adopt more neutral or even positive feelings about what's true.

And for some people, it's not so simple as just releasing those attitudes. They know what's true. They notice their judgment about what's true. And their bodies, minds, and hearts seem to cling to that judgment for dear life, refusing to abandon the old ideas and instead embrace what's true.

Why?

Our scripts or maps include clear ideas about what the goal, effort, and timelines of our sexuality "should" be—easily orgasmic, with spontaneous desire, all of those myths. And what does it mean if we don't function the way we "should"? It means we're broken. Sometimes, for some people, having a sexuality that doesn't match the map doesn't just mean you're different, it means you're a failure. A freak. "Abnormal." Diseased, disgusting, inadequate, all these terrible words that mean we are not normal. We tie our identities to our sexuality, our sense of whether we're a "good woman" or a "good girl." If that's you, letting go of the myths may feel similar to letting go of self-criticism, as I described in chapter 5. On some level, we feel that letting go of those goals is giving up hope; it feels like failure. This is as true for sex-related goals like desire style, orgasm, and pleasure as it is for goals in the rest of life—ending a relationship, deciding not to complete a degree or go to grad school, accepting that your body shape doesn't match the cultural ideal.

Letting go of "shoulds"—feelings and thoughts like, "I shouldn't be this way" and, "I wish my sexuality were different"—requires that your little monitor recognize that your previous goal is unattainable and then . . . fall into the pit of despair we encounter when our monitor decides a goal is not attainable. In short, it requires a kind of "failure," accepting that you will probably never be the sexual person you were taught to be your whole life.

This is what can make changing your map so difficult, and it may be the single greatest obstacle standing between women and their own optimal sexual wellbeing. Embracing pleasure may require that we acknowledge desires and curiosities and sensations that we were taught all our lives were shameful. Embracing responsive desire may require that we abandon all hope that we'll ever conform to the model of sexual relationships we have always believed is the one and only "right" kind of sexual relationship. Once you know what's true, can you let go of what's false? Can you abandon the goals to which you have tied aspects of your identity? It requires a journey through the pit of despair, grieving for the map that was wrong and all the places you missed as a result.

How can people survive that kind of apparent "failure"? Where do they go, once they're in that pit?

The way to get through is to stay very still, to notice all the aspects of your identity that were tied to the lies you were told, to notice all the grief you feel in letting go of the self you spent your life trying to be. Notice, too, the anger you feel at having been lied to for so long. Notice all of these with nonjudgment. Allow them to be true.

As we saw in chapter 4, emotions are tunnels: You have to go through the darkness to get to the light at the end. Sometimes that's fairly easy, but sometimes it hurts like hell. Sometimes letting go of a particular goal feels like you have to let go of your entire identity. It's not an easy process; parts of it are downright uncomfortable. But it's so, so worth it, because at the end of the tunnel is the ultimate reward: you.

"to feel normal"

Let's return to Ms. B. from the beginning of the chapter. What do you think her goal is? Is it pleasure? Connection with her partner? Self-discovery?

From what little we know of her (and from what we know of the way women are socialized around sex), it seems likely that her unconscious goal is to conform to the expected ideal. To have desire come spontaneously, to have orgasms during intercourse. In short, to feel "normal."

We know by now that there's no such thing as normal—or rather, that we're all normal. We're all made of the same parts as everyone else, organized in a unique way. No two alike.

And yet what most of us want is to feel normal.

(In fact, one of the normal things about your sexuality is to worry sometimes about whether you're normal. Yes, being worried about being normal is . . . normal.)

But why is "normal" the goal? What do people want, when they want to be normal?

I don't have direct scientific evidence for what I'm about to say—I'm not even sure what that evidence would look like—but I'll tell you what I know based on decades of interactions with students, clinicians, journalists, and strangers from across the globe: I think that to feel normal is to feel that you *belong*. Remember what Camilla said way back in chapter 1: "We're all just trying to belong somewhere." We want to know that we are safe within the bounds of shared human experience, that what's on our map is the same as what is on other people's maps.

If we find ourselves in a place that we can't find on our map—that is, if we have an experience for which we have no frame of reference, no script—we feel lost. Unknown territory feels risky, unsafe—remember from chapter 4: "I am lost/I am home." In unknown territory, we feel, "I am at risk!" Our stress response kicks in and we're like that Iggy Pop rat: Everything seems like a potential threat.

But then if someone comes along and says, "You're okay—see, I've got this place here on my map. This is definitely part of the territory," we can relax. We know we're still at home, safe within bounds. We belong here.

When people ask me, "Am I normal?" they're asking, "Do I belong?"

The answer is yes. You belong in your body. You belong in the world. You've belonged since the day you were born, this is your home. You don't have to earn it by conforming to some externally imposed sexual standard.

If you change your goal from "normal" to "wherever I belong," then you're always successful because you're already there.

For many years, I kept a small comic taped to my office door. It shows an old Buddhist monk sitting next to a young Buddhist monk. The older monk is saying, "Nothing happens next. This is it."

Being more nerd than nun, I see it as a commentary on the discrepancy-reducing feedback loop and criterion velocity, on the importance of training your little monitor to enjoy the present rather than constantly push toward the future. What if . . . this is a radical idea, but just go with me: What if you felt that way—"This is it"—about your sexual functioning? What if the sexuality you have right now is the sexuality you get? What if this is it?

When I pose that question, women have a tremendously wide range of responses, from radiantly beaming smiles to sudden waves of sobbing despair.

If you beam radiantly at the idea that your sexuality, as it is now, is it, *awesome*. I hope the science in this book will help to expand and enliven your sexual wellbeing.

If you would feel grief, shame, despair, rage, uncertainty, frustration, or fear if the sexuality you have today were it for your sexuality, it might be that before you can explore your own sexuality with joy, you must move through the fear or rage or grief that is standing between you and the warm light of compassion. And that's not easy. But it is possible—and I believe it is worth it. Always remember this:

The day you were born, the world had a choice about what to teach you about your body. It could have taught you to live with confidence and joy inside your body. It could have taught you that your body and your sexuality are beautiful gifts. But instead, the world taught you to feel critical of and dissatisfied with your sexuality and your body. You were taught to value and expect something from your sexuality that does not match what your sexuality actually is. You were told a story about what would happen in your sexual life, and that story was false. You were lied to. I am pissed, on your behalf, at the world for that lie. And I'm working to create a world that doesn't lie to women about their bodies anymore.

I can't change the injury that the world inflicted on you, and neither can you.

What you *can* do is heal.

Like your genitals, your sexuality is perfect and beautiful exactly as it is. You are normal. Beautiful. So when you notice yourself feeling dissatisfied with your sexuality, when you notice shame or frustration or grief, allow yourself to direct those feelings away from yourself and instead focus the emotions toward the culture that told you the wrong story. Rage not against yourself but against the culture that lied to you. Grieve not for your discrepancy from a fictitious "ideal" that is at best arbitrary and at worst an act of oppression and violence; grieve for the compassionate world you were born deserving . . . and did not get.

The purpose of allowing yourself to feel those Feels is not to change something out in the world. Feel your Feels so that they can discharge, release, and create space for something new inside you. When you allow that grief to move through you, you are letting go of the sexual person you were told you "should be," a phantom self that has taken up space in your mind for too long. And letting go of that phantom creates spaces for the sexual person you *are*. And when we all practice this, the world does change, person by person.

The sexuality you have right now *is it*. And it's beautiful, even— especially!—if it's not what you were taught it should be.

I don't know if you're more like Olivia or Camilla or Merritt or Laurie, or nothing at all like anyone I've ever met. I don't know how easily you discover and create contexts that generate pleasure and desire. I don't know how at home you feel in your sexuality, your own private garden. But I know that you are the gardener. And I know that the more you work *with* the innate characteristics of your garden, the healthier and more abundant it will grow. I know you are beautiful just as you are, fully capable of confident, joyful sex. I know you are normal.

Laurie and Johnny lived happily ever after—or most of the time ever after. Life is complicated and Laurie still has times when she gets sucked into exhaustion and overwhelm, times when her body seems to shut out all potential sources of pleasure. But three things changed permanently.

First, she practiced paying nonjudgmental attention to sensations, which taught her to be as kind and generous with herself as she was with everyone else she loved. She learned to notice and celebrate pleasure and joy, granting herself permission to feel good.

Second, though there wasn't much she could do to reduce the actual stressors *in her life, she reduced her* stress *by taking more deliberate effort to decompress and complete the stress response cycles that life activated. She let herself cry. She slowed down her showers, paid attention to the sensation of the water on her skin, and instead of slapping on body lotion like she was greasing a loaf pan, she paid attention to how nice it felt and how healthy her skin was. As she exercised, she visualized her stress as that orange monster in the Bugs Bunny cartoon—the one Bugs gives a manicure—and imagines herself running away from the monster, through her front door, and into Johnny's arms. She started experiencing the discharge of stress as pleasurable—or at least not a source of suffering.*

And finally, she became much gentler with herself when she noticed herself being self-critical about her body or feeling guilty about pleasure. She didn't say to herself, "Stop it!" She just thought, "Yup. There are the self-critical thoughts again." She practiced nonjudgment.

Perhaps these three changes would not have lasted as they have if it weren't for Johnny recognizing the opportunity in all of this.

Once he clicked onto the idea of turning off her offs, he started noticing more and more things he could do to help Laurie let go of the brakes. Sometimes it was a simple thing like doing the dishes and wiping down the kitchen counters. Sometimes it was, "Let's take a night off of worrying about whether we're going to have sex and just lie together and talk." Sometimes it was setting up a date night with plenty of time for her to unwind.

Higher-desire partners might think, "She should just be able to want it as much as I do!" They have negative feelings about their partner's sexual feelings. But Johnny realized it's not about just wanting sex, it's about creating a context—really, it's about creating a life—that makes space for both people's needs. He brought a sense of curiosity to the puzzle of turning off the offs. He brought a sense of wonder to the surprising way Laurie's sexuality can spring and blossom from fallow winter ground. He brought a sense of awe to the ecstatic way her passion overflows the garden walls, under the loving warm rain and sun of the right context.

Joy is the hard part. As a matter of fact, even writing this chapter about joy has been the hardest part of writing this book. Joy isn't obvious or simple. It isn't a destination you arrive at and it isn't "the journey." It's how you feel about your journey toward your truest erotic self. You are allowed to love your sexuality as it is right now, even—especially—if it's not what somebody else says it "should" be.

I am a creature of evidence and method; I want to understand the brain mechanism underlying joy—and I found some science about that, don't get me wrong. If you, too, need evidence, I've done all I can to offer it here. But the science can only lead us as far as to the edge of what is known. What I have learned in a quarter century as a sex educator is that joy is what happens when you jump off the edge of what is known, into the adventure of what is true.

I've said it over and over in this book: Trust your body. Trust it so completely you're willing to jump with it into the unknown. That jump is joy.

tl;dr

- The most important thing you can do to have a great sex life is to welcome your sexuality as it is, right now—even if it's not what you wanted or expected it to be.
- Letting go of old, bogus cultural standards requires a grieving process, going through the little monitor's pit of despair.
- To facilitate that letting go, develop the skill of "nonjudging."
- When you give yourself permission to be and feel whatever you are and feel, your body can complete the cycle, move through the tunnel, and come out to the light at the end.

conclusion

YOU ARE THE SECRET INGREDIENT

So what have we learned?

We've learned that we're all made of the same parts, organized in different ways—no two alike. That sexual response is the process of both turning on the ons and turning off the offs. That context—your environment and your mental state—influences how and when the ons and offs activate.

We've learned that genital response and being "turned on" aren't always the same thing. That desire can be spontaneous or responsive, and both are normal. That some women orgasm pretty reliably from intercourse, most don't, both are normal, and neither is a bigger deal than you want it to be.

Above all, we've learned that it's not how your sexuality functions that determines whether your sex life is characterized by worry and distress . . . or by confidence and joy. It's your capacity to welcome your sexuality as it is right now.

To get there, we've discussed anatomy, physiology, behavioral and comparative psychology, evolutionary psychology, health psychology, moral psychology, gender studies, media studies, and more. I've used metaphors, stories, my quarter century of experience as an educator, and a century or more of science.

The depth and complexity of women's sexuality demands all this, and more.

why I wrote this book

Like many of you, I was taught all the wrong things as I was growing up. Then as I reached adulthood, I made all the mistakes. And I spent many years stumbling with unspeakably good fortune into settings where I could learn how to get it "right"—settings like the Kinsey Institute and one of only a handful of Ph.D. programs with a formal concentration in human sexuality.

I wrote this book to share what I've learned—what has helped me and what I've seen help other women. I wrote it for my sister and my mother, for my sister's stepdaughters, for my nieces, and most of all for my students. I wrote it to share the science that taught me that I and my sister and my mother and my friends are all normal and healthy. I wrote it to grant us all permission to be different from one another.

I wrote it because I am done living in a world where women are lied to about their bodies; where women are objects of sexual desire rather than subjects of sexual pleasure; where sex is used as a weapon against women; and where women believe their bodies are broken, simply because those bodies are not male. And I am done living in a world where women are trained from birth to treat their bodies as the enemy.

I wrote this book to teach women to live with confidence and joy.

If you can remember even one of the ideas in this book—no two alike, brakes and accelerator, context, nonconcordant arousal, responsive desire, any of them—and use it to improve your relationship with your own sexuality, you'll be helping me with that goal. And if you share any of these ideas with even one other person, you'll be expanding the global space in which women can live with confidence and joy.

In a way, it's a small goal. I'm not trying to prevent cancer or solve the climate crisis or build peace in the Middle East. I'm just trying to help people live with confidence and joy inside their bodies—and maybe, just maybe, if enough people learn to live with confidence and joy, we can ultimately live in a world where everyone's sexual autonomy is respected.

Do I think that living with confidence and joy and respecting everyone's sexual autonomy could play a role in preventing cancer, solving the climate crisis, or building world peace? Yes, actually. But that's another story.

where to look for more answers

I don't have all the answers—I don't even have half the answers. The science is constantly growing and expanding, so more insight, more clarity will come. In this book I've presented some of the answers that I've seen help women, and I hope I've done it in a way that heals and renews and expands your sexuality.

All of us are engaged in the ongoing process of cultivating our gardens—digging out the weeds and nurturing the plants we hope will flourish. Often it's a joyful experience; sometimes it's painful; always it's deeply personal. And as we tend our gardens, all of us look outside ourselves for confirmation that what we are experiencing is normal. We look to our community for comfort when we're distressed. We look to experts for answers we can't find on our own. Everyone does it, from the toddler who falls down while they're learning to walk to the gifted meditator feeling their way through recovery from a sexual assault. We all look up from our own experience, look out to the world, and say, "That hurt. Am I okay? Am I doing this right?"

(You are doing it right. You are okay. When you hurt, you heal.)

And in the same way that our stress response physiology made a lot of sense when our typical stressors had sharp teeth and claws, so this practice of looking outside ourselves for confirmation that we're okay may have made more sense when "outside ourselves" meant our local community and people we actually knew in real life, rather than people we know only through mass media.

We live in a world of Top 5 Tips, where there are twelve new techniques for mind-blowing fellatio each month, followed by six sexy new positions he's always wanted to try. This world is full of fun, exciting, entertaining things that draw and hold our attention.

But the structure of the truth is quieter, slower, more personal, and *so* much more interesting than mere entertainment. And it lives exclusively *inside you*, in the quiet moments of joy, in the jarring moments of worry, in the torn moments when the flock that is you is trying simultaneously to fly away from a threat and toward a pleasure.

So when you notice something unexpected inside yourself and you want to look outward to check if it's normal, if you're okay, remember me saying this: *You are okay*. Let this book be a mirror: When you look up, see yourself. And you are beautiful.

Trust your body.

Listen to the small, quiet voice inside you that says, "Yes. Yes, more," or "No. Stop." Listen especially when that voice is saying both at once. When that happens, be compassionate with yourself. Go slow.

When you look "out there," you'll find inspiration and entertainment and amazing science and support, too. But you won't find the truth of your own sexual wellbeing—what *you* want, what *you* like, what *you* need. To find that, look inside.

I think very often people attend workshops like the ones I teach, or read a book like this one, hoping to find the "secret ingredient," the hidden all-powerful something or other that will put the apparent chaos of their sex lives into some kind of meaningful order.

So, what is the secret ingredient?

Well.

Have you seen the movie *Kung Fu Panda?*

It's about a cartoon panda named Po, who becomes a kung fu master through diligent effort, the support of his teacher, and the wisdom of the Dragon Scroll, which contains "the key to limitless power"—in other words, the secret ingredient.

When Po first looks at the scroll, he is disappointed to find that there is nothing written on it. It's a mirror—it reflects his own face.

And then comes his epiphany: "There is no secret ingredient. It's just you."

So. One more time, for the record:

Yes, you are normal. In fact, you're not just normal. You're amazing. Beguiling. Courageous. Delectable. All the way down to yawping and zesty. Your body is *beautiful* and your desires are *perfect*, just as they are.

The secret ingredient is *you*.

The science says so.

And now you can prove it.

acknowledgments

Gratitude, first of all, to all the women who've talked to me about their sex lives, whose stories are woven into the narratives of Camilla, Olivia, Merritt, and Laurie, and throughout the book. I hope I have done justice to your stories.

Gratitude to the researchers, educators, and counselors who talked to me, read chunks of the book, told me I didn't sound like a nut, told me I did sound like a nut, and/or nodded sympathetically as I apologized about the difference between writing science itself and writing about science for a general audience. In alphabetical order: Kent Berridge, Charles Carver, Kristen Chamberlin, Meredith Chivers, Cynthia Graham, Robin Milhausen, Caroline Pukall, and Kelly Suchinsky. Let the record show that any mistakes in the science are my own fault, despite precise and clear feedback from these good people.

Gratitude to Ms. Erika Moen, who drew the genitals so beautifully.

Gratitude to the beta readers, especially Andrew Wilson and Sabrina Golonka, Patrick Kinsman, Ruth Cohen, Anna Cook, and Jan Morris.

Gratitude to readers of my blog, who read early drafts of the book, commented on posts for four years, kept me intellectually and emotionally honest, and kept me questioning what I thought I knew, so that I could be a better writer.

Gratitude to my students at Smith College, who asked questions I'd never considered ("What's the evolutionary origin of the hymen?") and pushed me to understand ever more deeply what I was teaching, so that I could be a better teacher.

To all of you: Thank you.

And then there's the gratitude where there just aren't any words anymore, all there is is this swollen feeling around your heart and no way to talk about it. You know that feeling? It's the one that tells you to go to the person, get on your knees, and cover your face with your hands, grateful, humble, bound.

I'm pretty sure that every person for whom I have this feeling would find it very, very awkward if I actually did that. So instead I'll just write a list.

Here, in approximate chronological order, are the people who helped me in ways I don't have words for:

Nancy Nutt-Chase
Cynthia Graham and John Bancroft
Erick Janssen
David Lohrmann
Richard Stevens
Lindsay Edgecombe
Sarah Knight
Julie Ohotnicky
Amelia Nagoski
Stephen Crowley

Grateful. Humble. Bound. Thank you.

appendix 1: therapeutic masturbation

If you are experiencing frustration around orgasm—whether you're learning to orgasm, learning to orgasm with a partner, or learning to have more control over your orgasms—I offer these instructions.

1. Find your clitoris (instructions in chapter 1).
2. Create a great context. You can use your worksheets from chapter 3 to help with this. In general, it'll be a context where you have no concern about being interrupted for about thirty minutes, where you feel safe and private and undistracted by outside worries.
3. Touch your body and notice how that feels. Touch your feet and legs and arms and hands and neck and scalp. At first, when you're learning to have an orgasm, stop here. Spend your thirty minutes just doing this. Do it a few times a week for a couple weeks. Gradually incorporate your breasts, lower abdomen, inner thighs.
4. Now stimulate your clitoris indirectly. The most indirect stimulation is simply to think about your clitoris. Just give it quiet, loving attention. Try rocking or rotating your hips, to bring your attention to your pelvis. You may or may not notice some emotions emerging as you attend to your clitoris. That's normal. Allow any feelings and practice feeling affectionate and compassionate toward yourself, your genitals, and all those feelings.

   When you feel ready (and you may not feel ready for days or weeks—that's okay), move to "distal" stimulation, which means indirect, round-about stimulation. Try any of these, or whatever else feels right:

- Gently pinch your labia between your thumbs and forefingers, stretch the labia out, and tug from side to side. This will put very indirect pressure on the clitoris and move the skin over the clitoris (the clitoral hood).
- With your palm over your mons, press down a little and pull upward, toward your abdomen. Again, this will put gentle pressure on the clit and move the skin around it. Try different pressures, different speeds of tugging (e.g., one long slow tug, several quick tugs in a row), or rotating your palm in a circle.
- Place your palms against your inner thighs, so that the outside edges of your thumbs are pressing against your labia, possibly even squeezing them together. Rock your hips against the pressure of your hands.

Some people prefer indirect stimulation over direct stimulation. You may notice as you try these techniques that the muscles in your arms, legs, butt, and/or abdomen get tense. That's a normal part of the body arousal process. You might even find yourself feeling like you don't want to stop doing a particular kind of stimulation. I humbly suggest you go with your gut; don't stop. Keep going for as long as it feels good, just keep paying attention to the pleasurable sensations without trying to change them or even understand them.

5. Try direct stimulation. For most people this is pleasurable only when arousal has already started up, so once you're feeling pretty pleasurable and warm, try any of these:

- With the flat of one or two or three fingertips, lightly touch the head of the clitoris with a steady back-and-forth motion. Try slow, fast, or anything in between that feels good, and with light, brushing touch, light pressure, deep pressure . . . try different combinations of speeds and pressures.
- With as many fingertips as feels comfortable, rub circles directly over your clitoris—fast or slow, light touch or deep pressure, or anything in between.
- Again with varying numbers of fingers, and with different pressures and speeds, tug upward on the clitoris, from the clitoral hood.
- With whatever variation on fingers, speed, and pressure you want to try, flick upward from just under the head of the clitoris.

As your arousal level changes, notice and observe what happens to your body. Don't try to make it change. If you notice that your brain starts whirring away at anxieties or fears, notice that, too, know that you can worry about all that some other time, release those thoughts, and return your attention to the sensations inside your body.

6. Keep breathing. As you experience sexual pleasure, your muscles will tense, and often people find themselves holding their breath or breathing more shallowly. Periodically check in with your breathing, relax your abdominal muscles, and allow yourself to breathe.

Don't try to make anything happen, just allow yourself to notice what it feels like and let your body do what it wants. If you feel worried that you're losing control of your body, relax into that fear, reassure yourself that you're safe, know that you can stop anytime you choose. And of course, if it gets to be too much, feel free to stop anytime you like. The more you keep going, the more the pleasure and tension will spread through your body, and it will cross some intense threshold, and explode . . . eventually.

If you're learning to orgasm with a partner, do all of this alone for a week (or three), then do it with a photo of your partner sitting beside you. Do that for a week (or three). Then do it with them maybe on the phone or in the next room. Then with them in the room but far away, in the dark, blindfolded, and facing the other way. Gradually increase their proximity and even the light.

Once you're orgasming with your partner on the bed with you, begin showing them what feels good to you. Move your partner's hands on your body to show them what you like.

And always, notice if you're getting frustrated and remember that you are already at the goal: pleasure.

appendix 2: extended orgasm

Extending and expanding your orgasms is a kind of meditation. If you've never meditated in nonsexual ways, it might be easiest if you begin by practicing outside the context of sexuality. Here's how.

Begin with a simple breathing exercise like the one I describe in the spectatoring section in chapter 8.

Inhale through your nose for five seconds.

Then exhale through your mouth for ten seconds.

Do that eight times, for a total of two minutes.

As you breathe, your mind will wander to other things. That is normal and healthy! The point is not to prevent your mind from wandering but to notice when that happens, let those thoughts go for the moment, and gently return your attention to your breathing.

The breathing is good for you, but the noticing that your mind wandered and returning your attention to your breath is the crucial skill.

Do this every day, and gradually you'll notice yourself noticing what you're paying attention to all the time. Once that's happening spontaneously, you're ready to begin moving toward extended orgasm.

When you're ready, create a context where you have lots of time on your own (or with a partner you trust) without interruption or distraction. You'll need an hour or two—and if you're thinking, "I don't have an hour or two to have an orgasm," that's totally fair! Extended orgasm is the sex equivalent of running a marathon. You can be as healthy as anyone needs to be and never run a marathon. Just jog a few times a week, that's great! But sometimes you have the opportunity to set an ambitious goal and dedicate some time and attention to it. Whether it's a marathon or ecstasy, it's always a choice you make, depending on what fits your life.

So. Create a context. And begin with the breathing exercise for two minutes, practicing returning your attention to your breath when it strays.

Then begin a little sensory exploration, paying attention to how your body feels, using all the techniques in the therapeutic masturbation approach (appendix 1).

Imagine that arousal happens on a scale of 0–10, where 0 is no arousal and 10 is orgasm. Start at 0 and allow your arousal to grow up to 5, which is definitely turned on, definitely interested.

Then back down to 1. Allow the tension in your muscles to dissipate.

Go up to 6, and then back down to 2.

Of course, as you go through this process, notice when your attention strays to outside thoughts, let those thoughts go, and return your attention to the sensations of your body. And don't forget to breathe.

Up to 7, down to 3.

7 is pretty aroused. By the time you get to 7, your body may become reluctant to stop moving toward orgasm. This is where the crucial skill of taking your foot off the accelerator without putting it on the brakes comes in. Just turn off the ons without turning on the offs. Allow your muscles to relax, allow the arousal to dissipate softly.

Up to 8, down to 4.

Up to 9, down to 5.

9 is a very, very high level of arousal, and your body is very much on the train at this point. It wants to move forward to its destination. So it may be difficult, on your first attempts, to relax your abdominal, thigh, and buttock muscles enough to ease your arousal down. When you do, you may experience a kind of spreading warmth or tingling. Whereas fast orgasms are generally focused right in the genitals, these slower orgasms spread out over your whole body. Let that happen.

Still notice when your thoughts stray and return your attention to the sensations in your body.

Up to 9½, down to 6.

9½ is the bittersweet screaming edge of orgasm. At first, it may be it difficult to take pressure off the accelerator. Feel free not to the first few times you try this—the worst that can happen is you'll have an orgasm!

But once you learn the knack, allow your arousal to reach 6, go back to 9½, then down to 7.

You'll need to make a deliberate effort to ease tension away from your abdomen, buttocks, and thigh muscles, because that tension can push you over the edge. As you relax, you'll sense the arousal spreading from your genitals, radiating into the rest of your body.

Back to 9½, down to 8.

Back to 9½, down to 9. By now, you're constantly hovering around orgasm, holding yourself at the peak sexual tension your body can contain. That's extended orgasm. Congratulations! With practice, you can stay there as long as you like, as long as your body can sustain, always noticing what you're paying attention to and gently nudging your attention toward your body sensations. You're a bit like a bathtub at this point, where the tension is trickling into you at exactly the same rate that it's draining out. If it begins to trickle just a little bit more quickly than it's draining out, you'll cross the threshold and overflow. If it begins to drain just a bit more quickly than it's trickling in, you'll drift away from the peak. There is no such thing as failure here, only different kinds of success, because it's all intense pleasure.

This whole process might take forty-five minutes or an hour, and there will be Feelings, make no mistake. And even if you don't have an extended orgasm, you'll still have loads of pleasure!

The great thing about ecstatic pleasure is that it cannot coexist with shame, stress, fear, anger, bitterness, rage, or exhaustion. Practicing ecstasy is practicing living outside all of those things, learning how to release them. It's as good for you as vegetables, jogging, sleep, and breathing.

notes

Part 1. The (Not-So-Basic) Basics
1. Anatomy: No Two Alike

1. Wallen and Lloyd, "Female Sexual Arousal." See also Emhardt, Siegel, and Hoffman, "Anatomic Variation and Orgasm," and Mazloomdoost and Pauls, "Comprehensive Review of the Clitoris." It's fascinating and important research, but I rarely teach about it because many (not all) such studies, including the second citation, fall into the trap of converting a myth-based narrative of sexual functioning—e.g., that orgasm from vaginal stimulation is "orgasmic success"—into reductionist descriptions of anatomical size, shape, and position. Indeed, in 2014, a copyeditor inserted a comment here: "So which is 'better'? Bigger distance or smaller?," which is exactly the sort of question I'm trying to help people not ask. Far from helping women live with confidence and joy, such misdirected analysis only makes people worry that their genitals are wrong. People have already been taught enough judgmental stuff about their genitals. My goal in recounting this conversation here at the start of the book is to show me making the mistake of being too interested in the science and not interested enough in the person in front of me. The theme of this chapter and the entire book is, "We're all made of the same parts, organized in different ways." None of those organizations is better or worse: they're just different. But if even the science sometimes attempts to frame some genital shapes as "better" than others, we can be forgiven for struggling to stay nonjudgmental about our own genitals.

2. Aristotle, *Aristotle's Compleat Master-Piece*, 16.

3. Drysdale, Russell, and Glover, "Labiaplasty."

4. Moran and Lee, "What's Normal?"

5. The reality of the hymen is finally beginning to be discussed in the mainstream in the form of documentaries such as *How to Lose Your Virginity* and the media coverage related to it (Feeney, "Living Myths about Virginity") and a segment on the video series *Adam Ruins Everything*.

6. Hegazy and Al-Rukban, "Hymen: Facts and Conceptions."

7. This was in Talbot House in the fall semester of 2012. Hi, Talbot!

8. Wickman, "Plasticity of the Skene's Gland."

9. Not everyone is comfortable with the term "intersex." Some people prefer "ambiguous genitals" and some prefer "disorders of sex development" or "DSD" (Dreger, "Why 'Disorders of Sex Development'?"). I use "intersex" here because it feels most appropriate for this nonmedical context.

10. Fausto-Sterling, *Sexing the Body*, 2000.

11. As obvious as this idea may seem, given the all-the-same-parts framework, it is actually a radical idea that intersex activists have been fighting hard to promote for several decades. It's the only view that makes biological sense, and again, it's only from a cultural point of view that anyone could think otherwise. And yet in too many places, standard medical practice is to perform surgery to "normalize" the genitals (ILGA-Europe, "Public Statement"). Note that in 2013 the United Nations' special rapporteur on torture included these surgeries in his report "on Torture and Other Cruel, Inhuman or Degrading Treatment or Punishment." The report condemned medically unnecessary "normalizing" surgeries because "they can cause scarring, loss of sexual sensation, pain, incontinence and lifelong depression and have also been criticized as being unscientific, potentially harmful and contributing to stigma" (UN Human Rights Council, *Report of the Special Rapporteur*, 18).

12. McDowell et al., "Anthropometric Reference Data."

13. She's right, according to International Society for the Study of Vulvovaginal Disease. Vieira-Baptista et al., "International Society for the Study of Vulvovaginal Disease Recommendations."

14. Operation Beautiful is responsible for this excellent phrase (www.operationbeautiful.com/).

2. The Dual Control Model: Your Sexual Personality

1. Masters and Johnson, *Human Sexual Response*.

2. Kaplan, "Hypoactive Sexual Desire."

3. Janssen and Bancroft, "Dual Control Model," 197.
4. Goldstein et al., "Hypoactive Sexual Desire," 117.
5. Velten et al., "Temporal Stability of Sexual Excitation."
6. Velten et al., "Sexual Excitation and Sexual Inhibition," and Rettenberger, Klein, and Briken, "Relationship between Hypersexual Behavior." See also Granados, Carvalho, and Sierra, "How the Dual Control Model Predicts Female Sexual Response."
7. A not-so-sensitive accelerator, on the other hand, regardless of brakes, is one predictor of asexuality—people who don't desire sexual contact (not "stones"—folks who only want to touch their partners but don't want to be touched themselves). In the handful of studies on people who identify themselves as asexual, it turns out that they have significantly less accelerator than their sexual counterparts (Prause and Graham, "Asexuality"). There is no difference in their brakes, however. So maybe part of asexuality is that these individuals' brains are not prone to noticing sexually relevant stimuli. Of course this is only one part of the story, since asexuals represent only about 1 percent of the general population, and about 5 to 10 percent of women score as low SE. Again, there's nothing broken or wrong. Asexual people's sexual response mechanisms are made of all the same parts as sexual people's; they're just organized in a different way.
8. Carpenter et al., "Women's Scores"; Carpenter et al., "Dual Control Model."
9. Adapted from Milhausen et al., "Validation of the Sexual Excitation/Sexual Inhibition Inventory" and Janssen et al., "The Sexual Inhibition/Sexual Excitation Scales—Short Form."
10. Carpenter et al., "Dual Control Model."
11. Mental state impact on sexual interest:

	Increase (%)	No Change (%)	Decrease (%)
Depression			
Men	10	55	35
Women	9.5	40	50.5
Anxiety			
Men	25	58	17
Women	23	43	34

From Lykins, Janssen, and Graham, "Relationship between Negative Mood and Sexuality." See also Janssen, Macapagal, and Mustanski, "Effects of Mood on Sexuality."

12. Pfaus, "Neurobiology of Sexual Behavior."

13. Pfaus, Kippin, and Coria-Avila, "Animal Models."

14. Pfaus and Wilkins, "Novel Environment."

15. Velten et al., "Temporal Stability of Sexual Excitation."

3. Context: And the "One Ring" (to Rule Them All) in Your Emotional Brain

1. Four percent in Carpenter et al., "Dual Control Model," and 8 percent in my considerably less science-y experience on my blog and in my classes.

2. McCall and Meston, "Cues Resulting in Desire" and "Differences between Pre- and Postmenopausal Women."

3. Graham et al., "Turning On and Turning Off."

4. Gottman, *The Science of Trust*, 254.

5. Bergner, *What Do Women Want?*, 68–73.

6. Graham, Sanders, and Milhausen, "Sexual Excitation/Sexual Inhibition Inventory."

7. BBC News, "Words Can Change What We Smell."

8. Aubrey, "Feeling a Little Blue."

9. Ariely, *Predictably Irrational*.

10. Nakamura and Csikszentmihalyi, "Flow Theory and Research," 195–206.

11. Flaten, Simonsen, and Olsen, "Drug-Related Information." Hat tip to Goldacre, "Nerdstock."

12. Reynolds and Berridge, "Emotional Environments."

13. Gottman, *Science of Trust*, 192.

14. There's increasing evidence that in a variety of ways, in both rats and humans, context changes how the midbrain responds to stimuli. Human brain imaging studies have found that uncertainty and risk can influence NAc response (Abler et al., "Prediction Error") and that the NAc's of people with chronic back pain respond differently to "noxious thermal stimulation" (i.e., burning) than people who don't live with pain (Baliki et al., "Predicting Value of Pain"). Something particularly interesting about the study of brain functioning in people with chronic back pain: When they directed their attention to the burning sensation on the skin of their back, they reported that the heat hurt; when they directed their attention to the pain in the muscles of their back, they reported that the heat felt good. Where we focus our attention is part of context.

15. Berridge and Kringelbach, "Neuroscience of Affect," 295.

16. Jaak Panksepp and Lucy Biven (*Archaeology of Mind*) include in their taxonomy of the limbic brain SEEKING, RAGE, FEAR, LUST, CARE, PANIC/

GRIEF, and PLAY. Frederick Toates includes, along with stress and sex, social behavior, aggression, and exploration (*Biological Psychology*). Paul Ekman, using research on universal facial expressions, theorizes the basic emotional categories of anger, disgust, fear, happiness, sadness, and surprise (*Emotions Revealed*). It says a lot that there isn't yet a universally agreed-on system for understanding the organization of our most basic emotions. Nor is there a universally agreed-on definition of what an emotion or a motivation is or if they're the same thing or different—though my references reveal my inclinations (Berridge and Winkielman, "What Is an Unconscious Emotion?"; Panksepp, "What Is an Emotional Feeling?").

17. Berridge, *Mechanisms of Self-Control*. The Harvard psychologist Daniel Gilbert described Berridge as "one of the best neuroscientists in the world" (Berridge, Davidson, and Gilbert, *Neuroscience of Happiness*), but I would distinguish him from other neuroscientists this way: As a source of both the Iggy Pop rat study and the One Ring metaphor, he is the one and only author of rat brain research who has made me LOL.

18. Authors resort to quotation marks (Berridge's "wanting" and "liking") and capitals (Panksepp and Biven's SEEKING, etc. system in *Archaeology of Mind*) in an effort to reinforce the distinction between conscious liking, wanting, and learning and mesolimbic *liking*, *wanting*, and *learning*.

     To make that distinction in this book, I use a shortcut metaphor throughout: When I talk about a person's experience of motivation, learning, and pleasure or suffering (what people use to describe what they want, know, or feel), I say "you want/know/feel." When I talk about affective motivation, learning, and feelings (*wanting*, *liking*, *learning*), I say "your brain wants/knows/feels."

19. Childress et al., "Prelude to Passion."

Part 2. Sex in Context
4. Emotional Context: Sex in a Monkey Brain

1. Porges, "Reciprocal Influences between Body and Brain."
2. Levine, *In an Unspoken Voice*, 55–56.
3. Lykins, Janssen, and Graham, "Relationship between Negative Mood and Sexuality"; ter Kuile, Vigeveno, and Laan, "Acute and Chronic Daily Psychological Stress"; Laumann et al., "Sexual Problems among Women and Men."
4. Hamilton and Meston, "Chronic Stress and Sexual Function."
5. Levine, *In an Unspoken Voice*, 8.

6. Inevitably, it's more complicated than that. There is a brake that, in a healthy nervous system, is linked with the autonomic gas pedal, so that when life hits the gas pedal, the brake disengages, and when life relaxes the gas pedal, the brake reengages—the neomammalian vagus, or "vagal brake" as Stephen Porges describes it. This is in contrast to the reptilian vagus, which slows the heart and is the brake of "freeze" (Porges, *Polyvagal Theory*, 92–93).

7. It shows up over and over again in both fact and fiction, such as Forrest Gump's "I just felt like running" and, memorably, in P. G. Wodehouse's *Performing Flea*: "The puppy was run over by a motor bike the other day and emerged perfectly unhurt but a bit emotional. We had to chase him half across London before he simmered down. He just started running and kept on running until he felt better."

8. If you know of some research on this, please do send me an email! enagoski@gmail.com.

9. Nearly everyone has them (Radomsky et al., "Part 1—You Can Run but You Can't Hide," and Berry and Laskey, "Review of Obsessive Intrusive Thoughts"). A quarter of those with OCD report sexual intrusions (Grant et al., "Sexual Obsessions and Clinical Correlates"), including among children and youths with OCD (Fernández de la Cruz et al., "Sexual Obsessions in Pediatric"). People's reluctance to disclose sexual intrusions is grounded, alas, in real stigma and social rejection in response to such disclosure (Cathey and Wetterneck, "Stigma and Disclosure of Intrusive Thoughts").

10. The World Health Organization reports that "35 percent of women world-wide have experienced either intimate partner violence or non-partner sexual violence in their lifetime" ("Violence Against Women" fact sheet). The US National Criminal Justice Reference Services reports that about 18 percent of women in America are raped in their lifetime; about 25 percent are raped, assaulted, or physically abused by their partner in their lifetime, compared with 8 percent of men (US Department of Justice, *Full Report*).

11. US Department of Education, Office for Civil Rights, Boston, "Title IX and Sexual Assault: Exploring New Paradigms for Prevention and Response," March 24–25, 2011.

12. Lisak and Miller, "Repeat Rape and Multiple Offending."

13. For a clinical version of this categorization, see Gaffney, "Established and Emerging PTSD Treatments."

14. Sensorimotor therapy: Ogden, Minton, and Pain, *Trauma and the Body*. Somatic Experiencing: Levine, *Waking the Tiger* and *In an Unspoken Voice*.

15. Khong, "Mindfulness."

16. Mitchell and Trask, "Origin of Love."

17. Hitchens, *Hitch-22*.

18. Acevedo et al., "Neural Correlates."

19. Glass and Blum, "317."

20. For comprehensive reviews of the sex-attachment link, see Dewitte, "Different Perspectives on the Sex-Attachment Link," and Dunkley et al., "Sexual Functioning in Young Women and Men."

21. Johnson, *Hold Me Tight*, 189.

22. Kinsale, *Flowers from the Storm*, 431, 362.

23. Johnson, *Love Sense*, 121.

24. Feeney and Noller, "Attachment Style"; Bifulco et al., "Adult Attachment Style."

25. Items taken with permission from the "Experiences in Close Relationships" questionnaire (Fraley, Waller, and Brennan, "Self-Report Measures of Adult Attachment").

26. Warber and Emmers-Sommer, "Relationships among Sex, Gender and Attachment," and Dunkley et al., "Sexual Functioning in Young Women and Men."

27. Stefanou and McCabe, "Adult Attachment and Sexual Functioning"; see also Birnbaum et al., "When Sex Is More Than Just Sex," Cooper et al., "Attachment Styles, Sex Motives, and Sexual Behavior," and La Guardia et al., "Within-Person Variation in Security of Attachment."

28. Davila, Burge, and Hammen, "Why Does Attachment Style Change?"

29. Taylor and Master, "Social Responses to Stress."

30. David and Lyons-Ruth, "Differential Attachment Responses."

31. Rumi, *Teachings of Rumi*.

32. Ibid.

5. Cultural Context: A Sex-Positive Life in a Sex-Negative World

1. van de Velde, *Ideal Marriage*, 145.

2. Hite, *The Hite Report*, 365.

3. Britton et al., "Fat Talk."

4. Might this be starting to change? In one study, college women (mostly white) reported that they would like a woman more if she talked positively about her body than if she criticized her body—though they also reported

that they expected other women to prefer a woman who self-criticized (Tompkins et al., "Social Likeability").

5. Woertman and van den Brink, "Body Image."
6. Pazmany et al., "Body Image and Genital Self-Image."
7. Kilimnik and Meston, "Role of Body Esteem."
8. Longe et al., "Having a Word with Yourself."
9. Powers, Zuroff, and Topciu, "Covert and Overt Expressions of Self-Criticism."
10. Gruen et al., "Vulnerability to Stress."
11. Dickerson and Kemeny, "Acute Stressors and Cortisol Response."
12. Besser, Flett, and Davis, "Self-Criticism, Dependency"; Cantazaro and Wei, "Adult Attachment, Dependence"; Reichl, Schneider, and Spinath, "Relation of Self-Talk."
13. Hayes and Tantleff-Dunn, "Am I Too Fat to Be a Princess?"
14. At a 2009 conference on eating disorders, I attended a talk on the cultural origins of the "thin ideal" (Gans, "What's It All About?"), and this is what I learned: It's all about social status—men's social status. The "thin ideal" in Western culture originates with notions of women as property and status symbols.

    In the seventeenth century, a softer, rounder, plumper female was the ideal because it was only rich women who could afford the buttery, floury food and the sedentary lifestyle that allowed them to accumulate the abundant curves of the women in Rubens's paintings. Around the mid-nineteenth century, coinciding with the Industrial Revolution and the rise of the middle class, it became fashionable for a man to advertise how rich he was by marrying a woman who was too weak to work. It was a status symbol to have a wife who was small, thin, and weak, barely able to totter daintily around the house, who not only didn't but couldn't contribute to the household income. This is in contradiction to everything evolution would have a woman be: robust, healthy, strong, tall, and able healthfully to conceive, gestate, give birth to, and breast-feed multiple offspring.

    In the twenty-first century, body shape is still a marker of social status—rich women can afford real food (rather than processed crap) and have the leisure time for exercise. But, as always, these fashions around what shape a woman's body "should" be are about social class. They have nothing to do with fertility (on the contrary), nothing to do with an "evolved preference"—except insofar as we have an evolved preference for higher social status—and nothing to do with promoting women's health.

So can you trust what your culture taught you about what your body should look like?

15. Bacon, "HAES Manifesto."

16. Haidt's website, moralfoundations.org, describes the foundations in more detail. But for an important critique, see Suhler and Churchland's "Can Innate, Modular 'Foundations' Explain Morality?"

17. See, just for a start, Yeshe, *Introduction to Tantra*.

18. It is not, however, identical. There are different categories of stimuli, such as "body boundary violations," which are about body-envelope damage and often relate to blood and physical pain, and "core disgust," related to digestion. These two kinds of disgust produce distinguishable reactions (Shenhav and Mendes, "Aiming for the Stomach").

19. Mesquita, "Emoting: A Contextualized Process."

20. Borg and de Jong, "Feelings of Disgust."

21. Tybur, Lieberman, and Griskevicius, "Microbes, Mating, and Morality."

22. Graham, Sanders, and Milhausen, "Sexual Excitation/Sexual Inhibition Inventory."

23. de Jong et al., "Disgust and Contamination Sensitivity"; Borg, de Jong, and Schultz, "Vaginismus and Dyspareunia"; for a review, see de Jong, van Overveld, and Borg, "Giving In to Arousal."

24. Neff, "Self-Compassion, Self-Esteem, and Well-Being."

25. Adapted from www.self-compassion.org/self_compassion_exercise.pdf.

26. Stice, Rohde, and Shaw, *Body Project*, 95.

27. Germer, *Mindful Path to Self-Compassion*, 150.

28. Hawkins et al., "Thin-Ideal Media Image."

29. Becker et al., "Eating Behaviours and Attitudes."

30. Becker, *Body, Self, and Society*, 56.

31. In Becker et al., "Validity and Reliability," 35 percent of participants reported purging in the last twenty-eight days, using a traditional herbal purgative, but Thomas et al., in "Latent Profile Analysis," report only 74 percent of those using the traditional purgative said they did so specifically for weight loss, as opposed to, for example, medical reasons.

32. The aliveness of the simultaneous pressures of the moral model and the media model in particular are observable in the perpetuation of the "Madonna-whore" construction of women's sexuality. To witness how this is enacted in young women's sexuality, I recommend Tolman's *Dilemmas of Desire*.

Part 3. Sex in Action

6. Arousal: Lubrication Is Not Causation

1. Suschinsky, Lalumière, and Chivers, "Patterns of Genital Sexual Arousal"; Bradford and Meston, "Impact of Anxiety on Sexual Arousal."

2. Peterson, Janssen, and Laan, "Women's Sexual Responses to Heterosexual and Lesbian Erotica." Why are men and women different? The best available hypothesis, though not yet proven, is the "preparation hypothesis," which suggests that female genitals respond to more or less any sex-related stimuli in order to prepare for sexual activity, which prevents injury, while penile erection is better served by occurring in response to more specific stimuli (Lalumière et al., "Preparation Hypothesis").

3. If you run the same experiment but use a thermistor (a little clip that attaches to the inner labia and measures its temperature as a proxy for blood flow) instead of the photoplethysmograph, you'll get slightly more overlap (Henson, Rubin, and Henson, "Consistency of Objective Measures"). If you use magnetic resonance imaging (MRI) to get very precise measurements of changes in blood flow to the pelvis, you'll get slightly less overlap (Hall, Binik, and Di Tomasso, "Concordance between Physiological and Subjective Measures"). If you get really high tech and measure not just vaginal blood flow and subjective arousal but also brain activity using functional magnetic resonance imaging (fMRI), you'll find out that genital response does not overlap with women's brain activity (Arnow et al., "Women with Hypoactive Sexual Desire Disorder").

4. Bergner, "Women Who Want to Want"; Bergner, *What Do Women Want?*; Ryan and Jethá, *Sex at Dawn*, 272–73, 278; Magnanti, *The Sex Myth*, 14.

5. Angier, "Conversations/Ellen T. M. Laan."

6. Both, Everaerd, and Laan, "Modulation of Spinal Reflexes"; Laan, Everaerd, and Evers, "Assessment of Female Sexual Arousal."

7. Suschinsky, Lalumière, and Chivers, "Patterns of Genital Sexual Arousal." Hat tip to Kelly Suchinsky and Meredith Chivers for actually sitting down with me and letting me see the clips.

8. Velten, Chivers, and Brotto, "Does Repeated Testing."

9. Velten et al., "Investigating Female Sexual Concordance."

10. Suschinsky, Dawson, and Chivers, "Assessing the Relationship."

11. It's growing increasingly clear that women classified as having any degree of "gynephilia"—i.e., those who identify as something other than straight—have greater concordance than straight women (ibid.).

12. A special issue of *Biological Psychology* was devoted to concordance

research, and none of it was sex research (Hollenstein and Lanteigne, "Models and Methods of Emotional Concordance").

13. Benedek and Kaernbach, "Physiological Correlates."

14. Kring and Gordon, "Sex Differences in Emotion"; Schwartz, Brown, and Ahern, "Facial Muscle Patterning."

15. Gottman and Silver, *What Makes Love Last?*

16. Hess, "Women Want Sex."

17. James, *Fifty Shades of Grey*, 275.

18. Ibid.

19. Ibid., 293.

20. Koehler, "From the Mouths of Rapists."

21. Toulalan, *Imagining Sex*.

22. Moore, "Rep. Todd Akin." Akin initially apologized for the statement but in 2014 wrote that he regretted the apology because stress—which rape certainly causes—interferes with fertility and that is what he meant by "shut the whole thing down" (Eichelberger, "Todd Akin Is Not Sorry for His Insane Rape Comments"). To be clear, then: His opinion as a former (and potentially future) lawmaker is that if a woman doesn't have a miscarriage, she can't have been "legitimately" raped.

23. This has been replicated for the last two decades, but the first evidence was Morokoff and Heiman, "Effects of Erotic Stimuli on Sexually Functional and Dysfunctional Women," and has been explored in more detail by Velten and Brotto, "Interoception and Sexual Response." For crucial commentary see Meston and Stanton, "Desynchrony between Subjective and Genital." Also, in a nonclinical population, sexual distress predicted *greater* concordance (Suschinsky et al., "Relationship between Sexual Functioning and Sexual Concordance").

24. Bobby Henderson, Church of the Flying Spaghetti Monster, "Open Letter to Kansas School Board," www.venganza.org/about/open-letter/.

25. Bloemers et al., "Induction of Sexual Arousal in Women."

26. Velten et al., "Investigating Female Sexual Concordance."

27. Jozkowski et al., "Women's Perceptions about Lubricant Use."

7. Desire: Spontaneous, Responsive and Magnificent

1. What proportion of people have which desire style?

It may be that a small proportion of people—for example, about 6 percent of women, in one study (Hendrickx, Gijs, and Enzlin, "Prevalence Rates of Sexual Difficulties")—lack both spontaneous and responsive desire. Beyond that, I have yet to find useful statistics about who has which desire style. It would be a helpful number to have, because people find it reassuring to hear "X percent of people have responsive desire," but, despite numerous studies, among many different populations, using a varieties of methodologies, over many decades, science does not have an answer (Garde and Lunde, "Female Sexual Behaviour"; Michael et al., *Sex in America*; Beck, Bozman, and Qualtrough, "Experience of Sexual Desire"; Bancroft, Loftus, and Long, "Distress about Sex"; Cain et al., "Sexual Functioning"; Carvalheira, Brotto, and Leal, "Women's Motivations for Sex"; Štulhofer, Carvalheira, and Træen, "Insights from a Two-Country Study"). Based on what's available, I can only offer a best guess that about a third of women experience primarily or exclusively responsive desire.

Two new lines of research I know of may produce a formal measure of responsive desire. The first effort (Velten et al., "Development and Validation") is, unfortunately, a revision of a scale developed to study changes in women's mating "tactics" across the menstrual cycle (Gangestad, Thornhill, and Garver, "Changes in Women's Sexual Interests"), an endeavor that has been rejected in primatology in favor of a model based on sexual proceptivity, receptivity, and attraction (Dixson, *Sexual Selection*, chapter 6). Grounded as it is in a faulty understanding of human female sexual functioning, this line of inquiry thus seems unlikely to lead to clear insight.

The second line of inquiry (Mark and Lasslo, "Maintaining Sexual Desire") is more clinically oriented and offers not statistics on who experiences which desire style, but rather a framework for understanding the predictors of satisfactory sexual desire in long-term relationships. This forms the foundation of a growing elaboration of couples' approaches to coping with desire differential (Vowels and Mark, "Strategies for Mitigating").

But regardless of (what I see as) the shortcomings in the research assessing responsive desire, the more research I read and the more people I talk to about desire, the more I think the basic concept of desire should be, if not quite discarded altogether, certainly set aside as a marginal factor in understanding and developing sexual confidence and joy in individuals and relationships. My goals are to normalize the variety of experiences people have with sexual desire and increase readers' motivation to prioritize pleasure over desire, per se.

These goals seem to align better with a European than North American approach to sexual desire. The European Society for Sexual Medicine's position statement on sexual desire discrepancy includes as its suggestions, among other things: normalizing and depathologizing variation in sexual desire; challenging the myth of spontaneous sexual desire; and dealing with relationship issues and unmet relationship needs (Dewitte et al., "Sexual Desire Discrepancy").

tl;dr: What proportion of people have which desire style? Who cares? It's like asking what proportion of people have labia minora that extend beyond their labia majora. It is not predictive of any domain of sexual satisfaction; it only shows who conforms with the culturally constructed ideal.

2. In the research, you'll find this described as "arousal first, then desire," and the first edition of *Come As You Are* used this language. But many journalists were confused and troubled by "arousal first, then desire," as this language falls perilously close to the long-standing rape myth that if you just start having sex with a woman, she won't be able to help herself, and to the advice that women should "just do it," on the (faulty) assumption that she won't be "just" having sex she neither wants nor likes. One reader told me that her husband's understanding of the "arousal first" language led him to stick his hands down her pants out of the blue, and when she said, "No, I'm not turned on," he replied, "But you will be." Which is the opposite of what I'm trying to teach.

Because of these misunderstandings, within months of *CAYA*'s publication I changed the way I taught from "arousal first, then desire," to "pleasure first, then desire." Research-driven clinicians have asked me why I use the alternative language, and this is the reason. It's actually more accurate and is less easily misconstrued through the lens of rape culture.

3. Of course, it varies from individual to individual as well. Scenario 1 might feel spontaneous for a person with a brake that is less sensitive to stress, and Scenario 3 might feel responsive for a person with an accelerator that requires more stimulation before pleasure stoked from a distance finally sparks into desire. But the general process is the same for everyone. Pleasure plus the right context—the right external circumstances and internal state—equals desire.

4. Ryan, "Women's Lived Experiences Seeking and Using Adaptation Strategies."

5. There are some cases when hormones might be involved in desire issues, mostly involving medical issues. For example, some women who have double oophorectomies (removal of the ovaries) before the age of forty-five may be more likely to experience low desire. And there may be a subgroup of women—about 15 percent—whose sexual arousability is testosterone dependent, primarily while taking hormonal contraception; specifically,

their sexual response mechanism may have low sensitivity to testosterone, so they require more of it before their sexual interest kicks in (Bancroft and Graham, "Varied Nature of Women's Sexuality").

About a third of women experience a decrease in sexual interest when they're on the birth control pill, about a fifth of women experience an increase in their interest in sex, and the remaining half experience no particular change (Sanders et al., "Prospective Study"). So if your interest in sex went down when you started on hormonal contraception and you'd like it to go back up, switch to a different pill, or try the ring, IUD, implant, or any other hormonal birth control method. Every woman's body responds differently to different hormone combinations.

It has also been found that the much-touted decrease in women's interest in sex as they age is associated with age itself, not with hormones (Erekson et al., "Sexual Function in Older Women"). It's complicated, and there are exceptions of course, but a good rule of thumb is that hormones can help with genital/peripheral issues—pain, dryness, sensation, etc.—but not with brain/central issues, and desire is a brain issue (Basson, "Hormones and Sexuality").

6. Basson, "Biopsychosocial Models of Women's Sexual Response"; Brotto et al., "Predictors of Sexual Desire Disorders."

7. Beach, "Characteristics of Masculine 'Sex Drive.'" For a brief discussion of the history of the conceptualization of sex as a drive, see Heiman and Pfaff, "Sexual Arousal and Related Concepts."

8. It's not sexual drive that makes people panic when they're "deprived" of sex. Instead it is, at least in part, loneliness. Connection *is* a drive (Nagoski, "I'm Sorry You're Lonely").

9. Toates, *How Sexual Desire Works*, chapter 4.

10. Note that curiosity and play are as innate to humans (and other social mammals) as hunger or thirst (Toates, *Biological Psychology*). This is important because the "you don't need sex" perspective in sex education, offered in the laudable hope that it would protect women from the sexual entitlement of men (see Manne, *Down Girl* and *Entitled*), has sometimes unfortunately swayed to the opposite extreme, advocating absolute abstinence (Duffey, *Relations of the Sexes*; Foster, *Social Emergency*). Sex is an innate motivation in humans, and in my view the only prerequisites are mutual, free consent and absence of unwanted pain. This is easier said than done, precisely because of men's sexual entitlement.

11. Perel, "Secret to Desire in a Long-Term Relationship."

12. Gottman, *Science of Trust*, 257.

13. Charles Carver has suggested that pleasure could be a signal that we can stop paying attention to one thing and shift it to something more dissatisfying ("Pleasure as a Sign"). See discrepancy reducing feedback loop, chapter 8 of this book, note 21.

14. Dwyer and Sobhan, "Statistical Review and Evaluation," accessed September 11, 2020, at https://www.accessdata.fda.gov/drugsatfda_docs/nda/2015/022526Orig1s000StatR.pdf.

15. Ng, "Risk Assessment and Risk Mitigation Review(s)." Number of "satisfying sexual events" is the secondary key endpoint and it "failed to meet statistical significance between treatment groups" (p. 8).

16. Filipovic, "Can 1 Little Pill Save Female Desire?"

17. Sole-Smith, "Pleasure in a Pill?" (Note the article's headline conflates pleasure and desire.)

18. E.g., Stein, "Female Libido Pill Fires Up Debate," and Adams, "For Sexual Dysfunction, 'Men Get a Pill and Women Need Therapy.'" (Note the second headline conflates women's sexual desire difficulties with men's erectile/arousal difficulties.)

19. Nagoski, "World Cup of Women's Sexual Desire."

20. Meston and Buss, "Why Humans Have Sex."

21. For example, Clayton et al., "International Society for the Study of Women's Sexual Health," but for a counterexample, see Tiefer, "Sex Therapy as a Humanistic Enterprise."

22. Kleinplatz et al., "Components of Optimal Sexuality."

23. Rosen, "How Do Women Survivors."

24. Fahs and Plante, "On 'Good Sex' and Other Dangerous Ideas."

25. Kleinplatz and Ménard, *Magnificent Sex*, 185.

Part 4. Ecstasy for Everybody
8. Orgasm: Pleasure Is the Measure

1. Kinsey, Pomeroy, and Martin (*Sexual Behavior in the Human Male*, 158) defined orgasm as "a sudden release which produces local spasms or more extensive or all-consuming convulsions." Masters and Johnson's (*Human Sexual Response*, 6) "orgasmic phase" was "those few seconds during which the vasoconcentration [constriction of blood vessels] and myotonia [muscle constriction] developed from sexual stimuli are released. This involuntary climax is reached at any level that represents maximum sexual tension increment for the particular occasion." You'll notice these are

more inclusive than the twenty-first-century "consensus that a woman's orgasm involves a transient peak of intense sexual pleasure associated with rhythmic contractions of the pelvic circumvaginal musculature, often with concomitant uterine and anal contractions" (Bianchi-Demicheli and Ortigue, "Toward an Understanding of the Cerebral Substrates," 2646). This "consensus" definition contradicts the research on nonconcordance and on the contextual absence of pleasure with orgasm.

2. Levin and Wagner, "Orgasm in Women in the Laboratory."

3. Bohlen et al., "Female Orgasm." Researcher Nicole Prause measured orgasm in the laboratory and found that half of women reporting orgasm were not exhibiting physiological signs of it. She said in an interview, "This is real: a lot of women think they're having orgasms when they're not" (Rowland, *The Pleasure Gap*, chapter 2). I would argue that, rather than gaslighting women and telling them they don't know their own bodies, we ask ourselves what orgasm is, since it is evidently not what we're measuring. My own conclusion is that orgasm is the spontaneous, involuntary release of sexual tension (see note 1, this chapter).

4. Alzate, Useche, and Villegas, "Heart Rate Change."

5. And there is a lot happening in your brain. For a review, see Georgiadis and Kortekaas, "Sweetest Taboo."

6. Herbenick and Fortenberry, "Exercise-Induced Orgasm."

7. Levin and van Berlo, "Sexual Arousal and Orgasm." My guest lecture was the foundation of my TED talk (Emily Nagoski, "The Truth about Unwanted Arousal," filmed April 13, 2018, in Vancouver, Ontario, TED video, 15:08, http://go.ted.com/emilynagoski).

8. Research has found that approximately 30 percent of women experience nocturnal orgasm (Mah and Binik, "Nature of Human Orgasm").

9. LoPiccolo and LoPiccolo, eds., *Handbook of Sex Therapy*.

10. It's also true that different parts of the brain "light up" during vaginal stimulation compared to clitoral stimulation (Komisaruk et al., "Women's Clitoris, Vagina, and Cervix"). Different parts of your brain map onto different parts of your body. But we don't call them "vaginal somatosensory cortex orgasms" and "clitoral somatosensory cortex orgasms." Women with spinal cord injuries may even bypass the spine altogether and generate orgasm through stimulation of a cranial nerve that travels directly between the cervix and the brain (Komisaruk et al., "Brain Activation"). And those aren't "cranial nerve orgasms"; they're orgasms, no qualifier necessary.

11. This number has been replicated multiple times, using multiple methodologies, in multiple studies, including Kinsey's female volume and *The
Hite Report*. The highest rate of penetration during masturbation I've seen
comes from a 2007 study where women responded to the statement "I use
vibrators or introduce some objects into the vagina"; 21.4 percent said yes
at least sometimes (Carvalheira and Leal, "Masturbation among Women").
It's important to note that vibrators are typically used externally; Davis et
al. ("Characteristics of Vibrator Use among Women") found that 3 percent
(3 out of 115) of women masturbated with a vibrator "primarily" in their
vaginas and 24 percent (36/115) with the vibrator on "various genital
sites," which might include the vagina; 14 percent (11 out of 79) reported
primarily an "in and out" movement of the vibrator; and 79 percent of
women reported that clitoral-vibrator stimulation during solo masturbation "usually or always resulted in orgasm" and 30 percent reported that
vaginal-vibrator stimulation did so.

   In addition, according to Hite (1976), 1.5 percent of women masturbate exclusively with vaginal penetration; 5 percent of women always
enter their vaginas during masturbation; 1 percent penetrate the vagina
at orgasm, with one hand also stimulating the vulva; another 1 percent
penetrate the vagina to obtain lubrication. Kinsey et al. (1953, 161) note an
anatomical distinction between the vagina and the introitus:

   > Many of those who reported "vaginal penetrations" in mastur-
   > bation failed to distinguish the vestibule of the vagina (which is
   > well equipped with nerve endings) from the vagina itself (which
   > is poorly equipped or devoid of nerve endings). In many in-
   > stances, the female's fingers had been inserted only far enough
   > beyond the musculature ring which lives at the vaginal entrance
   > (the introitus) to provide a firm hold for the rest of her hand
   > while it was stimulating the outer portions of her genitalia.

12. This is another number that has been replicated using multiple methodologies for the better part of a century. For a thorough review, see Lloyd, *Case
of the Female Orgasm*, and Levin, "Human Female Orgasm."

13. Wallen and Lloyd, "Female Sexual Arousal," but see also note 1 from
chapter 1. These kinds of studies can help us understand, little by little,
something of the evolutionary history of human sexuality, but they offer
absolutely no insight into how we "should" experience our sexuality in our
daily lives. Wallen and Lloyd do not make this mistake, but other researchers do. When reading studies about anatomical morphology, beware of

language that equates particular anatomical morphology with "health," "dysfunction," or "success," unless they are discussing infection or unwanted pain.

14. Nagoski, "Definitive Answer."

15. Graham, "DSM Diagnostic Criteria." In a study of a random sample of Australian women, 8 percent reported "difficulty plus distress" (Hayes et al., "'True' Prevalence of Female Sexual Dysfunctions"); in a study of a large population sample, 10 percent of women reported "difficulty plus distress" (Witting et al., "Correlated Genetic and Non-Shared Environmental Influences"); of seventeen thousand Flemish women, 6.5 percent reported "orgasm dysfunction" (Hendrickx, Gijs, and Enzlin, "Prevalence Rates of Sexual Difficulties").

16. Armstrong, England, and Fogarty, "Accounting for Women's Orgasms." What was the best kind of stimulation for orgasm with a new partner? Stimulating your clitoris with your own hand.

17. Stroupe, "How Difficult Is Too Difficult?"

18. Read, King, and Watson, "Sexual Dysfunction in Primary Medical Care," found 7 percent in a general clinical sample.

19. Simons and Carey, "Prevalence of Sexual Dysfunctions," found 7–10 percent in their review of research. Note that 80 percent of women with "lifelong" anorgasmia are effectively treated with psychological interventions (Heiman, "Psychologic Treatments for Female Sexual Dysfunction"), which is one of several reasons that I suspect that the number of women with truly lifelong anorgasmia is substantially less than 5–10 percent.

20. Kingsberg et al., "Characterization of Orgasmic Difficulties."

21. For a more precise and scientific description of the little monitor (for example, that there isn't actually a little monitor), see Carver and Scheier, "Self-Regulation of Action and Affect." In comparative psychology, the phenomenon of curiosity is studied as "Exploration," per Toates, *Biological Psychology*, 404–6, or "SEEKING," per Panksepp and Biven, *Archaeology of Mind*, chapter 3.

22. It could also be to avoid something—these are "antigoals" and they are the targets of discrepancy enlarging, rather than reducing, feedback loops (Carver and Scheier, "Cybernetic Control Processes").

23. Schwarzer and Frensch, eds., *Personality, Human Development, and Culture*, chapter 1.

24. Wrosch et al., "Importance of Goal Disengagement," 370. This parallels the three coping strategies in Mitchell et al., "Managing Sexual

Difficulties": changing goals to fit circumstances, changing circumstances to fit goals, and living with a gap between goals and circumstances.

25. Herbenick et al., "Prevalence and Characteristics of Vibrator Use."

26. Marcus, "Changes in a Woman's Sexual Experience."

27. Haller, "The 5 Craziest Sex Studies EVER." Half of the research participants not wearing socks achieved orgasm, but that number went up to 80 percent when they kept their socks on.

28. Toates, *Motivational Systems*, 151–2.

9. Love What's True: The Ultimate Sex-Positive Context

1. Ellin, "More Women Look Over the Counter."

2. Sakaluk et al., "Dominant Heterosexual Sexual Scripts."

3. Our different paths to welcoming our sexualities as they are happen to parallel the different "pathways toward magnificent sex" outlined by Kleinplatz and Ménard (*Magnificent Sex*, chapter 12).

4. Baer, "Construct Validity of the Five Facet Mindfulness Questionnaire"; Van Dam, Earleywine, and Danoff-Burg, "Differential Item Function"; Baer et al., "Using Self-Report Assessment Methods"; Silverstein et al., "Effects of Mindfulness Training." (This last paper concludes, unaccountably, that interoception—awareness of one's body—is what made the difference, even though the "observe" factor did not change significantly and the "nonjudge" factor changed the most significantly.)

5. Hoge et al., "Mindfulness and Self-Compassion in Generalized Anxiety Disorder." In a similar study of both anxiety and depression, this one comparing the Mindful Attention Awareness Scale (MAAS) and the Self-Compassion Scale referred to in chapter 5, self-compassion was a better predictor than mindfulness—awareness alone, that is—of quality of life (Van Dam et al., "Self-Compassion Is a Better Predictor").

6. Mize and Iantaffi, "Place of Mindfulness in a Sensorimotor Psychotherapy Intervention."

7. Leavitt, Lefkowitz, and Waterman, "Role of Sexual Mindfulness."

8. Suschinsky and Lalumière, "Is Sexual Concordance Related."

9. The power of nonjudgment in sexual functioning also helps me understand the relationship between sexual desire issues and arousal nonconcordance. Researchers suggested that women with greater concerns about their sexual functioning might worry more about their genital sensations, which could reduce both their subjective arousal and their genital blood flow, even while increasing their attention to their genital blood flow (Velten

et al., "Investigating Female Sexual Concordance"). If that's true, then awareness itself isn't good or bad; it's the quality of the awareness that matters. Worried awareness, it seems, can hit the brakes. We can't change the sensitivity of the brakes, but we can change the context. We can shift worried awareness to nonjudging awareness. This would also explain why greater awareness of genital arousal in sexually distressed women was related to more arousal concordance, as mentioned in chapter 6, note 23 (Suschinshy et al., "The Relationship between Sexual Functioning and Sexual Concordance").

10. Moseley and Butler, *Explain Pain Supercharged*; Tracey, "Getting the Pain You Expect."

11. Pierce et al., "Vaginal Hypersensitivity and Hypothalamic-Pituitary-Adrenal Axis Dysfunction."

references

Abler, Birgit, Henrik Walter, Susanne Erk, Hannes Kammerer, and Manfred Spitzer. "Prediction Error as a Linear Function of Reward Probability Is Coded in Human Nucleus Accumbens." *NeuroImage* 31, no. 2 (2006): 790–95. doi:10.1016/j.neuroimage.2006.01.001.

Acevedo, Bianca P., Arthur Aron, Helen E. Fisher, and Lucy L. Brown. "Neural Correlates of Long-Term Intense Romantic Love." *Social Cognitive and Affective Neuroscience* 7, no. 2 (2011): 145–59. doi:10.1093/scan/nsq092.

Adams, Rebecca. "For Sexual Dysfunction, 'Men Get a Pill and Women Need Therapy.' What Gives?" Huffington Post, June 3, 2015. Accessed June 22, 2020. https://www.huffpost.com/entry/sexual-dysfunction-pill_n_6677502.

Alzate, H., B. Useche, and M. Villegas. "Heart Rate Change as Evidence for Vaginally Elicited Orgasm and Orgasm Intensity." *Annals of Sex Research* 2 (1989): 345–57.

Angier, Natalie. "Conversations/Ellen T. M. Laan; Science Is Finding Out What Women Really Want." *New York Times*, August 13, 1995. www.nytimes.com/1995/08/13/weekinreview/conversations-ellen-tm-laan-science-is-finding-out-what-women-really-want.html.

Ariely, Dan. *Predictably Irrational: The Hidden Forces That Shape Our Decisions.* Rev. ed. New York: Harper, 2009.

Aristotle [pseud.]. *Aristotle's Compleat Master-Piece in Three Parts Displaying the Secrets of Nature in the Generation of Man.* 1728.

Armstrong, Elizabeth A., Paula England, and Alison C. K. Fogarty. "Accounting for Women's Orgasms and Sexual Enjoyment in College Hookups and Relationships." *American Sociological Review* 77, no. 3 (2012): 435–62. doi:10.1177/0003122412445802.

Arnow, B. A., L. Millheiser, A. Garrett, M. Lake Polan, G. H. Glover, K. R. Hill, and A. Lightbody, et al. "Women with Hypoactive Sexual Desire Disorder Compared to Normal Females: A Functional Magnetic Resonance Imaging Study." *Neuroscience* 158, no. 2 (2009): 484–502. doi:10.1016/j .neuroscience.2008.09.044.

Aubrey, Allison. "Feeling a Little Blue May Mask Our Ability to Taste Fat." National Public Radio, June 6, 2013. www.npr.org/blogs/thesalt /2013/06/04/188706043/feeling-a-little-blue-may-mask-our-ability-to -taste-fat?ft=1&f=1007.

Bacon, Lindo. "The HAES Manifesto." From *Health at Every Size: The Surprising Truth about Your Weight*. Dallas: BenBella Books, 2010. lindobacon .com/HAESbook/pdf_files/HAES_Manifesto.pdf.

Baer, Ruth A. "Construct Validity of the Five Facet Mindfulness Questionnaire in Meditating and Nonmeditating Samples." *Assessment* 15, no. 3 (2008): 329–42. doi:10.1177/1073191107313003.

Baer, Ruth A., Gregory T. Smith, Jaclyn Hopkins, Jennifer Krietemeyer, and Leslie Toney. "Using Self-Report Assessment Methods to Explore Facets of Mindfulness." *Assessment* 13, no. 1 (2006): 27–45. doi:10.1177/107319110 5283504.

Baliki, Marwan N., Paul Y. Geha, Howard L. Fields, and A. Vania Apkarian. "Predicting Value of Pain and Analgesia: Nucleus Accumbens Response to Noxious Stimuli Changes in the Presence of Chronic Pain." *Neuron* 66, no. 1 (2010): 149–60. doi:10.1016/j.neuron.2010.03.002.

Bancroft, John, and Cynthia A. Graham. "The Varied Nature of Women's Sexuality: Unresolved Issues and a Theoretical Approach." *Hormones and Behavior* 59, no. 5 (2011): 717–29. http://dx.doi.org/10.1016/j .yhbeh.2011.01.005.

Bancroft, John, Jeni Loftus, and J. Scott Long. "Distress about Sex: A National Survey of Women in Heterosexual Relationships." *Archives of Sexual Behavior* 32, no. 3 (2003): 193–208.

Basson, Rosemary. "Biopsychosocial Models of Women's Sexual Response: Applications to Management of 'Desire Disorders.'" *Sexual and Relationship Therapy* 18, no. 1 (2003): 107–15. doi:10.1080/1468199031000061308.

————. "Hormones and Sexuality: Current Complexities and Future Directions." *Maturitas* 57, no. 1 (2007): 66–70. doi:10.1016/j.maturitas.2007 .02.018.

BBC News. "Words Can Change What We Smell." September 26, 2005. news .bbc.co.uk/2/hi/health/4558075.stm.

Beach, Frank A. "Characteristics of Masculine 'Sex Drive.'" *Nebraska Symposium on Motivation*, vol. 4. Lincoln: University of Nebraska Press, 1956, 1–32.

Beck, J. Gayle, Alan W. Bozman, and Tina Qualtrough. "The Experience of Sexual Desire: Psychological Correlates in a College Sample." *Journal of Sex Research* 28, no. 3 (1991): 443–56.

Becker, Anne E. *Body, Self, and Society: The View from Fiji*. Philadelphia: University of Pennsylvania Press, 1995.

Becker, Anne E., Rebecca A. Burwell, David B. Herzog, Paul Hamburg, and Stephen E. Gilman. "Eating Behaviours and Attitudes Following Prolonged Exposure to Television among Ethnic Fijian Adolescent Girls." *British Journal of Psychiatry* 180 (2002): 509–14. doi:10.1192/bjp.180.6.509.

Becker, Anne E., Jennifer J. Thomas, Asenaca Bainivualiku, Lauren Richards, Kesaia Navara, Andrea L. Roberts, Stephen E. Gilman, and Ruth H. Striegel-Moore. "Validity and Reliability of a Fijian Translation and Adaptation of the Eating Disorder Examination Questionnaire." *International Journal of Eating Disorders* 43, no. 2 (2010): 171–78. doi:10.1002 /eat.20675.

Benedek, Mathias, and Christian Kaernbach. "Physiological Correlates and Emotional Specificity of Human Piloerection." *Biological Psychology* 86, no. 3 (2011): 320–29.

Bergner, Daniel. *What Do Women Want? Adventures in the Science of Female Desire*. New York: Harper, 2013.

———. "Women Who Want to Want." *New York Times*, November 24, 2009. www.nytimes.com/2009/11/29/magazine/29sex-t.html?pagewanted =all&_r=0.

Berridge, Kent. *The Mechanisms of Self-Control: Lessons from Addiction*. Video, The Science Network, May 13, 2010. http://thesciencenetwork .org/programs/the-mechanisms-of-self-control-lessons-from-addiction /kent-berridge.

Berridge, Kent, Richie Davidson, and Daniel Gilbert. *The Neuroscience of Happiness*. Video, Aspen Ideas Festival, 2011. https://youtu.be/8f-T7lgdLPI.

Berridge, Kent C., and Morten L. Kringelbach. "Neuroscience of Affect: Brain Mechanisms of Pleasure and Displeasure." *Current Opinion in Neurobiology* 23, no. 3 (2013): 294–303. http://dx.doi.org/10.1016/j.conb.2013.01.017.

Berridge, Kent, and Piotr Winkielman. "What Is an Unconscious Emotion?

(The Case for Unconscious 'Liking')." *Cognition and Emotion* 17, no. 2 (2003): 181–211.

Berry, Lisa-Marie, and Ben Laskey. "A Review of Obsessive Intrusive Thoughts in the General Population." *Journal of Obsessive-Compulsive and Related Disorders* 1, no. 2 (2012): 125–32.

Besser, Avi, Gordon L. Flett, and Richard A. Davis. "Self-Criticism, Dependency, Silencing the Self, and Loneliness: A Test of a Mediational Model." *Personality and Individual Differences* 35, no. 8 (2003): 1735–52. http://dx.doi.org/10.1016/S0191-8869(02)00403-8.

Bianchi-Demicheli, Francesco, and Stephanie Ortigue. "Toward an Understanding of the Cerebral Substrates of Woman's Orgasm." *Neuropsychologia* 45, no. 12 (2007): 2645–59. http://dx.doi.org/10.1016/j.neuropsychologia.2007.04.016.

Bifulco, A., P. M. Moran, C. Ball, and O. Bernazzani. "Adult Attachment Style. I: Its Relationship to Clinical Depression." *Social Psychiatry and Psychiatric Epidemiology* 37 (2002): 50–59.

Birnbaum, Gurit E., Harry T. Reis, Mario Mikulincer, Omri Gillath, and Ayala Orpaz. "When Sex Is More Than Just Sex: Attachment Orientations, Sexual Experience, and Relationship Quality." *Journal of Personality and Social Psychology* 91, no. 5 (2006): 929–43. doi:10.1037/0022-3514.91.5.929.

Bloemers, Jos, Jeroen Gerritsen, Richard Bults, Hans Koppeschaar, Walter Everaerd, Berend Olivier, and Adriaan Tuiten. "Induction of Sexual Arousal in Women under Conditions of Institutional and Ambulatory Laboratory Circumstances: A Comparative Study." *Journal of Sexual Medicine* 7, no. 3 (2010): 1160–76. doi:10.1111/j.1743-6109.2009.01660.x.

Bohlen, Joseph G., James P. Held, Margaret Olwen Sanderson, and Andrew Ahlgren. "The Female Orgasm: Pelvic Contraction." *Archives of Sexual Behavior* 11, no. 5 (1982): 367–86.

Borg, Charmaine, and Peter J. de Jong. "Feelings of Disgust and Disgust-Induced Avoidance Weaken following Induced Sexual Arousal in Women." *PLoS ONE* 7, no. 9 (2012). doi:10.1371/journal.pone.0044111.

Borg, Charmaine, Peter J. de Jong, and Willibrord Weijmar Schultz. "Vaginismus and Dyspareunia: Relationship with General and Sex-Related Moral Standards." *Journal of Sexual Medicine* 8, no. 1 (2011): 223–31. doi:10.1111/j.1743-6109.2010.02080.x.

Both, Stephanie, Walter Everaerd, and Ellen Laan. "Modulation of Spinal Reflexes by Aversive and Sexually Appetitive Stimuli." *Psychophysiology* 40, no. 2 (2003): 174–83. doi:10.1111/1469-8986.00019.

Bradford, Andrea, and Cindy M. Meston. "The Impact of Anxiety on Sexual Arousal in Women." *Behaviour Research and Therapy* 44, no. 8 (2006): 1067–77. doi:10.1016/j.brat.2005.08.006.

Briganti, Paul, dir. *Adam Ruins Everything*. Season 1, episode 10, "Adam Ruins Sex." Written by Caldwell Tanner. Aired December 8, 2015, on truTV.

Britton, Lauren E., Denise M. Martz, Doris G. Bazzini, Lisa A. Curtin, and Anni LeaShomb. "Fat Talk and Self-Presentation of Body Image: Is There a Social Norm for Women to Self-Degrade?" *Body Image* 3, no. 3 (2006): 247–54.

Brotto, Lori A., A. John Petkau, Fernand Labrie, and Rosemary Basson. "Predictors of Sexual Desire Disorders in Women." *Journal of Sexual Medicine* 8 no. 3 (2011): 742–53. doi:10.1111/j.1743-6109.2010.02146.x.

Cain, Virginia S., Catherine B. Johannes, Nancy E. Avis, Beth Mohr, Miriam Schocken, Joan Skurnick, and Marcia Ory. "Sexual Functioning and Practices in a Multi-Ethnic Study of Midlife Women: Baseline Results from SWAN." *Journal of Sex Research* 40, no. 3 (2003): 266–76.

Cantazaro, Amy, and Meifen Wei. "Adult Attachment, Dependence, Self-Criticism, and Depressive Symptoms: A Test of a Mediational Model." *Journal of Personality* 78, no. 4 (2010): 1135–62. wei.public.iastate.edu /manuscript/attachment dependence self-criticism.pdf.

Carpenter, Deanna L., Cynthia Graham, Erick Janssen, Harrie Vorst, and Jelte Wicherts. "The Dual Control Model: Gender, Sexual Problems, and Prevalence of Sexual Excitation and Inhibition Profiles." www.slideserve.com /phoebe/the-dual-control-model-gender-sexual-problems-and-preva lence-of-sexual-excitation-and-inhibition-profiles.

Carpenter, Deanna, Erick Janssen, Cynthia Graham, Harrie Vorst, and Jelte Wicherts. "Women's Scores on the Sexual Inhibition/Sexual Excitation Scales (SIS/SES): Gender Similarities and Differences." *Journal of Sex Research* 45, no. 1 (2008): 36–48. doi:10.1080/00224490701808076.

Carvalheira, Ana A., Lori A. Brotto, and Isabel Leal. "Women's Motivations for Sex: Exploring the Diagnostic and Statistical Manual, Fourth Edition, Text Revision Criteria for Hypoactive Sexual Desire and Female Sexual Arousal Disorders." *Journal of Sexual Medicine* 7, no. 4 (2010): 1454–63. doi:10.1111/j.1743-6109.2009.01693.x.

Carvalheira, Ana, and Isabel Leal. "Masturbation among Women: Associated Factors and Sexual Response in a Portuguese Community Sample." *Journal of Sex & Marital Therapy* 39, no. 4 (2013): 347–67. doi:10.1080/00926 23X.2011.628440.

Carver, Charles S. "Pleasure as a Sign You Can Attend to Something Else: Placing Positive Feelings within a General Model of Affect." *Cognition and Emotion* 17, no. 2 (2003): 241–61.

Carver, Charles S., and Michael F. Scheier. "Cybernetic Control Processes and the Self-Regulation of Behavior." In *The Oxford Handbook of Human Motivation*, edited by Richard M. Ryan, 28–42. New York: Oxford University Press, 2012.

———. "Self-Regulation of Action and Affect." In *Handbook of Self-Regulation: Research, Theory, and Applications*, 2nd ed., edited by Kathleen D. Vohs and Roy F. Baumeister, 3–21. New York: Guilford Press, 2013.

Cathey, Angela J., and Chad T. Wetterneck. "Stigma and Disclosure of Intrusive Thoughts about Sexual Themes." *Journal of Obsessive-Compulsive and Related Disorders* 2, no. 4 (2013): 439–43.

Childress, Anna Rose, Ronald N. Ehrman, Ze Wang, Yin Li, Nathan Sciortino, Jonathan Hakun, William Jens, et al. "Prelude to Passion: Limbic Activation by 'Unseen' Drug and Sexual Cues." *PLoS ONE* 3, no. 1 (2008). doi:10.1371/journal.pone.0001506.

Clayton, Anita H., Irwin Goldstein, Noel N. Kim, Stanley E. Althof, Stephanie S. Faubion, Brooke M. Faught, Sharon J. Parish, et al. "The International Society for the Study of Women's Sexual Health Process of Care for Management of Hypoactive Sexual Desire Disorder in Women." In *Mayo Clinic Proceedings* 93, no. 4, pp. 467–87. Amsterdam: Elsevier, 2018.

Cooper, Lynne M., Mark Pioli, Ash Levitt, Amelia E. Talley, Lada Micheas, and Nancy L. Collins. "Attachment Styles, Sex Motives, and Sexual Behavior: Evidence for Gender-Specific Expressions of Attachment Dynamics." In *Dynamics of Romantic Love: Attachment, Caregiving, and Sex*, edited by Mario Mikulincer and Gail S. Goodman, 243–74. New York: Guilford Press, 2006.

David, Daryn H., and Karlen Lyons-Ruth. "Differential Attachment Responses of Male and Female Infants to Frightening Maternal Behavior: Tend or Befriend versus Fight or Flight?" *Infant Mental Health Journal* 26, no. 1 (2005): 1–18. doi:10.1002/imhj.20033.

Davila, Joanne, Dorli Burge, and Constance Hammen. "Why Does Attachment Style Change?" *Journal of Personality and Social Psychology* 73, no. 4 (1997): 826–38. doi:10.1037/0022-3514.73.4.826.

Davis, Clive M., Joani Blank, Hung-Yu Lin, and Consuelo Bonillas. "Characteristics of Vibrator Use among Women." *Journal of Sex Research* 33, no. 4 (1996): 313–20.

de Jong, Peter J., Mark van Overveld, and Charmaine Borg. "Giving In to Arousal or Staying Stuck in Disgust? Disgust-Based Mechanisms in Sex and Sexual Dysfunction." *Journal of Sex Research* 50, no. 3 (2013): 247–62. doi:10.1080/00224499.2012.746280.

de Jong, Peter J., Mark van Overveld, Willibrord Weijmar Schultz, Madelon L. Peters, and Femke M. Buwalda. "Disgust and Contamination Sensitivity in Vaginismus and Dyspareunia." *Archives of Sexual Behavior* 38, no. 2 (2009): 244–52. www.ncbi.nlm.nih.gov/pubmed/17909958.

Dewitte, Marieke. "Different Perspectives on the Sex-Attachment Link: Towards an Emotion-Motivational Account." *Journal of Sex Research* 49, no. 2–3 (2012): 105–24.

Dewitte, Marieke, Joana Carvalho, Giovanni Corona, Erika Limoncin, Patricia Pascoal, Yacov Reisman, and Aleksandar Štulhofer. "Sexual Desire Discrepancy: A Position Statement of the European Society for Sexual Medicine." *Sexual Medicine* 8, no. 2 (2020): 121–31.

Dickerson, S. S., and M. E. Kemeny. "Acute Stressors and Cortisol Response: A Theoretical Integration and Synthesis of Laboratory Research." *Psychological Bulletin* 130, no. 3 (2004): 355–91.

Dixson, Alan F. *Sexual Selection and the Origins of Human Mating Systems.* Oxford: Oxford University Press, 2009.

Dreger, Alice Domurat. "Why 'Disorders of Sex Development'? (On Language and Life)." November 17, 2007. http://alicedreger.com/dsd.html.

Drysdale, Kirsten, Ali Russell, and Andrew Glover. "Labiaplasty: Hungry Beast." ABC TV Australia, 2010. http://vimeo.com/10883108.

Duffey, Eliza Bisbee. *The Relations of the Sexes.* 1876. New York: Arno Press, 1974.

Dunkley, Cara R., Silvain S. Dang, Sabrina C. H. Chang, and Boris B. Gorzalka. "Sexual Functioning in Young Women and Men: Role of Attachment Orientation." *Journal of Sex & Marital Therapy* 42, no. 5 (2016): 413–30.

Dwyer, Kate and Mahboob Sobhan. "Statistical Review and Evaluation of Application Number: 022526Orig1s000." Accessed September 11, 2020. https://www.accessdata.fda.gov/drugsatfda_docs/nda/2015/022526Orig1s000StatR.pdf.

Eichelberger, Erika. "Todd Akin Is Not Sorry for His Insane Rape Comments." *Mother Jones*, July 10, 2014. Accessed July 27, 2014. http://www.motherjones.com/mojo/2014/07/todd-akin-book-legitimate-rape.

Ekman, Paul. *Emotions Revealed: Recognizing Faces and Feelings to Improve Communication and Emotional Life.* 2nd ed. New York: Henry Holt, 2007.

Ellin, Abby. "More Women Look Over the Counter for a Libido Fix." *New York Times*, July 2, 2012. www.nytimes.com/2012/07/03/health/more-women -seek-over-the-counter-sexual-remedies.html.

Emhardt, E., J. Siegel, and L. Hoffman. "Anatomic Variation and Orgasm: Could Variations in Anatomy Explain Differences in Orgasmic Success?" *Clinical Anatomy* 29, no. 5 (2016): 665–72.

Erekson, Elisabeth A., Deanna K. Martin, Kejia Zhu, Maria M. Ciarleglio, Divya A. Patel, Marsha K. Guess, and Elena S. Ratner. "Sexual Function in Older Women after Oophorectomy." *Obstetrics & Gynecology* 120, no. 4 (2012): 833–42. doi:10.1097/AOG.0b013e31826af3d1.

Fahs, Breanne, and Rebecca Plante. "On 'Good Sex' and Other Dangerous Ideas: Women Narrate Their Joyous and Happy Sexual Encounters." *Journal of Gender Studies* 26, no. 1 (2017): 33–44.

Fausto-Sterling, Anne. *Sexing the Body: Gender Politics and the Construction of Sexuality*. New York: Basic Books, 2000.

Feeney, Judith A., and Patricia Noller. "Attachment Style as a Predictor of Adult Romantic Relationships." *Journal of Personality and Social Psychology* 58, no. 2 (1990): 281–91. doi:10.1037/0022-3514.58.2.281.

Feeney, Nolan. "Living Myths about Virginity." *Atlantic*, February 7, 2014. www.theatlantic.com/health/archive/2014/02/living-myths-about-vir ginity/283628.

Fernández de la Cruz, Lorena, Faye Barrow, Koen Bolhuis, Georgina Krebs, Chloe Volz, Eriko Nakatani, Isobel Heyman, and David Mataix-Cols. "Sexual Obsessions in Pediatric Obsessive-Compulsive Disorder: Clinical Characteristics and Treatment Outcomes." *Depression and Anxiety* 30, no. 8 (2013): 732–40.

Filipovic, Jill. "Can 1 Little Pill Save Female Desire?" *Cosmopolitan*, February 24, 2015. Accessed June 22, 2020. https://www.cosmopolitan.com /sex-love/news/a36745/can-a-pill-save-female-desire/.

Flaten, Magne Arve, Terje Simonsen, and Harald Olsen. "Drug-Related Information Generates Placebo and Nocebo Responses That Modify the Drug Response." *Psychosomatic Medicine* 61, no. 2 (1999): 250–55. www.psycho somaticmedicine.org/content/61/2/250.full.

Foster, William Trufant. *The Social Emergency: Studies in Sex Hygiene and Morals*. Boston: Houghton Mifflin, 1914.

Fraley, R. Chris, Neils G. Waller, and Kelly A. Brennan. "An Item Response Theory Analysis of Self-Report Measures of Adult Attachment."

Journal of Personality and Social Psychology 78, no. 2 (2000): 350–65. doi:10.1037/0022-3514.78.2.350.

Gaffney, D. "Established and Emerging PTSD Treatments." *Mental Health Clinician* 2, no. 7 (2013): 213–19.

Gangestad, Steven W., Randy Thornhill, and Christine E. Garver. "Changes in Women's Sexual Interests and Their Partner's Mate-Retention Tactics across the Menstrual Cycle: Evidence for Shifting Conflicts of Interest." *Proceedings of the Royal Society of London. Series B: Biological Sciences* 269, no. 1494 (2002): 975–82.

Gans, Margery. "What's It All About? Attending to the Meaning of Eating Disorders." Paper presented at the Collaborative Ways to Address Disordered Eating on Campus: It Takes a Village conference. Cambridge, MA, April 17–18, 2009.

Garde, K., and I. Lunde. "Female Sexual Behaviour: A Study in a Random Sample of 40-Year-Old Women." *Maturitas* 2, no. 3 (1980): 225–40.

Georgiadis, J. R., and Rudie Kortekaas. "The Sweetest Taboo: Functional Neurobiology of Human Sexuality in Relation to Pleasure." In *Pleasures of the Brain*, edited by Morten L. Kringelbach and Kent. C. Berridge, 178–201. New York: Oxford University Press, 2010.

Germer, Christopher K. *The Mindful Path to Self-Compassion: Freeing Yourself from Destructive Thoughts and Emotions.* New York: Guilford Press, 2009.

Glass, Ira, and Deborah Blum. "317: Unconditional Love Transcript." *This American Life*, Chicago Public Media. September 15, 2006. www.thisamericanlife.org/radio-archives/episode/317/transcript.

Goldacre, Ben. "Ben Goldacre at Nerdstock." YouTube video, 2010. www.youtube.com/watch?v=O1Q3jZw4FGs.

Goldstein, Andrew, Caroline F. Pukall, and Irwin Goldstein. *When Sex Hurts: A Woman's Guide to Banishing Sexual Pain.* Boston: Da Capo Press, 2011.

Goldstein, Irwin, Noel N. Kim, Anita H. Clayton, Leonard R. DeRogatis, Annamaria Giraldi, Sharon J. Parish, James Pfaus, et al. "Hypoactive Sexual Desire Disorder: International Society for the Study of Women's Sexual Health (ISSWSH) Expert Consensus Panel Review." In *Mayo Clinic Proceedings* 92, no. 1, pp. 114–28. Amsterdam: Elsevier, 2017.

Gottman, John M. *The Science of Trust: Emotional Attunement for Couples.* New York: W. W. Norton, 2011.

Gottman, John, and Nan Silver. *What Makes Love Last? How to Build Trust and Avoid Betrayal.* New York: Simon & Schuster, 2013.

Graham, Cynthia A. "The DSM Diagnostic Criteria for Female Orgasmic Disorder." *Archives of Sexual Behavior* 39, no. 2 (2010): 256–70. doi:10.1007/s10508-009-9542-2.

Graham, Cynthia A., Stephanie A. Sanders, and Robin R. Milhausen. "The Sexual Excitation/Sexual Inhibition Inventory for Women: Psychometric Properties." *Archives of Sexual Behavior* 35, no. 4 (2006): 397–409.

Graham, Cynthia A., Stephanie A. Sanders, Robin R. Milhausen, and Kimberly R. McBride. "Turning On and Turning Off: A Focus Group Study of the Factors That Affect Women's Sexual Arousal." *Archives of Sexual Behavior* 33, no. 6 (2004): 527–38.

Granados, Reina, Joana Carvalho, and Juan Carlos Sierra. "Preliminary Evidence on How the Dual Control Model Predicts Female Sexual Response to a Bogus Negative Feedback." *Psychological Reports* (2020): https://doi.org/10.1177%2F0033294120907310.

Grant, Jon E., Anthony Pinto, Matthew Gunnip, Maria C. Mancebo, Jane L. Eisen, and Steven A. Rasmussen. "Sexual Obsessions and Clinical Correlates in Adults with Obsessive-Compulsive Disorder." *Comprehensive Psychiatry* 47, no. 5 (2006): 325–29.

Gruen, Rand J., Raul Silva, Joshua Ehrlich, Jack W. Schweitzer, and Arnold J. Friedhoff. "Vulnerability to Stress: Self-Criticism and Stress-Induced Changes in Biochemistry." *Journal of Personality* 65, no. 1 (1997): 33–47. doi:10.1111/j.1467-6494.1997.tb00528.x.

Hall, Kathryn S., Yitzchak Binik, and Enrico Di Tomasso. "Concordance between Physiological and Subjective Measures of Sexual Arousal." *Behaviour Research and Therapy* 23, no. 3 (1985): 297–303.

Haller, Madeline. "The 5 Craziest Sex Studies EVER." *Men's Health*. September 22, 2012. Accessed September 11, 2020. https://www.menshealth.com/sex-women/a19534159/the-5-craziest-sex-studies-ever/.

Hamilton, Lisa Dawn, and Cindy M. Meston. "Chronic Stress and Sexual Function in Women." *Journal of Sexual Medicine* 10, no. 10 (2013): 2443–54.

Hawkins, Nicole, P. Scott Richards, H. Mac Granley, and David M. Stein. "The Impact of Exposure to the Thin-Ideal Media Image on Women." *Eating Disorders: The Journal of Treatment & Prevention* 12, no. 1 (2004): 35–50. doi:10.1080/10640260490267751.

Hayes, Richard D., Lorraine Dennerstein, Catherine M. Bennet, and Christopher K. Fairley. "What Is the 'True' Prevalence of Female Sexual Dysfunctions and Does the Way We Assess These Conditions Have an Impact?" *Journal of Sexual Medicine* 5, no. 4 (2008): 777–87.

Hayes, Sharon, and Stacey Tantleff-Dunn. "Am I Too Fat to Be a Princess? Examining the Effects of Popular Children's Media on Young Girls' Body Image." *British Journal of Developmental Psychology* 28, no. 2 (2010): 413–26. doi:10.1348/026151009X424240.

Hegazy, A. A., and M. O. Al-Rukban. "Hymen: Facts and Conceptions." *The Health* 3, no. 4 (2012): 109–15.

Heiman, Julia R. "Psychologic Treatments for Female Sexual Dysfunction: Are They Effective and Do We Need Them?" *Archives of Sexual Behavior* 31, no. 5 (2002): 445–50.

Heiman, Julia R., and Donald Pfaff. "Sexual Arousal and Related Concepts: An Introduction." *Hormones and Behavior* 59, no. 5 (2011): 613–15.

Hendrickx, Lies, Luk Gijs, and Paul Enzlin. "Prevalence Rates of Sexual Difficulties and Associated Distress in Heterosexual Men and Women: Results from an Internet Survey in Flanders." *Journal of Sex Research* 51, no. 1 (2014): 1–12. doi:10.1080/00224499.2013.819065.

Henson, Donald E., H. B. Rubin, and Claudia Henson. "Analysis of the Consistency of Objective Measures of Sexual Arousal in Women." *Journal of Applied Behavior Analysis* 12, no. 4 (1979): 701–11.

Herbenick, Debby, and J. Dennis Fortenberry. "Exercise-Induced Orgasm and Pleasure among Women." *Sexual and Relationship Therapy* 26, no. 4 (2011): 373–88. doi:10.1080/14681994.2011.647902.

Herbenick, Debra, Michael Reece, Stephanie Sanders, Brian Dodge, Annahita Ghassemi, and J. Dennis Fortenberry. "Prevalence and Characteristics of Vibrator Use by Women in the United States: Results from a Nationally Representative Study." *Journal of Sexual Medicine* 6 no. 7 (2009): 1857–66.

Hess, Amanda. "Women Want Sex, but Men Don't Want Them to Know It." Slate, June 4, 2013. www.slate.com/articles/double_x/doublex/2013/06/what_do_women_want_sex_according_to_daniel_bergner_s_new_book_on_female.html.

Hitchens, Christopher. *Hitch-22: A Memoir*. New York: Grand Central Publishing, 2010.

Hite, Shere. *The Hite Report: A Nationwide Study of Female Sexuality*. New York: Macmillan, 1976.

Hoge, Elizabeth A., Britta K. Hölzel, Luana Marques, Christina A. Metcalf, Narayan Brach, Sara W. Lazar, and Naomi M. Simon. "Mindfulness and Self-Compassion in Generalized Anxiety Disorder: Examining Predictors of Disability." *Evidence-Based Complementary and Alternative Medicine* (2013). http://dx.doi.org/10.1155/2013/576258.

Hollenstein, Tom, and Dianna Lanteigne. "Models and Methods of Emotional Concordance." *Biological Psychology* 98 (2014): 1–5. doi:10.1016/biopsy cho.2013.12.012.

ILGA-Europe. "Public Statement." https://ilga-europe.org/resources/ilga -europe-reports-and-other-materials/protecting-intersex-people-europe -toolkit.

James, E. L. *Fifty Shades of Grey.* New York: Vintage Books, 2012.

Janssen, Erick, and John Bancroft. "The Dual Control Model: The Role of Sexual Inhibition and Excitation in Sexual Arousal and Behavior." In *The Psychophysiology of Sex*, edited by Erick Janssen, 197. Bloomington: Indiana University Press, 2007.

Janssen, Erick, Deanna Carpenter, Cynthia Graham, Harrie Vorst, and Jelte Wicherts. "The Sexual Inhibition/Sexual Excitation Scales—Short Form." *Handbook of Sexuality-Related Measures*, 77. New York: Routledge, 2019.

Janssen, Erick, Kathryn R. Macapagal, and Brian Mustanski. "Individual Differences in the Effects of Mood on Sexuality: The Revised Mood and Sexuality Questionnaire (MSQ-R)." *Journal of Sex Research* 50, no. 7 (2013): 676–87.

Johnson, Sue. *Hold Me Tight: Seven Conversations for a Lifetime of Love.* New York: Little, Brown, 2008.

———. *Love Sense: The Revolutionary New Science of Romantic Relationships.* New York: Little, Brown, 2013.

Jozkowski, Kristen N., Debby Herbenick, Vanessa Schick, Michael Reece, Stephanie A. Sanders, and J. Dennis Fortenberry. "Women's Perceptions about Lubricant Use and Vaginal Wetness during Sexual Activities." *Journal of Sexual Medicine* 10, no. 2 (2013): 484–92. doi:10.1111/jsm.12022.

Kaplan, Helen Singer. "Hypoactive Sexual Desire." *Journal of Sex & Marital Therapy* 3, no. 1 (1977): 3–9.

Khong, Belinda Siew Luan. "Mindfulness: A Way of Cultivating Deep Respect for Emotions." *Mindfulness* 2, no. 1 (2011): 27–32. doi:10.1007 /s12671-010-0039-9.

Kilimnik, Chelsea D., and Cindy M. Meston. "Role of Body Esteem in the Sexual Excitation and Inhibition Responses of Women with and without a History of Childhood Sexual Abuse." *Journal of Sexual Medicine* 13, no. 11 (2016): 1718–28.

Kingsberg, Sheryl A., Natalia Tkachenko, Johna Lucas, Amy Burbrink, Wayne Kreppner, and Jodi B. Dickstein. "Characterization of Orgasmic Difficulties by Women: Focus Group Evaluation." *Journal of Sexual Medicine* 10, no. 9 (2013): 2242–50. doi:10.1111/jsm.12224.

Kinsale, Laura. *Flowers from the Storm*. New York: Harper, 1992.

Kinsey, Alfred Charles, Wardell Baxter Pomeroy, and Clyde E. Martin. *Sexual Behavior in the Human Male*. Philadelphia: W. B. Saunders, 1948.

Kinsey, Alfred C., Wardell B. Pomeroy, Clyde E. Martin, and Paul H. Gebhard. *Sexual Behavior in the Human Female*. Philadelphia: W. B. Saunders, 1953.

Kleinplatz, Peggy J., and A. Dana Ménard. *Magnificent Sex: Lessons from Extraordinary Lovers*. New York: Routledge, 2020.

Kleinplatz, Peggy J., A. Dana Ménard, Marie-Pierre Paquet, Nicolas Paradis, Meghan Campbell, Dino Zuccarino, and Lisa Mehak. "The Components of Optimal Sexuality: A Portrait of 'Great Sex.'" *Canadian Journal of Human Sexuality* 18, no. 1–2 (2009): 1–13.

Koehler, Sezin. "From the Mouths of Rapists: The Lyrics of Robin Thicke's Blurred Lines." *The Society Pages*, September 17, 2013. http://thesociety pages.org/socimages/2013/09/17/from-the-mouths-of-rapists-the-lyrics -of-robin-thickes-blurred-lines-and-real-life-rape/.

Komisaruk, Barry R., Beverly Whipple, Audrita Crawford, Sherry Grimes, Wen-Ching Liu, Andrew Kalnin, and Kristine Mosier. "Brain Activation during Vaginocervical Self-Stimulation and Orgasm in Women with Complete Spinal Cord Injury: fMRI Evidence of Mediation by the Vagus Nerves." *Brain Research* 1024, no. 1–2 (2004): 77–88.

Komisaruk, Barry R., Nan Wise, Eleni Frangos, Wen-Ching Liu, Kachina Allen, and Stuart Brody. "Women's Clitoris, Vagina, and Cervix Mapped on the Sensory Cortex: fMRI Evidence." *Journal of Sexual Medicine* 8, no. 10 (2011): 2822–30. doi:10.1111/j.1743-6109.2011.02388.x.

Kring, Ann M., and Albert H. Gordon. "Sex Differences in Emotion: Expression, Experience, and Physiology." *Journal of Personality and Social Psychology* 74, no. 3 (1998): 686–703.

Laan, Ellen, and Stephanie Both. "What Makes Women Experience Desire?" *Feminism & Psychology* 18, no. 4 (2008): 505–14.

Laan, Ellen, Walter Everaerd, and Andrea Evers. "Assessment of Female Sexual Arousal: Response Specificity and Construct Validity." *Psychophysiology* 32, no. 5 (1995): 476–85.

La Guardia, Jennifer G., Richard M. Ryan, Charles E. Couchman, and Edward L. Deci. "Within-Person Variation in Security of Attachment: A Self-Determination Theory Perspective on Attachment, Need Fulfillment, and Well-Being." *Journal of Personality and Social Psychology* 79, no. 3 (2000): 367–84.

Lalumière, Martin L., Megan L. Sawatsky, Samantha J. Dawson, and Kelly D.

Suschinsky. "The Empirical Status of the Preparation Hypothesis: Explicating Women's Genital Responses to Sexual Stimuli in the Laboratory." *Archives of Sexual Behavior* 49, no. 2 (2020): 1–20.

Laumann, E. O., A. Nicolosi, D. B. Glasser, A. Paik, C. Gingell, E. Moreira, and T. Wang. "Sexual Problems among Women and Men Aged 40–80 Y: Prevalence and Correlates Identified in the Global Study of Sexual Attitudes and Behaviors." *International Journal of Impotence Research* 17 (2005): 39–57. doi:10.1038/sj.ijir.3901250.

Leavitt, Chelom E., Eva S. Lefkowitz, and Emily A. Waterman. "The Role of Sexual Mindfulness in Sexual Wellbeing, Relational Wellbeing, and Self-Esteem." *Journal of Sex & Marital Therapy* 45, no. 6 (2019): 497–509.

Levin, Roy J. "The Human Female Orgasm: A Critical Evaluation of Its Proposed Reproductive Functions." *Sexual and Relationship Therapy* 26, no. 4 (2011): 301–14. doi:10.1080/14681994.2011.649692.

Levin, Roy J., and Willy van Berlo. "Sexual Arousal and Orgasm in Subjects Who Experience Forced or Non-Consensual Sexual Stimulation—a Review." *Journal of Clinical Forensic Medicine* 11, no. 2 (2004): 82–88.

Levin, Roy J., and Gorm Wagner. "Orgasm in Women in the Laboratory—Quantitative Studies on Duration, Intensity, Latency, and Vaginal Blood Flow." *Archives of Sexual Behavior* 14, no. 5 (1985): 439–49.

Levine, Peter A. *In an Unspoken Voice: How the Body Releases Trauma and Restores Goodness.* Berkeley, CA: North Atlantic Books, 2010.

———. *Waking the Tiger: Healing Trauma.* Berkeley, CA: North Atlantic Books, 1997.

Lisak, David, and Paul M. Miller. "Repeat Rape and Multiple Offending among Undetected Rapists." *Violence and Victims* 17, no. 1 (2002): 73–84.

Lloyd, Elisabeth A. *The Case of the Female Orgasm: Bias in the Science of Evolution.* Cambridge, MA: Harvard University Press, 2005.

Longe, Olivia, Frances A. Maratos, Paul Gilbert, Gaynor Evans, Faye Volker, Helen Rockliff, and Gina Rippon. "Having a Word with Yourself: Neural Correlates of Self-Criticism and Self-Reassurance." *NeuroImage* 49, no. 2 (2010): 1849–56. doi:10.1016/j.neuroimage.2009.09.019.

LoPiccolo, Joseph, and Leslie LoPiccolo, eds. *Handbook of Sex Therapy.* New York: Plenum, 1978.

Lykins, Amy D., Erick Janssen, and Cynthia A. Graham. "The Relationship between Negative Mood and Sexuality in Heterosexual College Women and Men." *Journal of Sex Research* 43, no. 2 (2006): 136–43.

Magnanti, Brooke. *The Sex Myth: Why Everything We're Told Is Wrong*. London: Weidenfeld & Nicolson, 2012.

Mah, Kenneth, and Yitzchak M. Binik. "The Nature of Human Orgasm: A Critical Review of Major Trends." *Clinical Psychology Review* 21, no. 6 (2001): 823–56.

Manne, Kate. *Down Girl: The Logic of Misogyny*. Oxford: Oxford University Press, 2017.

Manne, Kate. *Entitled: How Male Privilege Hurts Women*. New York: Crown, 2020.

Marcus, Bat Sheva. "Changes in a Woman's Sexual Experience and Expectations Following the Introduction of Electric Vibrator Assistance." *Journal of Sexual Medicine* 8, no. 12 (2011): 3398–3406. doi:10.1111/j.1743-6109.20 10.02132.x.

Mark, Kristen P., and Julie A. Lasslo. "Maintaining Sexual Desire in Long-Term Relationships: A Systematic Review and Conceptual Model." *Journal of Sex Research* 55, no. 4–5 (2018): 563–81.

Masters, William H., and Virginia E. Johnson. *Human Sexual Response*. Boston: Little, Brown, 1966.

Mazloomdoost, Donna, and Rachel N. Pauls. "A Comprehensive Review of the Clitoris and Its Role in Female Sexual Function." *Sexual Medicine Reviews* 3, no. 4 (2015): 245–63.

McCall, Katie, and Cindy Meston. "Cues Resulting in Desire for Sexual Activity in Women." *Journal of Sexual Medicine* 3, no. 5 (2006): 838–52. doi:10.1111/j.1743-6109.2006.00301.x.

———. "Differences Between Pre- and Postmenopausal Women in Cues for Sexual Desire." *Journal of Sexual Medicine* 4 no. 2 (2007): 364–71. doi:10.1111/j.1743-6109.2006.00421.x.

McDowell, Margaret A., Cheryl D. Fryar, Cynthia L. Ogden, and Katherine M. Flegal. "Anthropometric Reference Data for Children and Adults: United States, 2003–2006." National Health Statistics Report no. 10 (October 2008).

Mesquita, Batja. "Emoting: A Contextualized Process." In *The Mind in Context*, edited by Batja Mesquita, Lisa Feldman Barrett, and Eliot R. Smith, 83–104. New York: Guilford Press, 2010.

Meston, Cindy M., and David M. Buss. "Why Humans Have Sex." *Archives of Sexual Behavior* 36, no. 4 (2007): 477–507.

Meston, Cindy M., and Amelia M. Stanton. "Desynchrony between

Subjective and Genital Sexual Arousal in Women: Theoretically Interesting but Clinically Irrelevant." *Current Sexual Health Reports* 10, no. 3 (2018): 73–75.

Michael, Robert T., John H. Gagnon, Edward O. Laumann, and Gina Kolata. *Sex in America: A Definitive Survey.* Boston: Little, Brown, 1994.

Milhausen, Robin R., Cynthia A. Graham, Stephanie A. Sanders, William L. Yarber, and Scott B. Maitland. "Validation of the Sexual Excitation/Sexual Inhibition Inventory for Women and Men." *Archives of Sexual Behavior* 39, no. 5 (2010): 1091–1104.

Mitchell, John Cameron, and Stephen Trask. "The Origin of Love" from *Hedwig and the Angry Inch: Original Cast Recording.* Atlantic Compact Disc 13766. 1999.

Mitchell, Kirstin Rebecca, Michael King, Irwin Nazareth, and Kaye Wellings. "Managing Sexual Difficulties: A Qualitative Investigation of Coping Strategies." *Journal of Sex Research* 48, no. 4 (2011): 325–33.

Mize, Sara J. S., and Alex Iantaffi. "The Place of Mindfulness in a Sensorimotor Psychotherapy Intervention to Improve Women's Sexual Health." *Sexual and Relationship Therapy* 28, no. 1 (2013): 63–76. doi:10.1080/14681994.2013.770144.

Moore, Lori. "Rep. Todd Akin: The Statement and the Reaction." *New York Times*, August 20, 2012. www.nytimes.com/2012/08/21/us/politics/rep-todd-akin-legitimate-rape-statement-and-reaction.html?_r=0.

Moran, C., and C. Lee. "What's Normal? Influencing Women's Perceptions of Normal Genitalia: An Experiment Involving Exposure to Modified and Nonmodified Images." *BJOG: An International Journal of Obstetrics and Gynaecology* 121, no. 6 (2013): 761–66. doi:10.1111/1471-0528.12578.

Morokoff, Patricia J., and Julia R. Heiman. "Effects of Erotic Stimuli on Sexually Functional and Dysfunctional Women: Multiple Measures before and after Sex Therapy." *Behaviour Research and Therapy* 18, no. 2 (1980): 127–37.

Moseley, G. Lorimer, and David S. Butler. *Explain Pain Supercharged.* Adelaide, Australia: NOI, 2017.

Nagoski, Emily. "I'm Sorry You're Lonely but It's Not My Job to Help You: The Science of Incels." *Medium*, May 5, 2018. Accessed June 23, 2020. https://medium.com/@enagoski/im-sorry-you-re-lonely-but-it-s-not-my-job-to-help-you-the-science-of-incels-25bf83e2aaa0.

———. "The Definitive Answer to the Question, 'Does the G-Spot Exist?'" *Medium*, July 6, 2014. Accessed September 11, 2020. https://medium

.com/@enagoski/the-definitive-answer-to-the-question-does-the-g-spot-exist-5d962de0c34c.

———. "The Truth about Unwanted Arousal." Filmed April 13, 2018, in Vancouver, Ontario. TED video, 15:08. http://go.ted.com/emilynagoski.

———. "The World Cup of Women's Sexual Desire." *Medium*, August 11, 2015. Accessed June 23, 2020. https://medium.com@enagoski/the-world-cup-of-women-s-sexual-desire-9a085617495e.

Nakamura, J., and M. Csikszentmihalyi. "Flow Theory and Research." In *The Handbook of Positive Psychology*, edited by C. R. Snyder and S. J. Lopez, 195–206. Oxford: Oxford University Press, 2009.

Neff, Kristin D. "Self-Compassion, Self-Esteem, and Well-Being." *Social and Personality Psychology Compass* 5, no. 1 (2011): 1–12. doi:10.1111/j.1751-9004.2010.00330.x.

Ng, Theresa. "Risk Assessment and Risk Mitigation Review(s) Application Number 210557Orig1s000." Accessed June 22, 2020. https://www.accessdata.fda.gov/drugsatfda_docs/nda/2019/210557Orig1s000RiskR.pdf.

Ogden, Pat, Kekuni Minton, and Clare Pain. *Trauma and the Body: A Sensorimotor Approach to Psychotherapy.* New York: W. W. Norton, 2006.

Panksepp, Jaak. "What Is an Emotional Feeling? Lessons about Affective Origins from Cross-Species Neuroscience." *Motivation and Emotion* 36, no. 1 (2012): 4–15.

Panksepp, Jaak, and Lucy Biven. *The Archaeology of Mind: Neuroevolutionary Origins of Human Emotions.* New York: W. W. Norton, 2012.

Pazmany, Els, Sophie Bergeron, Lukas Van Oudenhove, Johan Verhaeghe, and Paul Enzlin. "Body Image and Genital Self-Image in Pre-Menopausal Women with Dyspareunia." *Archives of Sexual Behavior* 42, no. 6 (2013): 999–1010. doi:10.1007/s10508-013-0102-4.

Perel, Esther. *Mating in Captivity: Unlocking Erotic Intelligence.* New York: Harper, 2006.

———. "The Secret to Desire in a Long-Term Relationship." TED video, February 2013. www.ted.com/talks/esther_perel_the_secret_to_desire_in_a_long_term_relationship.

Peterson, Zoë D., Erick Janssen, and Ellen Laan. "Women's Sexual Responses to Heterosexual and Lesbian Erotica: The Role of Stimulus Intensity, Affective Reaction, and Sexual History." *Archives of Sexual Behavior* 39, no. 4 (2010): 880–97. doi:10.1007/s10508-009-9546-y.

Pfaus, James G. "Neurobiology of Sexual Behavior." *Current Opinion in Neu-*

robiology 9, no. 6 (1999): 751–58. https://pubmed.ncbi.nlm.nih.gov/1060 7643/.

Pfaus, James G., Tod E. Kippin, and Genaro Coria-Avila. "What Can Animal Models Tell Us about Human Sexual Response?" *Annual Review of Sex Research* 14 (2003): 1–63.

Pfaus, James G., and Mark F. Wilkins. "A Novel Environment Disrupts Population in Sexually Naive but Not Experienced Male Rats: Reversal with Naloxone." *Physiology & Behavior* 57, no. 6 (1995): 1045–49.

Pierce, Angela N., Janelle M. Ryals, Ruipeng Wang, and Julie A. Christianson. "Vaginal Hypersensitivity and Hypothalamic-Pituitary-Adrenal Axis Dysfunction as a Result of Neonatal Maternal Separation in Female Mice." *Neuroscience* 263 (2014): 216–30.

Porges, Stephen W. *The Polyvagal Theory: Neurophysiological Foundations of Emotions, Attachment, Communication, and Self-Regulation.* New York: W. W. Norton, 2011.

———. "Reciprocal Influences between Body and Brain in the Perception and Expression of Affect: A Polyvagal Perspective." In *The Healing Power of Emotion* edited by Diana Fosha, Daniel J. Siegel, and Marion Solomon, 27–54. New York: W. W. Norton, 2009.

Powers, Theodore A., David C. Zuroff, and Raluca A. Topciu. "Covert and Overt Expressions of Self-Criticism and Perfectionism and Their Relation to Depression." *European Journal of Personality* 18, no. 1 (2004): 61–72. doi:10.1002/per.499.

Prause, Nicole, and Cynthia A. Graham. "Asexuality: Classification and Characterization." *Archives of Sexual Behavior* 36, no. 3 (2007): 341–56. doi:10.1007/s10508-006-9142-3.

Radomsky, Adam S., Gillian M. Alcolado, Jonathan S. Abramowitz, Pino Alonso, Amparo Belloch, Martine Bouvard, David A. Clark, et al. "Part 1—You Can Run but You Can't Hide: Intrusive Thoughts on Six Continents." *Journal of Obsessive-Compulsive and Related Disorders* 3, no. 3 (2014): 269–79.

Read, Simon, Michael King, and James Watson. "Sexual Dysfunction in Primary Medical Care: Prevalence, Characteristics and Detection by the General Practitioner." *Journal of Public Health Medicine* 19, no. 4 (1997): 387–91.

Reichl, Corinna, Johann F. Schneider, and Frank M. Spinath. "Relation of Self-Talk Frequency to Loneliness, Need to Belong, and Health in German Adults." *Personality and Individual Differences* 54, no. 2 (2013): 241–45. http://dx.doi.org/10.1016/j.paid.2012.09.003.

Rettenberger, Martin, Verena Klein, and Peer Briken. "The Relationship between Hypersexual Behavior, Sexual Excitation, Sexual Inhibition, and Personality Traits." *Archives of Sexual Behavior* 45, no. 1 (2016): 219–33.

Reynolds, Sheila M., and Kent C. Berridge. "Emotional Environments Retune the Valence of Appetitive versus Fearful Functions in Nucleus Accumbens." *Nature Neuroscience* 11 (2008): 423–25. doi:10.1038/nn2061.

Rosen, Lianne. "How Do Women Survivors of Childhood Sexual Abuse Experience 'Good Sex' Later in Life? A Mixed-Methods Investigation." PhD diss., University of Victoria, 2018.

Rowland, Katherine. *The Pleasure Gap: American Women and the Unfinished Sexual Revolution.* London: Hachette UK, 2020.

Rumi, Mevlana Jalaludin. *Teachings of Rumi (the Masnavi): The Spiritual Couplets of Jalaludin Rumi.* Translated by E. H. Whinfield. London: Octagon Press, 1994.

Ryan, Christopher, and Cacilda Jethá. *Sex at Dawn: The Prehistoric Origins of Modern Sexuality.* New York: Harper, 2010.

Ryan, Rebecca. "Women's Lived Experiences Seeking and Using Adaptation Strategies Aimed at Improving Subjective Low Sexual Desire with Their Current Male Sexual Partner." PhD diss., Indiana University Bloomington, 2019. ProQuest Dissertations Publishing (13814724).

Sakaluk, John K., Leah M. Todd, Robin Milhausen, Nathan J. Lachowsky, and Undergraduate Research Group in Sexuality. "Dominant Heterosexual Sexual Scripts in Emerging Adulthood: Conceptualization and Measurement." *Journal of Sex Research* 51, no. 5 (2013): 516–31. doi:10.1080/00224 499.2012.745473.

Sanders, Stephanie A., Cynthia A. Graham, Jennifer L. Bass, and John Bancroft. "A Prospective Study of the Effects of Oral Contraceptives on Sexuality and Well-Being and Their Relationship to Discontinuation." *Contraception* 64, no. 1 (2001): 51–8.

Schwartz, Gary E., Serena-Lynn Brown, and Geoffrey L. Ahern. "Facial Muscle Patterning and Subjective Experience during Affective Imagery: Sex Differences." *Psychophysiology* 17, no. 1 (1980): 75–82.

Schwarzer, Ralf, and Peter A. Frensch, eds. *Personality, Human Development, and Culture.* New York: Psychology Press, 2010.

Shenhav, A., and W. B. Mendes. "Aiming for the Stomach and Hitting the Heart: Dissociable Triggers and Sources for Disgust Reactions." *Emotion* 14, no. 2 (November 2013): 301–9. www.ncbi.nlm.nih.gov/pubmed/24219399.

Silverstein, R. Gina, Anne-Catharine H. Brown, Harold D. Roth, and

Willoughby B. Britton. "Effects of Mindfulness Training on Body Aware-ness to Sexual Stimuli: Implications for Female Sexual Dysfunction." *Psychosomatic Medicine* 73, no. 9 (2011): 817–25.

Simons, Jeffrey, and Michael P. Carey. "Prevalence of Sexual Dysfunctions." *Archives of Sexual Behavior* 30, no. 2 (2001): 177–219.

Sole-Smith, Virginia. "Pleasure in a Pill?" *Marie Claire*, September 16, 2015. Accessed June 22, 2020. http://www.marieclaire.com/sex-love/advice /a11640/pleasure-in-a-pill-female-viagra/.

Stefanou, Christina, and Marita P. McCabe. "Adult Attachment and Sexual Functioning: A Review of Past Research." *Journal of Sexual Medicine* 9, no. 10 (2012): 2499–507. doi:10.1111/j.1743-6109.2012.02843.x.

Stein, Rob. "Female Libido Pill Fires Up Debate about Women and Sex." *All Things Considered*, NPR, February 16, 2015. Accessed June 22, 2020. https://www.npr.org/sections/health-shots/2015/02/16/384043661 /female-libido-pill-fires-up-debate-about-women-and-sex.

Stice, Eric, Paul Rohde, and Heather Shaw. *The Body Project: A Dissonance-Based Eating Disorder Prevention Intervention*. New York: Oxford University Press, 2013.

Stopes, Marie. *Married Love*. 1918. Oxford: Oxford University Press, 2008.

Stroupe, Natalie N. "How Difficult Is Too Difficult? The Relationships among Women's Sexual Experience and Attitudes, Difficulty with Orgasm, and Perception of Themselves as Orgasmic or Anorgasmic." Master's thesis, University of Kansas, 2008. http://kuscholarworks.ku.edu/dspace/han dle/1808/4517.

Štulhofer, Aleksandar, Ana Alexandra Carvalheira, and Bente Træen. "Is Responsive Sexual Desire for Partnered Sex Problematic among Men? Insights from a Two-Country Study." *Sexual and Relationship Therapy* 28, no. 3 (2013): 246–58. doi:10.1080/14681994.2012.756137.

Suhler, Christopher L., and Patricia Churchland. "Can Innate, Modular 'Foundations' Explain Morality? Challenges for Haidt's Moral Foundations Theory." *Journal of Cognitive Neuroscience* 23, no. 9 (2011): 2103–16. doi:10.1162/jocn.2011.21637.

Suschinsky, Kelly D., Samantha J. Dawson, and Meredith L. Chivers. "Assessing the Relationship between Sexual Concordance, Sexual Attractions, and Sexual Identity in Women." *Archives of Sexual Behavior* 46, no. 1 (2017): 179–92.

Suschinsky, Kelly D., Jackie S. Huberman, Larah Maunder, Lori A. Brotto, Tom

Hollenstein, and Meredith L. Chivers. "The Relationship between Sexual Functioning and Sexual Concordance in Women." *Journal of Sex & Marital Therapy* 45, no. 3 (2019): 230–46.

Suschinsky, Kelly D., and Martin L. Lalumière. "Is Sexual Concordance Related to Awareness of Physiological States?" *Archives of Sexual Behavior* 41, no. 1 (2012): 199–208.

Suschinsky, Kelly D., Martin L. Lalumière, and Meredith L. Chivers. "Sex Differences in Patterns of Genital Sexual Arousal: Measurement Artifacts or True Phenomena?" *Archives of Sexual Behavior* 38, no. 4 (2009): 559–73. doi:10.1007/s10508-008-9339-8.

Taylor, Shelley E., and Sarah L. Master. "Social Responses to Stress: The Tend-and-Befriend Model." In *The Handbook of Stress Science: Biology, Psychology, and Health*, edited by Richard J. Contrada and Andrew Baum, 101–109. New York: Springer, 2011.

ter Kuile, Moniek M., Daan Vigeveno, and Ellen Laan. "Preliminary Evidence That Acute and Chronic Daily Psychological Stress Affect Sexual Arousal in Sexually Functional Women." *Behaviour Research and Therapy* 45, no. 9 (2007): 2078–89. http://dx.doi.org/10.1016/j.brat.2007.03.006.

Thomas, J. J., R. D. Crosby, S. A. Wonderlich, R. H. Striegel-Moore, and A. E. Becker. "A Latent Profile Analysis of the Typology of Bulimic Symptoms in an Indigenous Pacific Population: Evidence of Cross-Cultural Variation in Phenomenology." *Psychological Medicine* 41, no. 1 (2011): 195–206. http://dx.doi.org/10.1017/S0033291710000255.

Tiefer, Leonore. "Sex Therapy as a Humanistic Enterprise." *Sexual and Relationship Therapy* 21, no. 3 (2006): 359–75. doi:10.1080/14681990600740723.

Toates, Frederick. *Biological Psychology*. 3rd ed. New York: Prentice Hall/Pearson, 2011.

———. *How Sexual Desire Works: The Enigmatic Urge*. Cambridge: Cambridge University Press, 2014.

———. *Motivational Systems*. New York: Cambridge University Press, 1986, 151–59.

Tolman, Deborah L. *Dilemmas of Desire: Teenage Girls Talk about Sexuality*. Cambridge, MA: Harvard University Press, 2002.

Tompkins, K. Brooke, Denise M. Martz, Courtney A. Rocheleau, and Doris G. Bazzini. "Social Likeability, Conformity, and Body Talk: Does Fat Talk Have a Normative Rival in Female Body Image Conversations?" *Body Image* 6, no. 4 (2009): 292–98.

Toulalan, Sarah. *Imagining Sex: Pornography and Bodies in Seventeenth-Century England*. New York: Oxford University Press, 2007.

Tracey, Irene. "Getting the Pain You Expect: Mechanisms of Placebo, Nocebo and Reappraisal Effects in Humans." *Nature Medicine* 16 (2010): 1277–83. doi:10.1038/nm.2229.

Tybur, Joshua M., Debra Lieberman, and Vladas Griskevicius. "Microbes, Mating, and Morality: Individual Differences in Three Functional Domains of Disgust." *Journal of Personality and Social Psychology* 97, no. 1 (2009): 103–22. doi:10.1037/a0015474.

UN Human Rights Council. *Report of the Special Rapporteur on Torture and Other Cruel, Inhuman or Degrading Treatment or Punishment*. February 1, 2013. A/HRC/22/53.

US Department of Justice. *Full Report of the Prevalence, Incidence, and Consequences of Violence against Women*. November 2000. www.ncjrs.gov/pdf files1/nij/183781.pdf.

Van Dam, Nicholas T., Mitch Earleywine, and Sharon Danoff-Burg. "Differential Item Function across Mediators and Non-Mediators on the Five Facet Mindfulness Questionnaire." *Personal and Individual Differences* 47, no. 5 (2009): 516–21.

Van Dam, Nicholas T., Sean C. Sheppard, John P. Forsyth, and Mitch Earleywine. "Self-Compassion Is a Better Predictor Than Mindfulness of Symptom Severity and Quality of Life in Mixed Anxiety and Depression." *Journal of Anxiety Disorders* 25, no. 1 (2011): 123–30.

van de Velde, T. H. *Ideal Marriage: Its Physiology and Technique*. Translated by Stella Browne. New York: Random House, 1926.

Velten, Julia, and Lori A. Brotto. "Interoception and Sexual Response in Women with Low Sexual Desire." *PloS ONE* 12, no. 10 (2017).

Velten, Julia, Meredith L. Chivers, and Lori A. Brotto. "Does Repeated Testing Impact Concordance between Genital and Self-Reported Sexual Arousal in Women?" *Archives of Sexual Behavior* 47, no. 3 (2018): 651–60.

Velten, Julia, Samantha J. Dawson, Kelly Suschinsky, Lori A. Brotto, and Meredith L. Chivers. (2020) "Development and Validation of a Measure of Responsive Sexual Desire." *Journal of Sex & Marital Therapy* 46, no. 2 (2020): 122–40. doi:10.1080/0092623X.2019.1654580.

Velten, Julia, Saskia Scholten, Cynthia A. Graham, Dirk Adolph, and Jürgen Margraf. "Investigating Female Sexual Concordance: Do Sexual Excitation and Sexual Inhibition Moderate the Agreement of Genital and Subjective

Sexual Arousal in Women?" *Archives of Sexual Behavior* 45, no. 8 (2016): 1957–71.

Velten, Julia, Saskia Scholten, Cynthia A. Graham, and Jürgen Margraf. "Sexual Excitation and Sexual Inhibition as Predictors of Sexual Function in Women: A Cross-Sectional and Longitudinal Study." *Journal of Sex & Marital Therapy* 43, no. 2 (2017): 95–109.

Velten, Julia, Lisa Zahler, Saskia Scholten, and Jürgen Margraf. "Temporal Stability of Sexual Excitation and Sexual Inhibition in Women." *Archives of Sexual Behavior* 48, no. 3 (2019): 881-89.

Vieira-Baptista, Pedro, Gutemberg Almeida, Fabrizio Bogliatto, Tanja Gizela Bohl, Matthé Burger, Bina Cohen-Sacher, Karen Gibbon, et al. "International Society for the Study of Vulvovaginal Disease Recommendations regarding Female Cosmetic Genital Surgery." *Journal of Lower Genital Tract Disease* 22, no. 4 (2018): 415–34.

Vowels, Laura M., and Kristen P. Mark. "Strategies for Mitigating Sexual Desire Discrepancy in Relationships." *Archives of Sexual Behavior* 49, no. 3 (2020): 1017–28.

Wallen, Kim, and Elisabeth A. Lloyd. "Female Sexual Arousal: Genital Anatomy and Orgasm in Intercourse." *Hormones and Behavior* 59, no. 5 (2011): 780–92. doi:10.1016/j.yhbeh.2010.12.004.

Warber, Katie M., and Tara M. Emmers-Sommer. "The Relationships among Sex, Gender and Attachment." *Language and Communications Quarterly* 1 (2012): 60–81.

Wickman, D. "Plasticity of the Skene's Gland in Women Who Report Fluid Ejaculation with Orgasm." *Journal of Sexual Medicine* 14, no. 1 (2017): S67.

Witting, K., P. Santtila, F. Rijsdijk, M. Varjonen, P. Jern, A. Johansson, B. von der Pahlen, K. Alanko, and N. K. Sandnabba. "Correlated Genetic and Non-Shared Environmental Influences Account for the Co-Morbidity between Female Sexual Dysfunctions." *Psychological Medicine* 39, no. 1 (2009): 115–27.

Woertman, Liesbeth, and Femke van den Brink. "Body Image and Female Sexual Functioning and Behavior: A Review." *Journal of Sex Research* 49, no. 2 (2012): 184–211. doi:10.1080/00224499.2012.658586.

World Health Organization. "Violence against Women: Intimate Partner and Sexual Violence against Women." Fact sheet. November 29, 2017. https://www.who.int/news-room/fact-sheets/detail/.

Wrosch, Carsten, Michael F. Scheier, Charles S. Carver, and Richard Schulz. "The Importance of Goal Disengagement in Adaptive Self-Regulation: When Giving Up Is Beneficial." *Self and Identity* 2 (2003): 1–20.

Yeshe, Lama Thubten. *Introduction to Tantra: The Transformation of Desire.* ReadHowYouWant.com, 2010.

index

Page numbers in *italics* refer to illustrations.

about the author

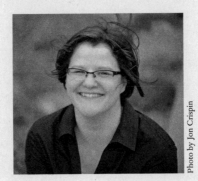

Photo by Jon Crispin

EMILY NAGOSKI is the award-winning author of the *New York Times* bestseller *Come As You Are: The Surprising New Science That Will Transform Your Sex Life* and *The Come As You Are Workbook,* and coauthor, with her sister, Amelia, of *New York Times* bestseller *Burnout: The Secret to Unlocking the Stress Cycle.* She began her work as a sex educator at the University of Delaware, where she volunteered as a peer sex educator while studying psychology with minors in cognitive science and philosophy. She went on to earn a M.S. in Counseling and a Ph.D. in Health Behavior, both from Indiana University, with clinical and research training at the Kinsey Institute. Now she combines sex education and stress education to teach women to live with confidence and joy inside their bodies.

Emily lives in western Massachusetts with two dogs, two cats, and a cartoonist.

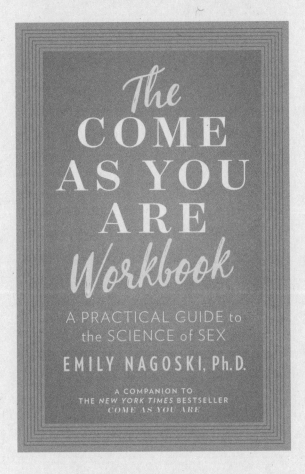
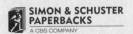